Aging and the Immune Response

IMMUNOLOGY SERIES

1. Mechanisms in Allergy: Reagin-Mediated Hypersensitivity
   Edited by Lawrence Goodfriend, Alec Sehon and Robert P. Orange
2. Immunopathology: Methods and Techniques
   Edited by Theodore P. Zacharia and Sidney S. Breese, Jr.
3. Immunity and Cancer in Man: An Introduction
   Edited by Arnold E. Reif
4. *Bordetella pertussis:* Immunological and Other Biological Activities
   J.J. Munoz and R.K. Bergman
5. The Lymphocyte: Structure and Function (in two parts)
   Edited by John J. Marchalonis
6. Immunology of Receptors
   Edited by B. Cinader
7. Immediate Hypersensitivity: Modern Concepts and Development
   Edited by Michael K. Bach
8. Theoretical Immunology
   Edited by George I. Bell, Alan S. Perelson, and George H. Pimbley, Jr.
9. Immunodiagnosis of Cancer (in two parts)
   Edited by Ronald B. Herberman and K. Robert McIntire
10. Immunologically Mediated Renal Diseases: Criteria for Diagnosis and Treatment
    Edited by Robert T. McCluskey and Giuseppe A. Andres
11. Clinical Immunotherapy
    Edited by Albert F. LoBuglio
12. Mechanisms of Immunity to Virus-Induced Tumors
    Edited by John W. Blasecki
13. Manual of Macrophage Methodology: Collection, Characterization, and Function
    Edited by Herbert B. Herscowitz, Howard T. Holden, Joseph A. Bellanti, and Abdul Ghaffar
14. Suppressor Cells in Human Disease
    Edited by James S. Goodwin
15. Immunological Aspects of Aging
    Edited by Diego Segre and Lester Smith

16. Cellular and Molecular Mechanisms of Immunologic Tolerance
Edited by Tomáš Hraba and Milan Hašek

17. Immune Regulation: Evolution and Biological Significance
Edited by Laurens N. Ruben and M. Eric Gershwin

18. Tumor Immunity in Prognosis: The Role of Mononuclear Cell Infiltration
Edited by Stephen Haskill

19. Immunopharmacology and the Regulation of Leukocyte Function
Edited by David R. Webb

20. Pathogenesis and Immunology of Treponemal Infection
Edited by Ronald F. Schell and Daniel M. Musher

21. Macrophage-Mediated Antibody-Dependent Cellular Cytotoxicity
Edited by Hillel S. Koren

22. Molecular Immunology: A Textbook
Edited by M. Zouhair Atassi, Carel J. van Oss, and Darryl R. Absolom

23. Monoclonal Antibodies and Cancer
Edited by George L. Wright, Jr.

24. Stress, Immunity, and Aging
Edited by Edwin L. Cooper

25. Immune Modulation Agents and Their Mechanisms
Edited by Richard L. Fenichel and Michael A. Chirigos

26. Mononuclear Phagocyte Biology
Edited by Alvin Volkman

27. The Lactoperoxidase System: Chemistry and Biological Significance
Edited by Kenneth M. Pruitt and Jorma O. Tenovuo

28. Introduction to Medical Immunology
Edited by Gabriel Virella, Jean-Michel Goust, H. Hugh Fudenberg, and Christian C. Patrick

29. Handbook of Food Allergies
Edited by James C. Breneman

30. Human Hybridomas: Diagnostic and Therapeutic Applications
Edited by Anthony J. Strelkauskas

31. Aging and the Immune Response: Cellular and Humoral Aspects
Edited by Edmond A. Goidl

32. Complications of Organ Transplantation
Edited by Luis H. Toledo-Pereyra

33. Monoclonal Antibodies: Hybridoma Techniques
Edited by Lawrence B. Schook

Additional Volumes in Preparation

Aging and the Immune Response

Cellular and Humoral Aspects

edited by

Edmond A. Goidl

The University of Maryland School
of Medicine
Baltimore, Maryland

MARCEL DEKKER, INC. New York and Basel

Library of Congress Cataloging-in-Publication Data

Aging and the immune response.

(Immunology series; 31)
Includes index.
1. Immune system--Aging. 2. Aging--Immunological aspects. I. Goidl, Edmond A. II. Series : Immunology series ; v. 34. [DNLM: 1. Aging. 2. Antibody Formation--in old age. 3. Immunity, Cellular--in old age. W1 IM53K v.34 / QW 568 A267]
QR182.A37 1987 618.97'079 86-24236
ISBN 0-8247-7635-6

MARCEL DEKKER, INC.
270 Madison Avenue, New York, New York 10016

Current printing (last digit):
10 9 8 7 6 5 4 3 2 1

PRINTED IN THE UNITED STATES OF AMERICA

For my mother
and in memory of my father

Preface

By the end of the century we shall observe a dramatic increase in the percentage of the population of developed countries reaching their sixth and seventh and later decades. It is therefore crucial that our knowledge of the aging process continues to grow. This volume focuses on the recent developments in the relationship between aging and the immune response. I have tried to bring together the most recent research accomplished by laboratories around the world. The responsibility for any omission rests with me.

This book contains 17 chapters. They span different aspects of the aging immune response. The effect of aging on the functions of T-cell reactivity is covered by Richard A. Miller and David E. Harrison in Chapter 1. Takashi Makinodan et al. in the second chapter examine the vulnerability of T cells in aging. In Chapter 3, Rita B. Effros and Roy L. Walford discuss the increased susceptibility to infectious agents in aging. Risë Schwab and Marc E. Weksler have studied the proliferative capabilities of lymphocytes from aged human donors and they present their results in Chapter 4.

At the B-cell level, in Chapters 5 and 6, Dorith Zharhary and Norman R. Klinman review their analysis of the clonal repertoire. They are followed by Andrew W. Wade and Myron R. Szewczuk, who look at mucosal B-cell immunity. The loss of tolerance induction seen in the senescent immune response is described in Chapter 7 by Gail S. Habicht.

Two aspects of the effects of immunoregulatory thymic hormones are presented by Gino Doria and his group in Chapter 8 and by Raymond N.

Hiramoto et al. in Chapter 9. In Chapter 10, Marilyn L. Thoman and William O. Weigle discuss the functions of cytokines on the aging immune response.

Dietary manipulations and their consequences on the immune response and on development of autoimmunity are illustrated in Chapter 11 by Gabriel Fernandes.

The next two contributions focus on the nature of suppressor mechanisms in both mice and men: Chapter 12 by Susan R. S. Gottesman et al., and Chapter 13 by Diego Segre and Mariangela Segre. The metabolism of zinc and its relationship to the aging immune response are described in Chapter 14 by Richard A. Winchurch.

The last three chapters are devoted to several aspects of the immune network in maturation and aging: Sybille Müller et al. examine idiotypes; Audrey J. Manheimer et al. describe rheumatoid factors and their occurrence in aging; and Edmond A. Goidl looks at the regulation of autoimmunity by auto-anti-idiotypic antibody.

At a recent workshop the difficult task of exactly defining aging was attempted without much success; I hope that this book contributes data which will help in the further understanding of the relationship between the immune response and the aging process.

I am deeply grateful to Ms. Susan J. Martin for her efforts in this endeavor, to Ms. Linda Slater for her secretarial skills, and to the editorial staff of Marcel Dekker, Inc., for their support and patience.

Edmond A. Goidl

Contributors

Luciano Adorini, M.D. Senior Investigator, Laboratory of Pathology, ENEA, C.R.E. Casaccia, Rome, Italy

Blanche Bellon, Ph.D.* Visiting Fellow, Department of Microbiology, Mount Sinai School of Medicine, New York, New York

Constantin A. Bona, M.D., Ph.D. Professor, Department of Microbiology, Mount Sinai School of Medicine, New York, New York

Hui-chen Chang, M.S. Research Affiliate, Department of Molecular Immunology, Roswell Park Memorial Institute, Buffalo, New York

Mei-ping Chang, Ph.D. Research Microbiologist, Geriatric Research, Education and Clinical Center, West Los Angeles Veterans Administration Medical Center, and Research Immunologist, University of California at Los Angeles School of Medicine, Los Angeles, California

Gino Doria, M.D. Professor of Immunology, Laboratory of Pathology, ENEA, C.R.E. Casaccia, Rome, Italy

*Current affiliation: CNS ERA 48, INSERM U28, and Hôpital Broussais, Paris, France

Rita B. Effros, Ph.D. Adjunct Associate Professor, Department of Pathology, University of California at Los Angeles School of Medicine, Los Angeles, California

Gabriel Fernandes, Ph.D. Associate Professor, Department of Medicine, The University of Texas Health Science Center at San Antonio, San Antonio, Texas

Daniela Frasca Doctor in Biological Sciences, Senior Investigator, Laboratory of Pathology, ENEA, C.R.E. Casaccia, Rome, Italy

Vithal K. Ghanta, Ph.D. Research Associate Professor, Department of Biology and Microbiology, and Comprehensive Cancer Center, University of Alabama, Birmingham, Alabama

Edmond A. Goidl, Ph.D. Associate Professor, Department of Microbiology and Immunology, The University of Maryland School of Medicine, Baltimore, Maryland

Susan R. S. Gottesman, Ph.D., M.D. Research Assistant Professor, Department of Pathology, New York University School of Medicine, New York, New York

Gail S. Habicht, Ph.D. Associate Professor, Department of Pathology, State University of New York, Stony Brook, New York

David E. Harrison, Ph.D. Senior Staff Scientist, The Jackson Laboratory, Bar Harbor, Maine

Raymond N. Hiramato, Ph.D. Professor, Department of Microbiology, Veterans Administration Medical Center and Comprehensive Cancer Center, University of Alabama, Birmingham, Alabama

Jyh-Hsiung Huang, Ph.D. Research Affiliate, Department of Molecular Immunology, Roswell Park Memorial Institute, Buffalo, New York

Norman R. Klinman, M.D., Ph.D. Member, Department of Immunology, Scripps Clinic and Research Foundation, La Jolla, California

Heinz Köhler, M.D., Ph.D. Director, Department of Molecular Immunology, Roswell Park Memorial Institute, Buffalo, New York

Shun-cheng Li, M.D. Geriatric Research, Education and Clinical Center, West Los Angeles Veterans Administration Medical Center, and University of California at Los Angeles School of Medicine, Los Angeles, California

Takashi Makinodan, Ph.D. Director, Geriatric Research, Education and Clinical Center, West Los Angeles Veterans Administration Medical Center, and Professor in Residence, Department of Medicine, University of California at Los Angeles School of Medicine, Los Angeles, California

Audrey J. Manheimer-Lory, M.S., Ph.D. Graduate Student, Department of Microbiology, Mount Sinai School of Medicine, New York, New York

Richard A. Miller, M.D., Ph.D. Associate Professor, Department of Pathology, Boston University School of Medicine, Boston, Massachusetts

Sybille Müller, Ph.D. Cancer Research Scientist III, Department of Molecular Immunology, Roswell Park Memorial Institute, Buffalo, New York

Dean C. Norman, M.D. Associate Clinical Chief, Geriatric Research, Education and Clinical Center, West Los Angeles Veterans Administration Medical Center, and Assistant Professor of Medicine, University of California at Los Angeles School of Medicine, Los Angeles, California

Risë Schwab, Ph.D. Instructor in Immunology, Division of Geriatrics, Department of Medicine, Cornell University Medical College, New York, New York

Diego Segre, D.V.M., Ph.D. Professor, Department of Veterinary Pathobiology, University of Illinois, Urbana, Illinois

Mariangela Segre, D.Sc. Associate Professor, Department of Veterinary Pathobiology, University of Illinois, Urbana, Illinois

Sen-jaw Soong, Ph.D. Professor, Department of Biostatistics and Biomathematics and Comprehensive Cancer Center, University of Alabama, Birmingham, Alabama

Myron R. Szewczuk, M.Sc., Ph.D. Associate Professor, Department of Microbiology and Immunology, Queen's University, Kingston, Ontario, Canada

Marilyn L. Thoman, Ph.D. Assistant Member, Department of Immunology, Scripps Clinic and Research Foundation, La Jolla, California

G. J. Thorbecke, M.D., Ph.D. Professor, Department of Pathology, New York University School of Medicine, New York, New York

Andrew W. Wade, Ph.D. Postdoctoral Fellow, Department of Microbiology and Immunology, Queen's University, Kingston, Ontario, Canada

Roy L. Walford, M.D. Professor, Department of Pathology, University of California at Los Angeles School of Medicine, Los Angeles, California

Mary M. Ward, Ph.D. Cancer Research Scientist I, Department of Molecular Immunology, Roswell Park Memorial Institute, Buffalo, New York

Ronald E. Ward, Ph.D. Cancer Research Scientist III, Department of Molecular Immunology, Roswell Park Memorial Institute, Buffalo, New York

William O. Weigle, Ph.D. Member and Chairman, Department of Immunology, Scripps Clinic and Research Foundation, La Jolla, California

Marc E. Weksler, M.D. Wright Professor of Medicine, Division of Geriatrics, Department of Medicine, Cornell University Medical College, New York, New York

Richard A. Winchurch, Ph.D. Associate Professor of Surgery and Director of Research, Department of Surgery, Baltimore Regional Burn Center, Johns Hopkins University School of Medicine and Francis Scott Key Medical Center, Baltimore, Maryland

Dorith Zharhary, Ph.D.* Research Fellow, Department of Immunology, Scripps Clinic and Research Foundation, La Jolla, California

---

*Current affiliation: Weizmann Institute of Science, Rehovot, Israel

Contents

Aging and the Immune Response

1

Clonal Analysis of Age-Associated Changes in T-Cell Reactivity

Richard A. Miller

Boston University School of Medicine
Boston, Massachusetts

David E. Harrison

The Jackson Laboratory
Bar Harbor, Maine

I. INTRODUCTION

In principle, the net strength of an immune reaction may depend on the outcome of a complicated set of multicellular interactions. The generation of antigen-specific cytotoxic T lymphocytes (CTL), for example, can be affected by changes in the number of reactive precursors (pCTL) able to give rise to CTL effectors, changes in the number or intrinsic activity of the effectors that arise from each precursor that does respond, similar kinds of alteration in the lymphokine-producing helper T cells that promote CTL clonal expansion and maturation, and/or variation in suppressive cells that regulate the effectors and their precursors. It has become clear that aging brings about a loss in the net strength of immune responses tested in a number of ways (although there is great variation among the individual members of most elderly cohorts). We are, however, still far from a detailed, quantitative picture of the changes in cellular biology that must underlie age-associated loss of protective immune function.

In an effort to reduce some of the difficulties inherent in the analysis of complex, multicellular interactions, we have attempted to measure age-associated changes in one of the fundamental variables likely to influence net immune strength: the number of T lymphocytes able to respond to mitogenic or antigenic stimulation. We use a method, limiting dilution analysis (LDA), that can provide independent estimates of (a) the number of responding cells in a given sample and (b) the amount of functional effect (e.g., lymphokine production) attributable to each responding cell. We find, in general, that aging leads to a decrease in the frequency of T cells that are able to respond to stimulation by producing a measurable level of functional effect, but that the amount of effect attributable to the cells that do respond is not altered by age.

II. LIMITING DILUTION ANALYSIS: PRINCIPLES, ADVANTAGES, AND LIMITATIONS

The first systematic application of limiting dilution methods to cellular immunology came in the efforts of Lefkovits and his colleagues to estimate the number of B cells able to give rise to clones of antibody-secreting plasma cells under various conditions of stimulation (1). The "splenic focus" system developed by Klinman and his colleagues (2) provides a way to analyze clonal interactions in antibody formation in a more nearly "natural," in vivo situation. Extension of these methods to the estimation of pCTL came from the realization that optimal expansion of each pCTL could be obtained only in the presence of "helper factors" supplied in the form of T-cell-conditioned medium (3,4). Methods for the quantitation of helper T cell precursors, either through their supportive effect on B or CTL development (5,6), or more directly through their ability to elaborate lymphokines (7), have also been developed.

The success of each of these methods depends on the development of culture conditions that supply all the cellular, hormonal, and nutritional factors needed to support the clonal expansion and differentiation of the cell type under consideration, but devoid of these cells themselves. To quantitate pCTL, for example, one usually needs to provide a stimulus (e.g., alloantigen or mitogen), saturating levels of helper factors including (but probably not limited to) the T-cell growth factor interleukin 2 (IL-2), and "feeder" cells that may provide additional needed cofactors, a "sink" for toxic factors, or both. After an interval, one tests each of many culture wells, set up at several doses, for the presence of cytotoxic effectors. In culture wells that received high numbers of pCTL, every culture well will yield effectors, but titration of the responding population will enter a dose range at which some but not all wells have received a pCTL cell and thus score "positive" for CTL effect.

An illustration is provided in Figure 1, based on an experiment (7) to estimate the frequency of precursors for IL-2 secreting helper T cells (pHTL) in BALB/c mouse splenocytes reactive to H-2^b alloantigens. Each culture well contained 10^4 T-cell-depleted peritoneal stimulators of the (BALB/c $\times$ C57BL/6)F_1 genotype, as a source of both H-2^b alloantigen and "feeder" cells. BALB/c spleen cells were then titrated in at doses of 100–1600 per well, using 20 wells at each concentration. After 5 days of incubation we removed 100 μl of supernatant from each well to test for IL-2 accumulation. Each point in Figure 1

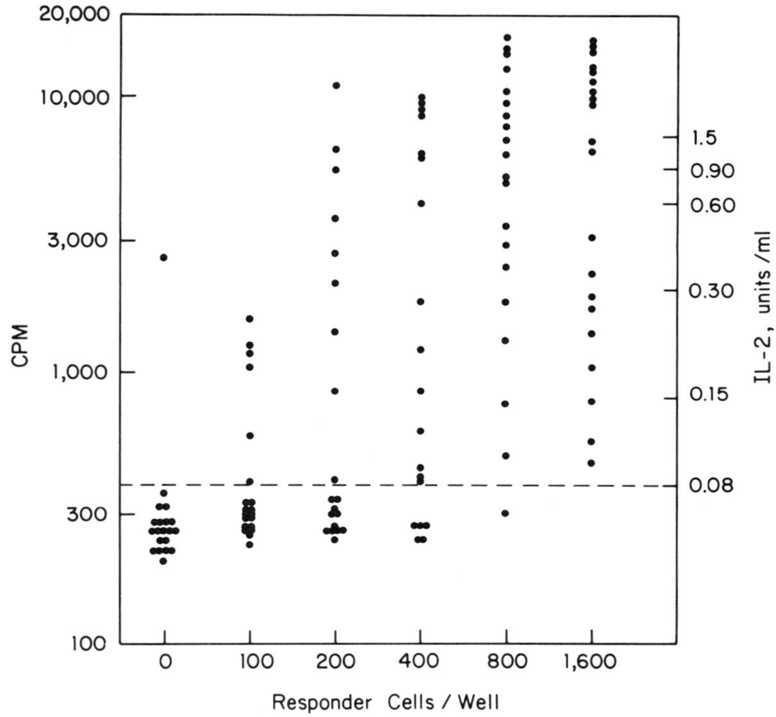

Figure 1 A representative pHTL titration. Each point represents IL-2 production in a single culture well set up with the indicated concentration of BALB/c spleen cells, together with 10^4 (BALB/c × C57BL/6)F_1 T-cell-depleted peritoneal cell stimulators. Supernatant from each well (20 wells at each responder cell concentration) was removed at day 5 and tested for IL-2 content by bioassay; the results are expressed both as crude counts per minute (left-hand axis) and as equivalent IL-2 concentration in arbitrary laboratory units per milliliter. The dashed line at 379 cpm is set 3 standard deviations above the mean level of the "no responder" background wells, which received only the peritoneal stimulator cells. (From Ref. 7.)

represents the IL-2 level in an individual culture well, both as crude counts per minute (left axis) and as equivalent amount of IL-2 (in arbitrary units per milliliter, right axis). A group of "background" wells is also set up containing all components except BALB/c responder cells, as a test for production of IL-2 by the stimulator cells themselves. An occasional background well is found to contain IL-2 (as in Figure 1); this probably represents a T cell that escaped destruction in the complement-mediated anti-Thy-1 treatment used for T-cell depletion of the stimulator cells. The dashed horizontal line represents the threshold value, set arbitrarily at 3 standard deviations above the mean background level of counts per minute, used to score the experimental wells as "positive" or "negative" for IL-2-producing helper cells. It is apparent that addition of as few as 200–800 BALB/c splenocytes per well leads to IL-2 production in most of the wells, and that an aliquot containing about 400 BALB/c spleen cells must, on average, contain at least one cell able to react to H-2^b antigens by producing IL-2 (or, more likely, by producing a clone of IL-2-secreting cells).

The statistical analysis of the distribution of positive wells as a function of the input cell dose is based on the Poisson distribution. The monograph of Lefkovits and Waldmann (8) contains a clear discussion of the principles involved, and Taswell (9) provides a useful and mathematically sophisticated evaluation of the available algorithms. Several useful results emerge from these analyses. First of all, the frequencies estimated are frequencies, not of the effector cells themselves, but more strictly of the immediate, stimulus-sensitive *precursors* of the cells whose effect we eventually measure. Second, the frequency estimates provide only minimum estimates; the "true" frequency could well be higher if the assay method were to miss some of the responsible cells because of insensitivity, asynchronous appearance of effectors, or other condition. Third, the key assumptions on which the statistical analysis is based—i.e., that the distribution of positive and negative wells depends only on the frequency of a single kind of cell, and that a single cell of this type will be sufficient to generate a detectable positive response—can be tested by a chi-square test comparing the observed distribution of negative wells to that predicted by the Poisson distribution (8,9).

When the data of Figure 1 are replotted to show the proportion of negative wells in each group as a function of the input dose of splenocytes, one obtains the graph shown in Figure 2. The closeness of the observed points to a straight line through the origin indicates a good fit to the Poisson distribution (in this case $p(\chi^2) = .97$) and is consistent with the idea that a single cell type is limiting in these culture conditions. The slope of the line is proportional to the frequency of the limiting cell type and is in this case 0.0034. In other words, 3.4 BALB/c spleen cells per thousand were able, under our culture conditions, to respond to H-2^b by producing a clone of IL-2-secreting cells.

Frequency estimates of this sort would be especially useful for the analysis of developmental changes in the immune response if they could be shown to reflect changes in the antigen-reactive pHTL themselves, and if they could be insensitive to parallel changes in regulatory cells. Although there are reports of systems in which regulatory interactions alter apparent frequency measurements (10–12), we have several reasons to believe that our own assays are suppressor independent.

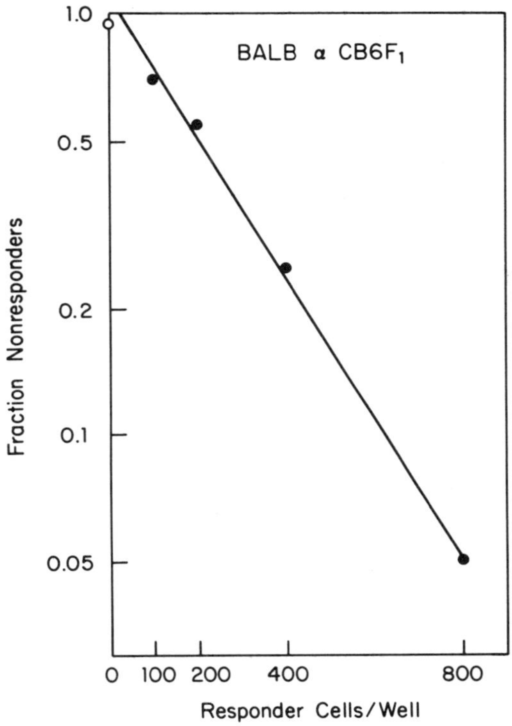

Figure 2 The data of Figure 1 replotted to show goodness of fit to the predicted one-hit Poisson model. The frequency of wells negative for IL-2 production is plotted as a function of the number of spleen cells originally added to each well in the group. The regression line has a slope, estimated by the chi-square minimization method (9), of 3.4 pHTL/10^3 spleen cells. (From Ref. 7.)

1. The amount of IL-2 that accumulates under limiting dilution conditions is 30–1000-fold higher than the amount produced, per reactive cell, under conventional culture conditions (7,13; and see Ref. 14 for an example involving pCTL). This suggests that accumulation of IL-2 in the usual "bulk culture" assays may be highly regulated and that IL-2 levels in LDAs are less so. Crowded bulk cultures in which each culture well is likely to receive adequate numbers of suppressor (and/or lymphokine-utilizing) cells, and in which regulatory actions that may require cell–cell contact are facilitated, may promote suppressive interactions unlikely to occur in more dilute cultures.

2. Most suppressor cell circuits involve Lyt-2^+ T cells, and yet the removal of Lyt-2^+ cells does not increase the measured pHTL frequency of the remaining Lyt-2^- T cells beyond that expected from enrichment (7,15). Similarly, adding back excess Lyt-2^+ cells does not diminish the measured pHTL frequency of the Lyt-2^- population.
3. The level of IL-2 accumulation in alloantigen-stimulated bulk cultures is 10-fold higher for CBA/H responder mice than for C57BL/6 mice; the pHTL frequencies for H-2-reactive cells are the same, however, for both strains (7,13). Similarly, CBA/H mice produce equal amounts of IL-2 in conventional cultures when stimulated with H-2 or with MLS determinants, despite a 10-fold higher pHTL frequency for the MLS antigens (7,13). Both findings suggest that the factors that regulate IL-2 accumulation in conventional mixed lymphocyte cultures fail to operate under LDA conditions and thus fail to influence measured precursor frequencies.
4. Analysis of pHTL frequencies in responses to influenza virus (16) have recently provided direct evidence that Lyt-2^+ suppressor T cells, able to block the expression of helper T-cell function in conventional in vitro reactions to influenza, do not alter the measured pHTL frequencies to these viral antigens.

These observations suggest that regulatory interactions have little effect on frequency estimates in our experimental conditions, and that our method therefore can provide information about age-associated changes in the antigen-reactive precursor cells themselves.

III. CHANGES WITH AGE IN THE PROPORTION OF T CELLS THAT REACT TO ANTIGENS AND MITOGENS

Several research groups have reported that splenocytes from old mice have a diminished ability to produce the helper T-cell growth factor IL-2 (17-20), and some of these have also found diminished function in the ability to respond to IL-2 either through proliferation or through development of CTL effectors (19, 20). To begin to analyze these results at the clonal level, we carried out LDA tests on mice at a variety of ages, using the method outlined in Figures 1 and 2. The results are shown in Figure 3, in which the frequencies represent the proportion of splenic T cells able to generate a clone of IL-2-producing helpers after stimulation across a complete H-2 haplotype. There is a statistically significant decline, with age, in alloreactive pHTL frequency ($p < .05$), but there is much variation within each age group, as well as overlap between the ranges from mice of widely differing ages.

These experiments were performed in such a way that old and young control mice were not always tested together, and day-to-day variation in the assay

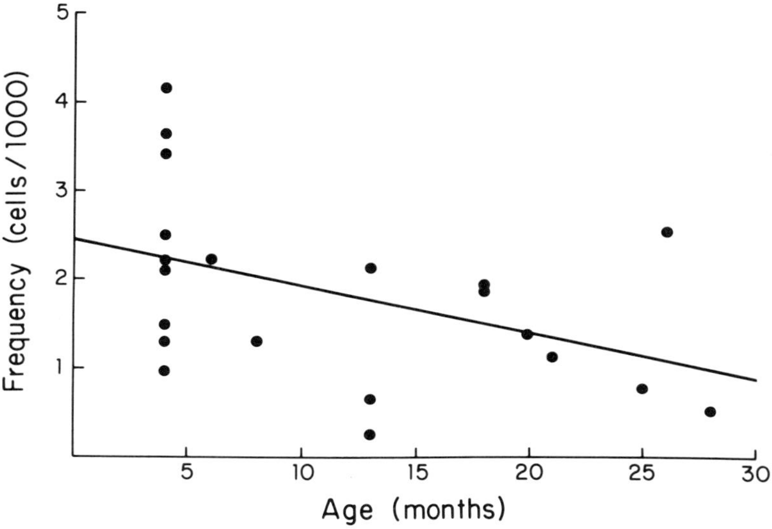

Figure 3 Change, with age, of H-2-reactive pHTL frequencies estimated by limiting dilution analysis. Frequencies were determined from titration of either spleen cells or splenic T cells and are expressed as pHTL per 10^3 T cells on the assumption that the spleen contains approximately 35% T lymphocytes. Of the 21 titrations shown, 12 were CBA anti-(B6 X CBA), 5 were B6 anti-(BALB/c X B6), and 4 were BALB/c anti-(BALB/c X B6). By linear regression, frequency = 2.45 - (age X 0.053), with $R = .436$ and $p < .05$. (From Ref. 13.)

method may have confounded our ability to detect more dramatic age-associated changes in precursor frequency. We therefore undertook a series of experiments in which each day's assay included at least one old and one young mouse. Furthermore, in view of the possibility that H-2 antigens might activate a non-representative subset of the entire T-cell pool, we decided to test for reactions to the mitogen concanavalin A (Con A), which had been shown (21) to stimulate a large fraction of both the Lyt-2^- helper and Lyt-2^+ killer T-cell subsets.

Figure 4 shows the frequency of Con-A-reactive pHTL, pCTL, and pPTL (precursors of proliferating T lymphocytes) in splenocytes of mice 4 or 18 months old. Each point represents one mouse. Points representing mice of different ages tested together are connected. Only experiments in which the data fit the expected Poisson distribution with a $p(\chi^2) > .10$ are included. In a few cases (3/30), only one of the pair of mice tested met this criterion, and data from these mice are also included in Figure 4 without a connecting line.

The left-hand panel of Figure 4 shows data from pHTL titrations (for IL-2 production). The mean value for young mice was 128 ±38 (SEM) pHTL per

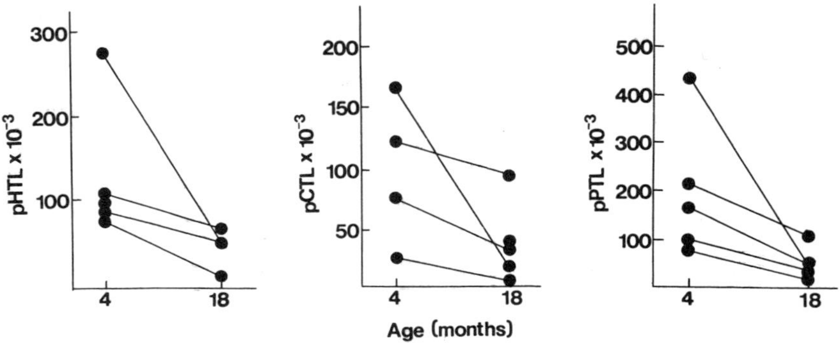

Figure 4 Age-associated changes in T-cell precursor frequencies in reactions to Con A: pHTL responses detected by IL-2 secretion (left), pCTL responses detected by lectin-facilitated reactions against P815 mastocytoma targets (middle), and pPTL proliferative frequencies estimated by thymidine incorporation (right). Each point represents a (BALB/c X C57BL/6)F_1 mouse of the indicated age. Points connected by a line were from mice assayed together. Only assays that fit the expected linear distribution with a $p(\chi^2) > .05$ are shown; 27 titrations of 30 met this criterion. Frequencies shown are per thousand spleen cells. (From Ref. 22.)

10^3 splenocytes. Since T cells are thought to make up about 35% of splenocytes, and about 60% of these are of the Lyt-2⁻, L3T4⁺ helper subset, the "expected" value, assuming 100% cloning efficiency, would be approximately $210/10^3$. Our method therefore seems to detect, in young mice, a substantial proportion (about 128/210 = 60%) of the maximum number of splenic helper cells predicted by theory.

In contrast, old mice have lower pHTL frequencies. In each experiment, the old mouse tested gave a lower pHTL value than the young control tested simultaneously. The mean ratio of young/old pHTL frequencies was 3.75:1, and the average for the old mice was 46 ±12 pHTL/10^3 splenocytes.

The middle panel of Figure 4 presents similar data for pCTL frequencies, using the method of Reference 23, in which clones are stimulated with Con A, encouraged to proliferate by addition of conditioned medium containing IL-2, and then tested for CTL effector function in a phytohemagglutinin (PHA)-facilitated assay for which recognition of specific target cell antigens is not required. Again, each old mouse had a lower pCTL frequency than a young control tested in parallel. The mean value for the young mice, 97 ±30, was close to the "theoretical" expectation of $140/10^3$, reassuring us that our method is able to activate a large fraction of the entire splenic cytotoxic T-cell pool. The mean ratio of young to old pCTL frequencies, averaged across experimental pairs, was 4.73:1.

The right-hand panel of Figure 4 shows that clonal proliferation in response to Con A plus IL-2 containing conditioned medium is similarly diminished with age. On average, $200/10^3$ (±63) splenocytes from young mice could generate a proliferating clone (theoretical value: $350/10^3$), and the average ratio of young to old was 4.24. Again, no old mouse generated pPTL at a higher frequency than its young control.

Figure 5 shows that a similar age-associated decline in precursor frequency applies to keyhole limpet hemocyanin (KLH)-specific helper T cells accumulated in lymph nodes draining a site of KLH injection in complete Freund's adjuvant. The left-hand panel depicts frequency results from limiting dilution analyses in cultures challenged with KLH at a dose of 20 μg/ml, and the right-hand panel presents results at a lower challenge dose, 0.20 μg/ml. Except for one experiment, the young mouse in each day's pair had a higher pHTL frequency to KLH in responses to either antigen concentration.

We thought it particularly important to see whether the age-related loss of precursor cells also applied to blood lymphocytes, since blood sampling might permit sequential, nondestructive testing of immune status at intervals throughout an animal's life. Furthermore, most experimentation on human T-cell function requires testing of blood cells, and data on murine blood cells is therefore

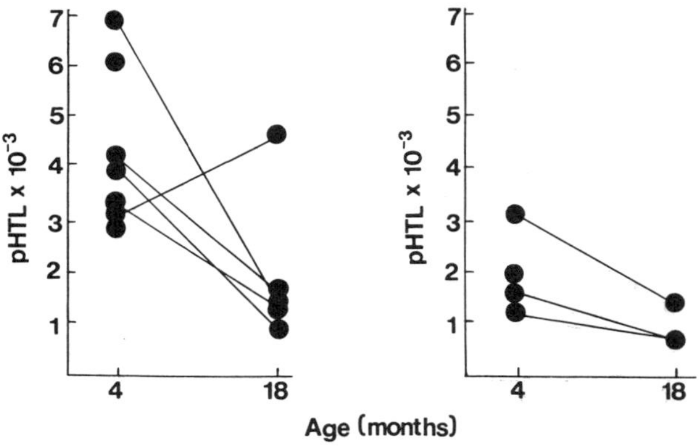

Figure 5 Effect of age on pHTL responses to KLH. Draining lymph node cells were removed from (BALB/c × C57BL/6)F_1 mice 4 days after priming with KLH in complete Freund's adjuvant and titered at varying doses into cultures containing 10^4 syngeneic T-cell-depleted peritoneal cells and KHL at either 20 μg/ml (left) or 0.02 μg/ml (right). Accumulation of IL-2 was tested at day 3, and wells scored as positive with respect to "background" wells set up in the absence of responder lymph node cells. As in Figure 4, each point represents an individual mouse of the age indicated, and lines connect mice assayed together. (From Ref. 22.)

Table 1 Precursor T-Cell Frequencies in Peripheral Blood Samples[a]

Age (months)	pHTL/10^3 PBL	pCTL/10^3 PBL	Mean ratio (N)
7–10	105 ±43	55 ±22	1.97 ±0.22 (4)
32–35	16 ±7	10 ±4	1.64 ±0.69 (6)

[a]Samples were taken from (B6 × CBA)F_1 mice of the ages indicated. Frequencies are expressed as cells per thousand peripheral blood leukocytes (PBL). In each day's assay, one old and one young mouse were tested in parallel, and the pHTL/pCTL ratio was calculated; the last column shows the mean value of this ratio.
Source: Ref. 24.

necessary to be able to compare results across species. The data in Table 1 show that helper and cytotoxic T-cell frequencies among murine blood T cells do indeed decline with age. Again, helper and killer cell subsets are affected by age to approximately equal degrees.

It is worth noting that the mice tested in this experiment were (C57BL/6 × CBA)F_1 animals housed at the Jackson Laboratories, in contrast to the (BALB/c × C57BL/6)F_1 mice used for the experiments in Figures 4 and 5, which had been raised in the National Aging Institute colony at the Charles River Breeding Laboratories. The observations on frequency loss therefore seem to be consistently demonstrable in spleen, lymph node, and blood samples taken from mice of different strains, bred and housed under different regimens, and challenged either with mitogens, soluble proteins, or alloantigens.

Investigations in other laboratories have suggested that age-related changes in absolute T-cell numbers, and in distribution of T cells among different subsets, while sometimes of statistical significance, are seldom large. In contrast, our data demonstrate that mice in the last third of their lifespan typically have three- to sixfold lower numbers of reactive helper and killer cells in comparison to young mice. Therefore precursor loss is not accompanied by a parallel loss of morphologically normal T cells, and seems instead to reflect an increasing number of cells that appear intact but do not respond to stimulation, at least under limiting dilution conditions.

IV. PRESERVATION, IN OLD MICE, OF THE AMOUNT OF EFFECTOR FUNCTION GENERATED PER REACTIVE CELL

The limiting dilution assay allows one to quantitate the level of functional effect (measured as IL-2 production, number of cytotoxic effectors, or degree of proliferation) attributable to each precursor cell that is able to respond under the assay conditions. Figure 6 shows data suggesting that there is no age-associated loss of effector function per reactive cell, at least for the precursors that react strongly enough to be detected at all. Each point in the figure represents a *group* of 12–16 wells set up together at a given cell concentration. The horizontal axis shows the number of precursor cells present in that well at the start of culture, as calculated from the frequency measured from the complete titration curve. The data from any single day's experiment have been normalized against the highest value (from old or young mouse) obtained during that day's experiment, to correct for day-to-day variation in assay sensitivity. Solid circles represent effector levels from old (18-month-old) mice, and open circles show data from 4-month-old controls.

For all three measures of function—IL-2 production, number of cytotoxic effectors, calculated (25) as $N \propto T$, and proliferation measured by radiothymidine incorporation—there is considerable variation at any given precursor concentration, but no consistent difference between old and young mice. The amount of functional effect tends to be less in wells set up with more than one clonal precursor, but old and young animals give similar results in wells receiving from 0 to 10 or more precursor cells. Figure 7 shows that a similar result emerges from analysis of KLH-stimulated cultures: there is no apparent age-related loss of functional effect generated per reactive cell.

V. EFFECT OF DIET-INDUCED LIFE SPAN EXTENSION ON T-CELL FREQUENCY LEVELS

If frequency changes are in fact "linked" to some more fundamental "clock" that influences the rate of age-related change in a wide range of physiological systems, one would expect alterations in the "rate of aging" to retard the rate at which T-cell frequencies decline. In rodent models, calorie restriction (especially when accompanied with adequate provision of specific nutrients), whether imposed at weaning or gradually imposed later in the life span, has been shown to lead both to increased longevity and to improved function well into what is chronologically old age (26-28). The strength of immune responses in calorie-restricted old mice has also been shown to be higher than in mice fed ad libitum (29,30). We tested (24) the frequencies of Con-A-responsive pHTL and pCTL cells in blood leukocytes of old mice 32-35 months old of the long-lived (C57BL/6 × CBA/H)F_1 hybrid strain, either fed ad lib or restricted from weaning to an amount of food approximately 60% of that consumed by conventional mice. Results of these assays (Figures 8 and 9) show that food-restricted mice retain relatively high levels of both pHTL and pCTL compared to conventionally fed mice of similar age. Food-restricted old mice have 3.5-fold higher pHTL levels and 4.5-fold higher pCTL levels compared to control-fed old mice. Restricted mice retain 50% of the pHTL cells, and 80% of the pCTL cells of young (7–10 month) control mice fed conventionally. Some mice were tested

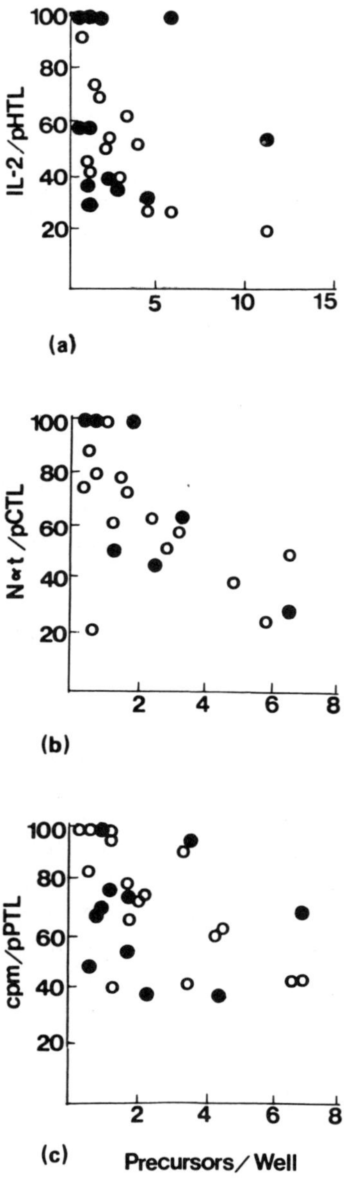

Figure 6 Level of effector function generated by T cells under limiting dilution conditions: lack of age effect (Con-A reactions). Each point represents the level of effector function—either IL-2 (a), cytotoxic activity calculated as N∝T as in Reference 25 (b), or counts per minute of thymidine incorporation(c)—obtained

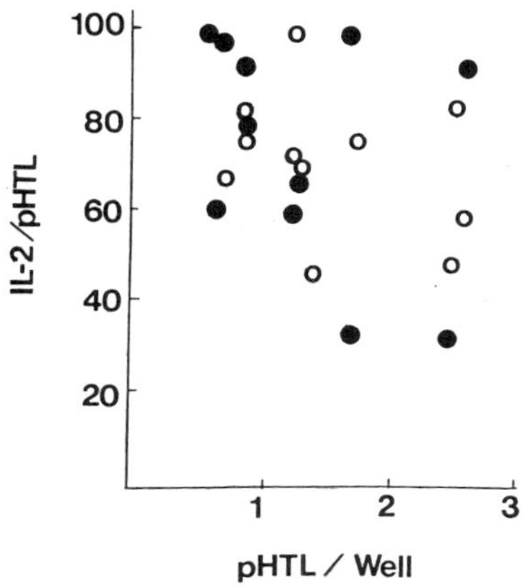

Figure 7 Production of IL-2 per number of reactive pHTL cells in limiting dilution reactions to KLH: lack of age effect. See legend to Figure 6 for details. (From Ref. 22.)

---

in a single group of 16 wells set up at one concentration from an individual mouse. Open circles represent young (4-month) mice, and solid circles represent old (18-month) mice. Results have been normalized as a percentage of the highest value obtained from old or young donors on a given day, to adjust for daily variation in assay sensitivity. (From Ref. 22.)

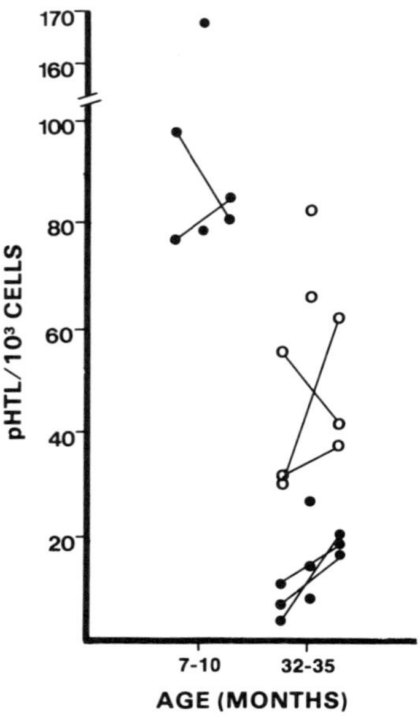

Figure 8 Preservation by food restriction of pHTL levels in peripheral blood samples of old mice. Values given represent frequencies of Con-A-reactive precursors (for IL-2 production) per thousand peripheral blood leukocytes in individual mice of the indicated ages. Open circles represent mice placed on a food-restricted diet from weaning. Solid circles represent mice fed a standard laboratory chow ad libitum. Some mice were tested twice (after an 8-week interval), and the corresponding values are connected by a line. (From Ref. 24.)

twice at intervals of 1-8 weeks (shown in the figures as connected points), to show that the low levels in the old mice fed ad lib were stable over time and therefore not attributable to the effects of acute ill health. It should be noted that about half the ad-lib-fed mice had died by the time these tests were carried out (32-35 months old), and it is possible that the survivors tended to be those with higher than average immune responses.

The ability of food restriction to slow the rate at which unresponsive helper and killer T cells accumulate in the immune system is consistent with the idea that this decline may be a key element in immunosenescence. In the same way, LDA tests, which can be carried out on as little as 5 μl of peripheral blood, provide a much-needed nondestructive test of age-associated changes in immune reactivity.

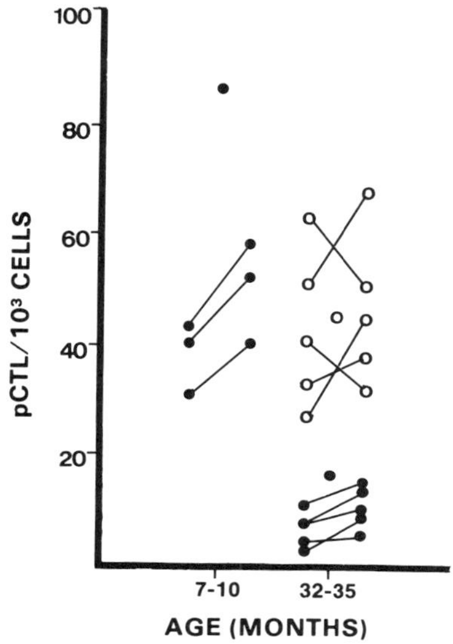

Figure 9 Preservation of pCTL frequencies by food restriction: Con-A reactions. Symbols are as in Figure 8, except that some mice were retested after an interval of only 1 week. (From Ref. 24.)

VI. EXPERIMENTAL MANIPULATION OF IMMUNE FUNCTION IN AGED MICE: ANALYSIS USING FREQUENCY MEASUREMENTS

Several experimental approaches to improving the immune reactivity of aged animals have been tested, and in some cases these have led to an increase in immune function. A common strategem has been to produce "heterochronic chimeras" by replacing some part of the immune system of old mice with cells taken from syngeneic young animals. The goal has been to define, in this way, the portions of the aged immune system that make the most significant contribution to diminished function.

Interpretation of these studies is difficult, because any improvement in immune reactivity that is seen might well be attributable, not to the "replacement" of some function missing from normal old mice, but rather to a compensatory alteration in some other element. One might, for example, be able to increase immune responsiveness in old mice either by an increase in pHTL frequency or by interfering with a suppressor cell circuit, regardless of whether these components are in fact altered by aging.

From this perspective, we decided to reinvestigate several models of immune "restoration" in aging mice. We expected to find that some forms of restoration might involve a genuine restoration of normal ("young") levels of antigen-reactive pHTL and pCTL and that other forms might involve instead a compensatory alteration (decline) in suppressive pathways, without any restoration of the effector cell populations. Our results, though still preliminary, suggest that while some models of immune rejuvenation (e.g., calorie restriction) may involve improvement of precursor numbers, others instead may bring about improved immune function through changes in regulatory circuitry.

A. T-Cell Frequencies in Hypophysectomized Mice

Scott et al. (31) have reported that removal of the pituitary from middle-aged rats (with endocrine supplementation) leads to a restoration of several indices of immune function. Harrison et al. (32) reinvestigated this phenomenon in hypophysectomized mice and found that surgerized mice did indeed have increased proliferative responses to PHA in vitro and increased delayed hypersensitivity (DTH) responses to sheep erythrocytes (SRBC) in vivo, as well as increased thymus weight and cortex/medullary ratio. Treated mice did not, however, regain youthful function in tests of their ability to mount antibody responses to SRBC, whether measured as levels of agglutinins or plaque-forming cells (PFC) in immunized mice. Hypophysectomized mice lived no longer than untreated controls, or sham-operated controls that received the same hormone supplementation as the mice in the hypophysectomized group.

To learn whether the increased mitogen and DTH responses reflected underlying increases in the proportion of helper T cells, we performed LDA estimates of Con-A-reactive pHTL in mice of this sort and also estimated pCTL frequencies in the same animals. The data are presented in Figure 10. As expected, old control mice have lower levels of both pHTL and pCTL than the young controls, and sham operation with endocrine supplementation has little effect on these frequencies. In contrast to the results (32) using conventional assays of immune function, hypophysectomized old mice do not have increased frequencies of pHTL or pCTL cells. If anything, hypophysectomy seems to lead to a slight decrease in both frequencies and decreases T-cell frequencies (especially pCTL) in young mice, as well.

The contrast between improved function in conventional assays and the absence of improvement in precursor frequencies leads us to propose that hypophysectomy may lead to better DTH and PHA reactions through an effect on cell types that regulate helper cells, rather than via an effect on the PHA and SRBC reactive helper cells themselves. This speculation must be considered tentative, of course, for several reasons. First of all, we have at this point acquired frequency data on only 5-8 mice in each group, and additional animals must be tested before we can be certain of the pattern of results suggested

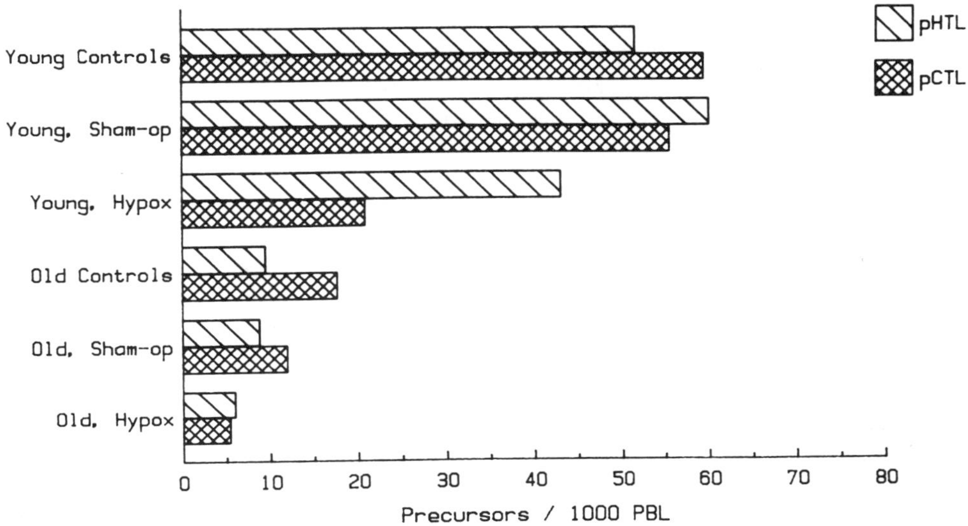

Figure 10 Frequencies of Con-A-responsive pHTL and pCTL in hypophysectomized young and old mice, and in controls. Values shown are precursors per thousand peripheral blood leukocytes. Young mice were 115–209 days old, and old mice were 641–739 days old when tested. Hypophysectomies and sham operations were performed 50–95 days before testing, and mice in these groups had received endocrine supplementation (32) from that time.

by our early data. Second, we need to acquire both conventional and frequency data on the same mice, and to the same antigens, rather than use "historical" controls for the conventional tests. Last, direct evidence of suppressor cells, in hypophysectomized mice, active in conventional assays but not under LDA conditions, would be better proof for our speculation than an indirect comparison between the results of two disparate assay systems. Nonetheless, the frequency data contradict the idea that improved immune response in hypophysectomized old mice results from a restoration of reactive T-cell precursors.

B. T-Cell Frequencies in Heterochronic Chimeras

Hirokawa and Makinodan (33) have demonstrated that immune responsiveness in old mice can be improved by treatment with a combination of irradiation, implantation of bone marrow cells from syngeneic young donors, and grafting of thymic gland tissue from syngeneic neonates. In these chimeras, termed "heterochronic" because they contain tissues from mice of different ages, marrow cells are thought to colonize the thymus gland and then to mature to peripheral T cells with the high level of function characteristic of cells in young mice. Similar results were obtained by Astle and Harrison (34), who found that improved responses to SRBC and to PHA were indeed obtained, although longevity was not thereby improved. This group also showed (34) that bone marrow derived from old mice was not sufficient, even together with a thymic implant, to restore immune reactivity in irradiated old recipients, in contrast to bone marrow from young mice. Restoration therefore seemed to require two components—marrow and thymic tissue—from young mice.

We have begun to reinvestigate heterochronic mice of this sort using the additional insights that can be obtained by limiting dilution methods. Our initial results, again relying on the estimation of Con-A-responsive pHTL and pCTL in reconstituted mice (6-9 mice per group), are presented in Figures 11 and 12. Irradiated young mice can indeed be repopulated by thymic tissue grafted together with marrow cells, and they recover nearly normal levels of both pHTL and pCTL; the age of the marrow donor does not seem to matter. Irradiated old mice do acquire improved numbers of pHTL cells (a result that parallels the suggestions of the conventional assays in Ref. 34), but they do *not* seem to regain comparable numbers of pCTL. In this context it would be of interest to test repopulated mice of this sort for cytotoxic function in conventional, high-

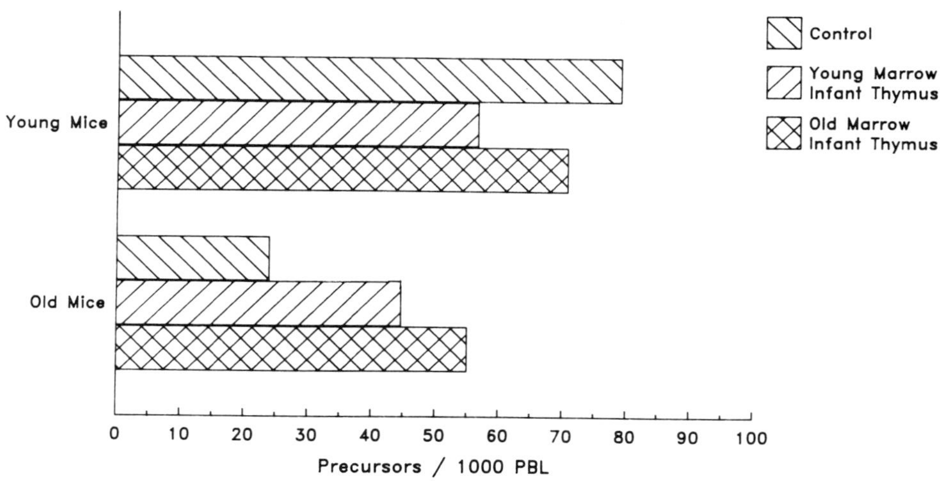

Figure 11 Con-A-reactive pHTL in peripheral blood of heterochronic irradiation chimeras and controls. Young mice were 204–254 days old when tested, and old mice were 613–838 days old. Mice in the experimental groups received, at least 90 days before test, treatment with 800–1000 rads of x-irradiation, 10^7 syngeneic unselected bone marrow cells from old or young donors intravenously, and a thymus gland from a donor 1–2 days old implanted under the kidney capsule, as described in more detail in Reference 34.

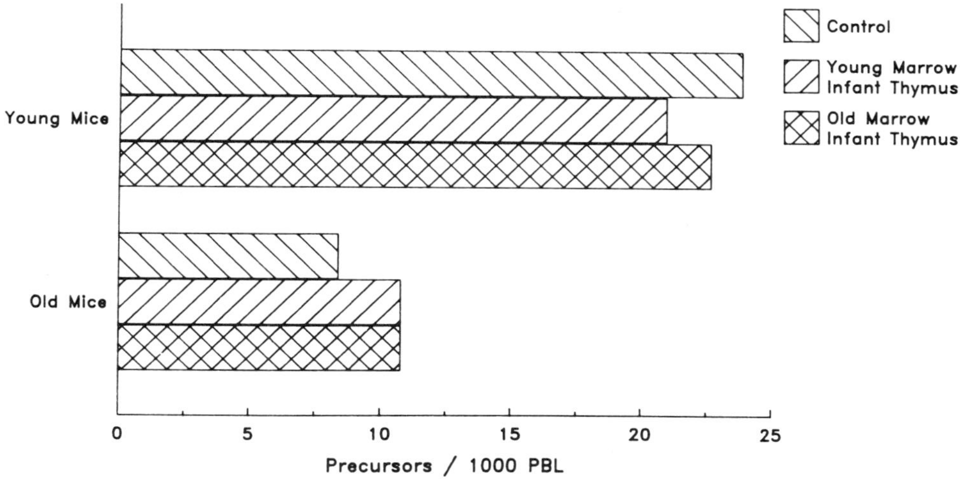

Figure 12 Con-A-reactive pCTL in peripheral blood of heterochronic chimeras. See legend to Figure 11 for additional details.

density assay cultures and in vivo. Interestingly, the poor performance of marrow from old donors in regenerating normal immune function in conventional assays (34) does *not* reflect a parallel disparity in the ability of this tissue to restore levels of either pHTL or pCTL. As in the hypophysectomy experiments, the disparity between the results of the conventional assays and the frequency data leads us to consider more complex, regulatory explanations. In this case, one could surmise that marrow from old mice contains (or gives rise to) cells that down-regulate the immune response, but that this down-regulation does not involve an effect on precursor cell frequencies. As in the case of the hypophysectomy experiments, however, this suggestion is supported only by tenuous evidence and is meant to be tested rather than believed.

C. T-Cell Frequencies in Parabiotic Chimeras

A second method for producing heterochronic, chimeric mice involves parabiotic connection between the circulatory systems of mice of different ages. Immune reactivity in mice of this sort was tested by Astle and Harrison (34), who found that the immune responses of old mice were only slightly improved by parabiosis to young animals. In contrast, the immune reactions of young mice linked surgically to old partners were substantially *decreased* compared to young controls. Similar findings have been reported by others for anti-SRBC reactions (35).

We subsequently measured pHTL and pCTL frequencies in parabiotic chimeras of this type, and the preliminary results (9-14 mice/group) are presented in Figures 13 and 14. The results are entirely consistent with the data from conventional assays of immune function (34): surgical linkage of an old mouse to a young mouse leads to little, if any, increase in pHTL and pCTL frequencies in comparison to the levels found in old mice linked to old partners (or to untreated old control mice). Linkage of an old mouse to a young animal, however, does depress reactive T-cell frequencies in the young mouse, in comparison to frequencies in young mice linked to young partners. The surgery itself does not lead to a depression of immune function; in fact, members of young-young pairs have higher levels of both pHTL and pCTL than do unmanipulated young controls.

These parabiotic mice, in essence, share a circulatory system. Radiolabeled erythrocytes injected into one partner equilibrate in the shared circulation with a $t_{1/2}$ of about 20 min (Astle and Harrison, unpublished). Assays of blood

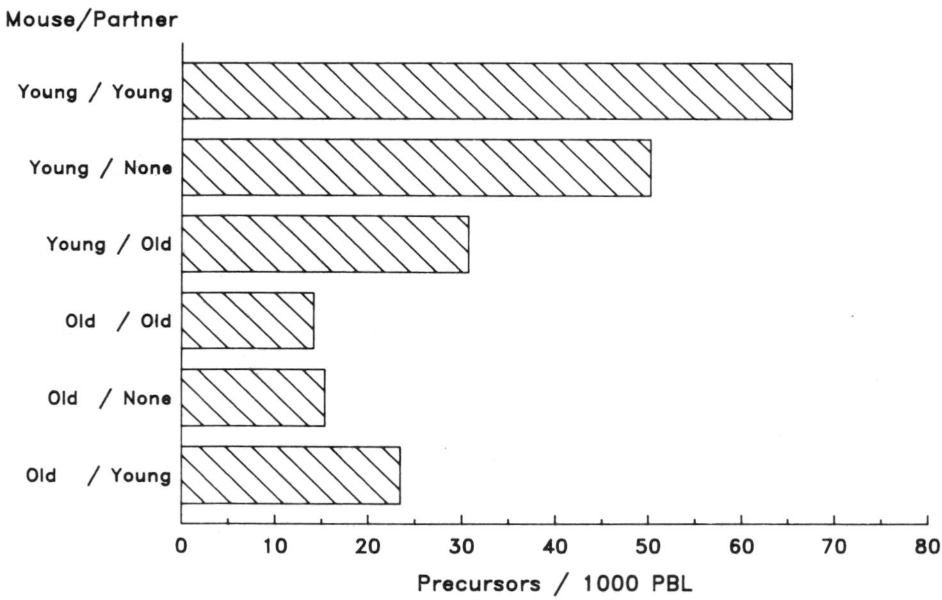

Figure 13 Con-A-reactive pHTL in peripheral blood of parabiotic chimeras. In the designation, the mouse whose blood is tested is listed first, followed by the surgically linked partner, if any. Young mice were 173-345 days old at the time of assay, and old mice were 668-775 days old. Parabiosis had been accomplished as in Reference 34, 103-173 days before the blood sampling.

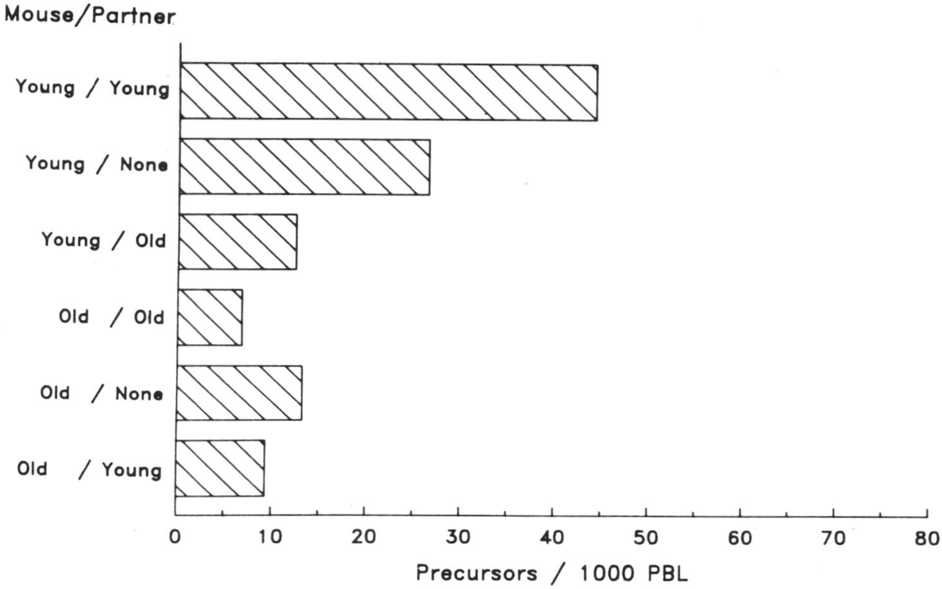

Figure 14 Con-A-reactive pCTL in peripheral blood of parabiotic chimeras. See legend to Figure 13 for further details.

lymphocyte responses from either member of an old-young pair are therefore likely to represent the weighted average of the T cells produced in the lymphoid systems of both animals together. If the immune system of a young mouse were to exert a beneficial influence on lymphopoiesis in the body of a connected old partner, either through soluble mediators or by "seeding" the immune system of the partner with migratory stem cells, one might expect the members of old-young pairs to have levels of precursor cells similar to those in members of young-young pairs. Clearly this does not occur. If the old member of an old-young pair were to produce factors or cells that could travel through the circulation to down-regulate lymphopoiesis in a young partner, one would expect to see the sort of data presented in Figures 13 and 14: low frequencies of both pHTL and pCTL in each member of an old-young pair. A third hypothesis, in which lymphopoiesis proceeds unaltered in both members of the heterochronic pair, and in which the "net" frequencies reflect simple admixture of the two contributions, cannot yet be eliminated by our data, since the small number of animals tested do not allow us to test, with much statistical confidence, the differences between the "suppression" hypothesis and the "simple mixture"

Table 2 Summary: Precursor Frequencies in Manipulated Old Mice

System	Conventional assays	Precursor frequencies
Food restriction	↑In many tests	↑pHTL and pCTL
Hypophysectomy	↑DTH, PHA	No increases
Irradiation chimera	↑PHA, PFC	↑pHTL?
Parabiotic chimera	No increases	No increases

idea. We may be able to distinguish these possibilities by testing larger numbers of mice, with greater age disparities.

Table 2 summarizes the results of our preliminary analysis of T-cell frequencies in old mice whose immune systems have been experimentally altered. Although some immune responses of old mice can be improved—as tested in conventional assays—by food restriction, by hypophysectomy, or by treatment with young marrow and an infant thymus, only in the first of these systems is there clear evidence for accompanying increases in both pHTL and pCTL cells. There is also some evidence for increased pHTL frequencies in the heterochronic chimeras. Parabiotic connection to a young partner does not seem to increase either frequencies or conventional measures. The increased function in hypophysectomized mice and in heterochronic chimeras may reflect changes in regulatory pathways, rather than in the mitogen-reactive precursors of CTL and lymphokine-producing helper T cells.

It is of interest to note that of the four experimental systems examined, food restriction is the only manipulation that increases longevity (29,32,34). Improved immune function, at least as measured by conventional assays, therefore seems not to lead by itself to life span extension in laboratory mice. Conversely, enhanced life span in food-restricted, genetically obese mice was not accompanied by improved immune function (29). Measurements of precursor frequencies, in their insensitivity to changes in regulatory leukocytes, may be more sensitive indicators of underlying changes in "biological age" than conventional measures of immune function.

VII. DISCUSSION AND PROSPECTS

Investigators in many laboratories have examined age-associated changes in precursor frequencies and have produced a remarkably consistent pattern: old mice are usually found to have a diminished number of precursor cells, but no loss in the amount of functional effect derived from each precursor cell that does respond. In addition to the evidence presented above, examples of this pattern may be seen for B cells stimulated in vitro with the mitogen lipopolysaccharide (LPS) (36), for antigen-reactive B cells in splenic focus assays (37), and for cytotoxic T cells reactive to alloantigens (38,39). A dissenting report (40) has, however, also appeared, on the question of age-associated loss of LPS-responsive B cells. Nor is it yet clear to what extent these studies of laboratory mice can be generalized to other species, and our preliminary evidence (Rozans and Miller, in preparation) suggests that age-dependent loss of pHTL and pCTL may be far less dramatic in humans than in mice.

What abnormalities, in metabolic and biochemical terms, are likely to underlie the "precursor loss" we detect in short-term in vitro clonal assays? Many successive activation events are now thought to take place between the initial reception of a mitogenic or antigenic signal and the production of a detectably large clone of effector lymphocytes. These events are likely to include changes in membrane permeability, RNA synthesis, lymphokine receptor expression, commitment to clonal expansion, and eventual differentiation into a mature effector. Age-associated defects at one or more of these stages might well produce the pattern of functional effects we and others have observed. Indeed, when mitogen-stimulated lymphocytes from old humans are subjected to analysis of cell cycle transitions (41), they exhibit defects at several different commitment points: entry into first S phase, entry into first mitosis, entry into subsequent mitoses, and so on. Acquisition of the interleukin-2 receptor, an event that precedes initiation of DNA synthesis, is also accomplished less frequently by mitogen-stimulated T cells from old mice and humans (Vie and Miller, in preparation). This line of evidence, though still very sketchy, suggests that individual T cells from old donors may "fail" at any of several stages in the activation pathway. A T cell that failed at any stage in the first several mitotic cycles after activation would probably escape detection as a pHTL or pCTL in our culture system.

The LDA methods discussed here can be useful in the analysis of other aspects of aging besides estimation of precursor numbers. The ability to detect an age-sensitive indicator of immune status using blood samples as small as 5 μl will permit longitudinal and crossover studies of normal and of experimentally manipulated aging mice. Since the LDA method facilitates the rapid screening of many individual T-cell clones without extensive prior selection for rapid growth in culture, it makes possible detailed analysis, at the clonal level, of age-dependent changes in patterns of lymphokine secretion, memory cell formation, antigen dose dependence, and receptor fine-specificity. A detailed understanding of immune senescence at the cellular level may help to guide the required analysis of genetic and biochemical changes that distinguish old from young lymphocytes.

ACKNOWLEDGMENTS

We wish to thank Osias Stutman, John Archer, C. M. Astle, Sandy Bristol, Bruce Jacobson, and Karen Derman for their contributions to the work described above. The research was supported by U.S. Public Health Service grants AG-03978, AG-01755, and AG-00595.

REFERENCES

1. Lefkovits, I. 1972. Induction of antibody-forming cell clones in microcultures. *Eur. J. Immunol.* 2:360.
2. Klinman, N. R. 1972. The mechanism of antigenic stimulation of primary and secondary precursor cells. *J. Exp. Med.* 136:241.
3. Fischer-Lindahl, K., and D. B. Wilson. 1977. Histocompatibility antigen-activated cytotoxic T lymphocytes. II. Estimates of the frequency and specificity of precursors. *J. Exp. Med.* 145:508.
4. Teh, H. S., E. Harley, R. A. Phillips, and R. G. Miller. 1977. Quantitative studies on the precursors of cytotoxic lymphocytes. I. Characterization of a clonal assay and determination of the size of clones derived from single precursors. *J. Immunol.* 118:1049.
5. Waldmann, H., I. Lefkovits, and J. Quintans. 1975. Limiting dilution analysis of helper T-cell function. *Immunology.* 28:1135.
6. Lutz, C. T., A. L. Glasebrook, and F. W. Fitch. 1981. Enumeration of alloreactive helper T lymphocytes which cooperate with cytolytic T lymphocytes. *Eur. J. Immunol.* 11:726.
7. Miller, R. A., and O. Stutman. 1982. Enumeration of IL-2 secreting helper T cells by limiting dilution analysis, and demonstration of unexpectedly high levels of IL-2 production per responding cell. *J. Immunol.* 128:2258.
8. Lefkovits, I., and H. Waldmann. 1979. Limiting Dilution Analysis of Cells in the Immune System. Cambridge University Press, Cambridge, England.
9. Taswell, C. 1981. Limiting dilution assays for the determination of immunocompetent cell frequencies. I. Data analysis. *J. Immunol.* 126:1614.
10. Stockinger, B. 1984. Cytotoxic T-cell precursors revealed in neonatally tolerant mice. *Proc. Natl. Acad. Sci. USA.* 81:220.
11. Weyand, C., J. Goronzy, and G. J. Hammerling. 1981. Recognition of polymorphic H-2 domains by T lymphocytes. I. Functional role of different H-2 domains for the generation of alloreactive cytotoxic T lymphocytes and determination of precursor frequencies. *J. Exp. Med.* 154:1717.
12. Eichmann, K., I. Falk, I. Melchers, and M. M. Simon. 1980. Quantitative studies on T cell diversity. I. Determination of the precursor frequencies for two types of *Streptococcus A*-specific helper cells in nonimmune, polyclonally activated splenic T cells. *J. Exp. Med.* 152:477.
13. Miller, R. A., and O. Stutman. 1982. Limiting dilution analysis of IL-2 production: Studies of age, genotype, and regulatory interactions. *Lymphokine Res. News.* 3:79.
14. Macphail, S., I. Yron, and O. Stutman. 1982. Primary in vitro cytotoxic T cell response to non-major histocompatibility complex alloantigens in normal mice. *J. Exp. Med.* 156:610.

15. Miller, R. A. 1983. IL-2 Production by mitogen-stimulated T cell subsets: Helper-precursors are predominantly Lyt-2⁻. *J. Immunol.* 131:2864.
16. Miller, R. A., and C. S. Reiss. 1984. Limiting dilution analysis reveals latent influenza virus-specific helper T cells in virus-primed mice. *J. Mol. Cell. Immunol.* 1:357.
17. Miller, R. A., and O. Stutman. 1981. Decline, in aging mice, of the anti-TNP cytotoxic response attributable to loss of Lyt-2⁻, IL-2-producing helper cell function. *Eur. J. Immunol.* 11:751.
18. Thoman, M. L., and W. O. Weigle. 1982. Cell-mediated immunity in aged mice: An underlying lesion in IL-2 synthesis. *J. Immunol.* 128:2358.
19. Gillis, S., R. Kozak, M. Durante, and M. E. Weksler. 1981. Immunological studies of aging. Decreased production of and response to T cell growth factor by lymphocytes from aged humans. *J. Clin. Inv.* 67:937.
20. Gilman, S. C., J. S. Rosenberg, and J. D. Feldman. 1982. T lymphocytes of young and aged rats. II. Functional defects and the role of interleukin-2. *J. Immunol.* 128:644.
21. Chen, W.-F., A. Wilson, R. Scollay, and K. Shortman. 1982. Limit-dilution assay and clonal expansion of all T cells capable of proliferation. *J. Immunol. Methods.* 52:307.
22. Miller, R. A. 1984. Age-associated decline in precursor frequency for different T cell-mediated reactions, with preservation of helper or cytotoxic effect per precursor cell. *J. Immunol.* 132:63.
23. Wilson, A., W.-F. Chen, R. Scollay, and K. Shortman. 1982. Semi-automated limit-dilution assay and clonal expansion of all T-cell precursors of cytotoxic lymphocytes. *J. Immunol. Methods.* 52:283.
24. Miller, R. A., and D. E. Harrison. 1985. Delayed reduction in T cell precursor frequencies accompanies diet-induced lifespan extension. *J. Immunol.* 134:1426.
25. Miller, R. G., and M. Dunkley. 1974. Quantitative analysis of the ^{51}Cr-release cytotoxicity assay for cytotoxic lymphocytes. *Cell. Immunol.* 14:284.
26. Weindruch, R., and R. L. Walford. 1982. Dietary restriction in mice beginning at 1 year of age: Effect on life span and spontaneous cancer incidence. *Science.* 215:1415.
27. Masoro, E. J., B. P. Yu, H. A. Bertrand, and F. T. Lynd. 1980. Nutritional probe of the aging process. *Fed. Proc.* 39:3178.
28. Everitt, A. V. 1971. Food intake, growth, and the ageing of collagen in rat tail tendon. *Gerontologia.* 17:98.
29. Harrison, D. E., J. R. Archer, and C. M. Astle. 1984. Effects of food restriction on aging: Separation of food intake and adiposity. *Proc. Natl. Acad. Sci. USA.* 81:1835.
30. Weindruch, R., S. R. S. Gottesman, and R. L. Walford. 1982. Modification of age-related immune decline in mice dietarily restricted from or after midadulthood. *Proc. Natl. Acad. Sci. USA.* 79:898.
31. Scott, W., R. Bolla, and W. D. Denckla. 1979. Age-related changes in im-

mune function of rats and the effect of long-term hypophysectomy. *Mech. Ageing Dev.* 11:127.

32. Harrison, D. E., J. R. Archer, and C. M. Astle. 1982. The effect of hypophysectomy on thymic aging in mice. *J. Immunol.* 129:2673.
33. Hirokawa, K., and T. Makinodan. 1975. Thymic involution: Effect on T cell differentiation. *J. Immunol.* 114:1659.
34. Astle, C. M., and D. E. Harrison. 1984. Effects of marrow donor and recipient age on immune responses. *J. Immunol.* 132:673.
35. Butenko, G. M., and I. B. Gubrii. 1980. Inhibition of the immune responses of young adult CBA mice due to parabiosis with their old partners. *Exp. Gerontol.* 15:605.
36. Andersson, J., A. Coutinho, and F. Melchers. 1977. Frequencies of mitogen-reactive B cells in the mouse. I. Distribution in different lymphoid organs from different inbred strains of mice at different ages. *J. Exp. Med.* 145: 1511.
37. Zharhary, D., and N. R. Klinman. 1983. Antigen responsiveness of the mature and generative B cell populations of aged mice. *J. Exp. Med.* 157: 1300.
38. Goodman, S. A., and T. Makinodan. 1972. Effect of age on cell-mediated immunity in long-lived mice. *Clin. Exp. Immunol.* 19:533.
39. Nordin, A. A., and G. D. Collins. 1983. Limiting dilution analysis of alloreactive cytotoxic precursor cells in aging mice. *J. Immunol.* 131: 2215.
40. Hooijkaas, H., A. A. Preesman, A. van Oudenaren, R. Benner, and J. J. Haaijman. 1983. Frequency analysis of functional immunoglobulin C and V gene expression in murine B cells at various ages. *J. Immunol.* 131:1629.
41. Hefton, J. M., G. J. Darlington, B. A. Casazza, and M. E. Weksler. 1980. Immunologic studies of aging. V. Impaired proliferation of PHA responsive human lymphocytes in culture. *J. Immunol.* 125:1007.

2

Vulnerability of the T-Cell Lineage to Aging

Takashi Makinodan, Mei-ping Chang, Dean C. Norman, and Shun-cheng Li

Geriatric Research, Education and Clinical Center
West Los Angeles Veterans Administration Medical Center
and University of California at Los Angeles School of Medicine
Los Angeles, California

I. INTRODUCTION

Thirty years ago, we first demonstrated that the ability to mount a T-cell-dependent primary antibody response to sheep red blood cell stimulation decreases with age in mice and that the decrease is due primarily to changes in the tissues making up the immune system and secondarily to changes in the systemic milieu (1,2). Since then, studies from various laboratories have established that other T-cell-dependent immunological activities are also vulnerable to aging (3) and that at the cellular level, the altered activities can be related to changes in the intrinsic properties of T cells (4).

To understand the basis of these changes in the T cells, we will need to resolve (a) whether T cells in certain stages of differentiation are more vulnerable to aging than those in other stages and (b) how aging causes these changes. Therefore, in this chapter, we first present evidence that T cells in only certain stages of the T-cell lineage manifest age-related changes and then discuss the possible causes for these changes.

II. T-CELL LINEAGE

The T-cell lineage contains at least seven stages (5-11): (a) the pluripotent lymphohematopoietic stem cell, (b) the lymphoid-committed oligopotent stem cell, (c) the unipotent prethymic stem cell, (d) the intrathymic T cell, (e) the

Table 1 A Proposed Schematic of the T-Cell Lineage[a]

Stages		Tissue site
I.	Pluripotent lymphohematopoietic stem cells	Bone marrow
II.	Lymphoid-committed oligopotent stem cells	Bone marrow
III.	Unipotent prethymic stem cells	Bone marrow
IV.	Intrathymic T cells	Thymus
V.	Postthymic T cells	Spleen, lymph nodes, circulation
VI.	Antigen/mitogen-responsive T cells	Spleen, lymph nodes, circulation
VII.	Effector T cells	Spleen, lymph nodes, circulation, inflammatory sites

[a]Pluripotent cells are mitotically quiescent, whereas oligopotent and unipotent stem cells are mitotically active. The self-renewing capacity decreases as the differentiation potential decreases. Most of the intrathymic T cells die. The thymus, the generator of diverse T cells, undergoes involution at around sexual maturity. Many of the antigen/mitogen-responsive T cells are mitotically quiescent.

postthymic T cell, (f) the antigen/mitogen-responsive T cell, and (g) the effector T-cell stages (Table 1).

The T-cell lineage has certain unique characteristics. One is that most of the T cells generated in the intrathymic stage die (12–14). We do not know whether they are killed or whether they suicide. An understanding of how they die may provide an insight as to why they die. Another characteristic is that many of the penultimately differentiated antigen/mitogen-responsive T cells are mitotically quiescent, similar to the pluripotent lymphohematopoietic stem cells, and thus are resistant to mitotic poisons over an extended period of time. For example, 40% of murine splenic T cells are mitotically inactive (15). This would suggest that if their capacity to repair DNA damages remains intact with age, these cells should be free of DNA damages. On the other hand, if their capacity to repair DNA damages decreases with age, as reflected by the decrease in their capacity to repair ultraviolet-light-induced DNA damage (16,17), then genetically altered T cells should accumulate with age, for they cannot be easily selected out of the system as long as they remain mitotically quiescent.

III. AGE-RELATED CHANGES IN BONE MARROW CELLS

To our knowledge, the only direct study that has examined the influence of age on mitotically quiescent, pluripotent stem cells was reported recently by Akagawa et al. (15). They subjected young and old BALB/c mice to continuous exposure to 6-thioguanine, which selectively kills normal mitotically active cells while sparing mitotically quiescent cells, and determined the number of stem cells that are resistant to 6-thioguanine. Old mice were found to possess 7 times more 6-thioguanine-resistant stem cells than young mice. The investigators then showed that these 6-thioguanine-resistant stem cells can become susceptible to 6-thioguanine killing by inducing them to become mitotically active colony-forming stem cells. These results would suggest that regulatory stromal cells, which are involved in stimulating mitotically quiescent stem cells to differentiate into mitotically active oligopotent stem cells, are vulnerable to aging.

All the experimental studies on the influence of age on oligopotent stem cells have used a heterogeneous population of stem cells because (a) the assays could not distinguish mitotically quiescent, pluripotent stem cells from mitotically active, oligopotent stem cells, and (b) there has been no practical method of separating them before their analysis. Be that as it may, the results of experiments using mixed stem cells show that most but not all parameters are resistant to aging. The parameters that are resistant to aging include the total number of stem cells (18,19), the ability of stem cells to differentiate into blood cells and immune cells (20,21), and the self-renewing ability of stem cells (22,23). One of the parameters that is vulnerable to aging is the ability to repair ionizing-radiation-induced DNA damage (24). Contradictory results have also been obtained from mixed stem cells studies; for example, results indicating a decrease (25,26) or no change (23,27) with age in the ability of stem cells to expand clonally in vivo and to generate cells in vitro. Differences in the methods of assay and in the proportion of the number of pluripotent stem cells to that of oligopotent stem cells in the test stem cell inoculum would appear to be primarily responsible for the contradictory results. In any event, the results indicating no change with age would suggest that both the pluripotent and oligopotent stem cells are resistant to aging, whereas those indicating a change with age would suggest that the pluripotent stem cells and/or oligopotent stem cells are vulnerable to aging.

Studies on the unipotent prethymic stem cells have been limited and, as with the studies on oligopotent stem cells, these investigations used a heterogeneous population of stem cells. The results suggest that the unipotent stem cells are more vulnerable to aging than the oligopotent stem cells. This is reflected by (a) a decrease in the ability to migrate into the thymus after injection of bone marrow cells of old donors into irradiated mice (28), (b) their cessation to migrate into the thymus of young parabiosed mice (29), (c) a decrease in the number that are responsive to ubiquitin, a thymic factor (30), and (d) a decrease in the repertoire of alloreactive cytolytic T cells in the spleen and thymus of irradiated mice transplanted with bone marrow cells of old donors (31).

In contrast to the effort expended in assessing the influence of age on parenchymal stem cells, that on stromal cells has been minimal. Moreover, with few exceptions, assessment of stromal cell activity has been indirect. This could be responsible for the contradictory results. Thus, support of the view that stromal cells are resistant to aging includes the observations that (a) the self-renewing ability of stromal cells of old mice is comparable to that of young mice (33) and (b) old mice repopulate their marrow as well as young mice after radiation ablation (23). Results supporting the view that stromal cells are susceptible to aging include the observations that (a) the proliferative capacity in vitro of bone marrow cells declines with age (26,33), (b) the ability to resynthesize stem cell regulator factors is decreased with age (23), (c) the number of mitotically quiescent pluripotent stem cells increases with age (15), and (d) the bone marrow of old but not young mice produces suppressor factors (34). On the other hand, observations that stromal cells of old mice produce in vitro a greater total nucleated cellularity and a greater number of splenic colony-forming stem cells than those of young mice (35) would support the view that aging enhances the activity of stromal cells. These contrasting results clearly emphasize the need for direct functional assessment of individual stromal cells.

IV. AGE-RELATED CHANGES IN THYMIC CELLS

As the generator of antigen/mitogen-responsive T cells, the thymus is involved in three key functions: (a) the formation and peripheralization of T cells, which occur during embryonic and early growth phases of life (36), (b) the production of chemotactic factors to attract prethymic stem cells to the gland (37), and (c) the production of hormones that act on intrathymic and postthymic immature T cells in the periphery (6). To date, four thymic peptides with hormonal activities have been chemically defined: thymic humoral factor (38), thymopoietin (39), thymosin α_1 (9,40), and thymulin (41). These hormones are found in the thymic epithelial cells (42,43) and therefore are presumed to be synthesized by them. However, very little is known of what role other stromal cells (fibroblasts, macrophages) play in the differentiation and regulation of the parenchymal T cells.

The thymus starts to involute at around sexual maturity in humans (44) and mice (45), which coincides with the cessation of prethymic stem cell migration into the thymus (29) and with the onset of age-related decline in T-cell-dependent antibody response (1). This and other related findings strongly suggest that thymic involution contributes to the decline in T-cell-dependent immunity with age.

Immunohistological studies by Hirokawa et al. (42) of thymic tissues of individuals aged from 1 day to 62 years established that thymosin α_1 is found in the epithelial cells of the cortical surface and the medulla and that aging selectively affects the epithelial cells in the medulla. Thus, they found that beginning at sexual maturity, the number of thymosin-α_1-containing epithelial cells in the medulla decreases progressively, so that only a fraction can be detected by the third decade of life. In contrast, those covering the cortical surface could still be detected in adequate numbers even in the atrophic thymus of a 62-year-old individual. In regard to thymosin α_1-containing epithelial cells of the cortical surface and medulla, it is interesting to note that Haynes et al. (43) found that these cortical and medullary epithelial cells obtained from an adult individual also contain thymopoietin and the human T-cell leukemia virus antigen p19.

To better understand the functional changes occurring in the involuting thymus, Hirokawa and co-workers (46–48) assessed the capacity of involuting thymic grafts to generate antigen/mitogen-responsive mature T cells. This was done by grafting thymic lobes from donor mice ranging in age from 1 day to 33 months into either experimentally induced (i.e., thymectomized, x-irradiated, and bone-marrow-reconstituted) T-cell-deficient young adult mice or naturally occurring T-cell-deficient athymic mice. The results revealed that the ability of thymic grafts to generate cytolytic T cells, for example, declines rapidly starting at birth, long before the thymus reaches its maximum size. On the other hand, the ability of thymic grafts to generate mitogen-sensitive T cells declines only slightly with age, with the decline beginning at midlife, long after the start of the involuting process. Bach and Beaurain (49) also found that the serum hormone level of thymectomized, thymulin-deficient young mice could be restored partially by grafting the thymus of adult mice that have no detectable thymulin in their blood. These results would suggest that (a) the intrathymic and post-thymic immature T cells could be the sole progenitor source of certain antigen/mitogen-responsive T cells after adulthood and (b) the atrophic changes occurring in the involuting thymus are due to factors both in the thymic organ and in the systemic milieu.

In other experiments, thymic adherent cells from mice ranging in age from 1 day to 20 months were analyzed by culturing them for a month in vitro and assessing the supernatants collected at weekly intervals for their ability to augment the antigen/mitogen responses of indicator thymocytes from 2- or 4-week-old mice and of indicator prethymic splenic cells from 3-month-old syngeneic nude mice (50). The results revealed that intrathymic but not prethymic T indicator cells are responsive to the supernatant. It is likely therefore that for the prethymic stem cells to undergo differentiation, a direct contact with the adherent cells would be necessary, as suggested by Stutman (6). The results of these experiments further revealed that the ability of thymic adherent cells to synthesize the augmenting factor declines drastically between 2.5 and 5 months of age, which is consistent with the findings derived from histological and thymic graft studies (42,46–48). Perhaps the most interesting findings in terms of homeostasis are those indicating that the thymic adherent cells can also synthesize an inhibitory factor, with the amount synthesized varying according to the age of the donor mouse. Thus, thymic adherent cells of newborn mice were shown to synthesize both the augmenting factor and the inhibitory factor, while those of young adult mice synthesize primarily the augmenting factor, and those of 20-month-old mice synthesize primarily the inhibitory factor. Mixture studies of the two factors would suggest that the target of the inhibitory factor is not the augmenting factor, but rather the augmentable thymocytes.

V. AGE-RELATED CHANGES IN PERIPHERAL T CELLS

A. Quantitative Changes

A decrease in the number of T cells has been detected in the blood of old humans and in the spleen and lymph nodes of aging mice (51). However, the pattern and magnitude of change in the number of T cells depend on the tissue and organ, i.e., whether they are in the blood, spleen, lymph nodes, or bone marrow (52,53). Nevertheless, the decreases can account for only a fraction of the functional changes.

B. Imbalance in T-Cell Subpopulations

Evidence for a shift in the proportion of regulatory T cells with enhancing and suppressive activities with age is abundant. Studies on T helper cells all showed a decrease (e.g., Refs. 54 and 55). The most recent evidence comes from the demonstration of a reduction in their ability to produce leukocyte migration inhibition factor (56) and interleukin 2 (57-61).

Information on T suppressor cells is less clear. Some investigators have seen an increase in suppressor activity with age in long-lived mice (62-66), while others have seen a decrease in suppressor activity in short-lived mice (67,68) and recently in one of the long-lived mice (69). The decrease in suppressor cell activity could account for the emergence of autoantibody and autoimmune disease in the older short-lived mice. However, it is perplexing to find autoantibody formation increasing with age in long-lived mice whose suppressor activity is also elevated. A possible explanation is that long-lived mice may be losing their sensitivity to suppression with age, as demonstrated by Doria et al. (66). Equally perplexing are the results obtained in humans. Thus, a decrease in suppressor activity has been observed by several investigators (70-72). In contrast, Gupta and Good (73) noted an increase in the number of T_γ suppressor cells. Moreover, Antel and Arnason (71) found that concanavalin-A-activated suppressor cells from elderly individuals produce less suppressor factors but suppress the mitogenic response of autologous cells to a greater extent than do those of the young. This would suggest that in contrast to old, long-lived mice, T cells of old humans are more sensitive to the suppressor factors. It is interesting to note that T cells of old individuals are also more sensitive to the suppressive actions of prostaglandins (74).

C. Changes at the Surface Membrane Level

At the surface membrane level, considerably fewer interleukin-2 (IL-2) receptors have been detected in antigen/mitogen-activated T blast cells of old than young humans (57), rats (60), and mice (61), as judged by the ability of activated T blast cells to absorb IL-2. Inasmuch as IL-2 is essential for activated T cells to proliferate, it is likely that the reduction in the number of IL-2 receptors with age is contributing to the age-related decline in the proliferative activity of T cells. In addition, the synthesis of IL-2 is diminished with age (57–61).

A decrease in the number of glucocorticoid and β-adrenergic receptors has also been reported in T cells of old humans (75) and rats (76). This could be contributing to the decrease in the rate at which T cells proliferate and differentiate in response to antigenic stimulation in old individuals. However, the findings on the reduced number of β-adrenergic receptors in old humans could not be confirmed by others (77,78). It was then demonstrated that the T cells of old humans with intact β-adrenergic receptors have reduced adenylate cyclase activity, which is due to a defect specifically in the catalytic activity of the enzyme complex, not in the nucleotide coupling activity (79).

In contrast to the age-associated decremental changes detected at the surface membrane level, new antigenic receptors have been observed indirectly. Thus, Callard et al. (80) showed that spleen cells of young mice can proliferate in response to cells from old syngeneic mice and young mice can synthesize cytotoxic antibodies when injected with cells from old syngeneic mice.

Finally, a change in membrane fluidity in T cells of old humans has been reported by Noronha et al. (81).

D. Changes at the Cytoplasmic Level

Morphologically, swollen mitochrondria containing myelinlike structures with reduced numbers of cristae have been observed in the cytoplasm of T cells of old, but not young, humans (82).

Metabolically, a variety of age-related changes have been detected at the cytoplasmic level. According to Kennes et al. (83), Ca^{2+} uptake, which plays a fundamental role in cellular activation, is decreased in T cells of old humans that have been stimulated by phytohemagglutinin (PHA). They also found that T cells of old individuals are more sensitive to Ca^{2+} loss than those of young individuals. Since the uptake of Ca^{2+} is restricted to the first 24 h after activation (84), these results suggest that the metabolic events occurring during the initial phase of T-cell activation are altered in old individuals. It is not surprising therefore that Tam and Walford (85) found an imbalance in the level of cyclic AMP and cyclic GMP in resting and mitogen-stimulated T cells of old mice. A similar age-related pattern of changes in the cyclic nucleotide levels of T cells was then found in humans (86), but this could not be confirmed by Mark and Weksler (87). The T cells of old individuals also display an impaired ability to produce nicotinamide adenine dinucleotide (NAD) in response to mitogenic stimulation (88), suggesting that age-related alteration in NAD(H)- or NADP(H)-dependent enzymes may also be contributing to the inability of T cells to proliferate.

E. Changes at the Nuclear Level

A variety of morphological changes have been detected at the nuclear level with age. Of the changes, the loss of chromosomes was first detected, with X and Y chromosomes being lost most frequently (89,90). This would suggest that loss of important genes in these chromosomes, especially those engaged in regulatory functions, could play an important role in aging. A decrease in the nuclear organizing region (91,92) has also been detected. This would indicate that a decrease in the ribosomal DNA content and/or the transcriptional activity of rDNA (93) may be occurring in the T cells of aging individuals, as seen in brain and heart tissues of old dogs (94) and humans (95,96). A decrease in the binding of actinomycin by mitogen-stimulated T blast cells has also been observed (97), which may reflect structural alterations in the chromatins. More recently, an increase in the frequency of T cells with micronuclei has been observed (98). It is not known whether these cells can proliferate in response to antigenic or mitogenic stimulation and generate functional progeny. If not, they could be contributing to the decline in circulating T-cell number in aging humans (51), as mentioned earlier.

Several functional changes have been detected in the nucleus of peripheral T cells of old individuals. They include (a) a decrease in the ability of T cells to repair ultraviolet-light-induced damages (16,17), (b) a decrease in the level of low molecular weight DNA polymerase, which presumably is involved in DNA repair (99), (c) presence of extrachromosomal inter-Alu DNA circles in certain T cells (100), which suggests that transpositional events may occur with age, (d) a decrease in the activity of purine nucleotide phosphorylase, a purine salvage enzyme whose absence can cause the level of toxic deoxyribonucleoside to increase (101), and (e) a possible defect in the ability of the nucleus of mitogen-stimulated T cells to respond to the cytoplasmic stimulatory factors (102). In addition, an age-related increase in the proportion of T cells that can proliferate in the presence of 6-thioguanine has been observed in humans (103,104) and in mice (105). The fact that these 6-thioguanine-resistant T cells possess levels of hypoxanthine guanine phosphoribosyl transferase (HGPRT) activity as low as those of HGPRT-deficient mutant cells and cannot grow in HAT (hypoxanthine-aminopterin-thymidine) medium would suggest that these metabolic changes are reflective of changes at the genomic level.

VI. POSSIBLE CAUSES FOR AGE-RELATED CHANGES IN T CELLS

It is clear that functional and/or morphological changes can be detected in antigen/mitogen-responsive T cells and in their precursors. Are these changes caused by extrinsic factors or by intrinsic factors? If the latter is the case, can they be passed on to their progeny cells? If so, where in the T-cell lineage do these changes originate? Answers to these questions are prerequisites for the development of experimental strategies to understand the molecular mechanism(s) of immunosenescence. Unfortunately, except for the preliminary studies on the influence of age on HGPRT-deficient T cells of humans (103,104) and mice (105), there has been no attempt to answer these questions. Consequently, we can only speculate at this time.

It would appear that many of the changes detected at the nuclear level of the antigen/mitogen-responsive T cells are genetic in origin. The changes detected at the cytoplasmic and surface membrane levels, on the other hand, could have been caused by either nongenetic or genetic factors. As to the nongenetic changes caused by extrinsic factors in the systemic milieu, they should be reversible and responsive to counteracting factors such as diet and certain drugs. As to genetic alterations, it should be noted that mitotically active cells are highly receptive to such alterations, as demonstrated in mitotically active tissue culture cells (106); moreover, a significant proportion of the antigen/mitogen-responsive T cells are mitotically quiescent, as demonstrated by their resistance to 6-thioguanine (15). Thus, it would seem reasonable to assume that the genetically induced changes detected in the antigen/mitogen-responsive T cells occurred earlier in their differentiation process.

Of the five percursors of the antigen/mitogen-responsive T cells, the most resistant to genetic changes should be the pluripotent stem cells because they are mitotically inactive in adult individuals (5,8). However, the oligopotent and unipotent presursor cells are mitotically active and they self-replicate extensively. Therefore, they should be vulnerable to genetic changes. The intrathymic and postthymic precursor cells should also be vulnerable to changes as they are mitotically active, but the extent to which the changes can accumulate with time will depend on their self-renewing activity, of which we know very little. Thus, it would appear that T cells in the middle of the differentiation vector are most vulnerable to stable genetic changes.

Although we do not yet understand the molecular mechanisms of immunosenescence, one picture that is emerging suggests that many control points exist along the path of gene expressions (107) that are vulnerable to aging. Thus, gene alterations caused by gene diminution, amplification, rearrangement or modification, and modulation of gene expression at the transcriptional, posttranscriptional, or translational level should be taken into consideration in analyzing how aging causes, for example, a diminution in IL-2 production by T cells.

VII. CONCLUSION

An attempt has been made to summarize our current knowledge of the vulnerability of T cells to aging with reference to their differentiation stages. Of the seven differentiation stages, age-related alterations have been detected in three: the unipotent stem stage, the intrathymic T-cell stage, and the antigen/mitogen-responsive T-cell stage. That the changes in the antigen/mitogen-responsive T cells are those engaged in the signal-receiving mechanisms is of particular importance. Thus, at the surface membrane level, we see changes in hormone receptors and in the receptor–enzyme complex. In the cytoplasm we see changes in calcium ion uptake and nucleotide activities, and in the nucleus we see changes at the chromosomal and DNA levels. We do not know whether these changes are due to changes occurring in the extrinsic milieu or to molecular aging processes occurring at the genetic level.

The penultimately differentiated, antigen/mitogen-responsive T cells are unique, since they are derived from mitotically active precursors and can exist in a noncycling state for years. They therefore should not be highly susceptible to stable genetic alterations but should be able to preserve genetic aberrations incurred earlier in differentiation. However, unlike other noncycling cells, these T cells may be called on at any moment in an individual's life to proliferate and differentiate in response to antigenic stimulation, thereby expressing their genetic aberrations. Thus, if the phenotypic changes observed in the antigen/mitogen-responsive T cells are genetic and can be transmitted to progeny effector cells, an equally important question is, Where in the T-cell lineage do these changes originate? The results of current studies suggest that they may have occurred in the intermediate stages of the T-cell lineage.

Based on these considerations and in view of recent advances in molecular biology, efforts must be expended to differentiate genetic from nongenetic changes, to pinpoint where in the T-cell lineage stable genetic changes occur, and to identify the control points in the expression of important T-cell functions that are affected by aging.

REFERENCES

1. Makinodan, T., and W. J. Peterson. 1962. Relative antibody-forming capacity of spleen cells as a function of age. *Proc. Natl. Acad. Sci. USA*. 48: 234.
2. Makinodan, T., and W. J. Peterson. 1964. Growth and senescence of the primary antibody-forming potential of the spleen. *J. Immunol.* 93:886.

3. Cinader, B. 1980. The immunobiology of aging. *In* Progress in Aging. V. Y. Yamamura and T. Tada, editors. Academic Press, Tokyo. 1519–1538.
4. Doria, G., D. Frasca, and L. Adorini. 1983. Immunoregulation of antibody response in aging. *In* Progress in Immunology. V. Y. Yamamura and T. Tada, editors. Academic Press, Tokyo. 1549–1561.
5. Rosse, C. 1976. Small lymphocyte and transitional cell populations of the bone marrow: Their role in the mediation of hemopoietic progenitor cell functions. *Int. Rev. Cytol.* 45:156.
6. Stutman, O. 1978. Intrathymic and extrathymic T cell maturation. *Immunol. Res.* 42:138.
7. Botnick, L. E., E. C. Hannon, and S. Hellman. 1979. Nature of the hemopoietic stem cell compartment and its proliferative potential. *Blood Cells.* 5:195.
8. Till, J. E., and E. A. McCulloch. 1980. Hemopoietic stem cell differentiation. *Biochem. Biophys. Acta.* 605:431.
9. Keller, G. M., and R. A. Phillips. 1982. Detection in vitro of a unique multipotent hemopoietic progenitor. *J. Cell. Physiol.* 1 (suppl.):31.
10. Nakahata, T., and M. Ogawa. 1982. Identification of a class of hemopoietic colony-forming units with extensive capability to self-renew and generate multipotential hemopoietic colonies. *Proc. Natl. Acad. Sci. USA.* 79:3843.
11. Scollay, R., and K. Shortman. 1983. Thymocyte subpopulations: An experimental review, including low cytometric cross-correlations between the major murine thymocyte markers. *Thymus.* 5:245.
12. Fitzgerald, P. H. 1964. The immunological role and long life span of small lymphocytes. *J. Theor. Biol.* 6:13.
13. Sprent, J., and A. Basten. 1973. Circulating T and B lymphocytes of the mouse. II. Life span. *Cell. Immunol.* 7:40.
14. McPhee, D., J. Pye, and K. Shortman. 1979. The differentiation of T lymphocytes. V. Evidence for intrathymic death of most thymocytes. *Thymus.* 1:151.
15. Akagawa, T., K. Onari, W. J. Peterson, and T. Makinodan. 1984. Differential effects of age on mitotically active and inactive bone marrow stem cells and splenic T cells in mice. *Cell. Immunol.* 86:53.
16. Lambert, B., U. Ringborg, and L. Skoog. 1979. Age-related decrease of ultraviolet light-induced DNA repair synthesis in human peripheral leukocytes. *Cancer Res.* 39:2972.
17. Niedermuller, H. 1982. Age dependency of DNA repair in rats after DNA damage by carcinogens. *Mech. Ageing Dev.* 19:259.
18. Coggle, J. E., and C. Proukakis. 1970. The effect of age on the bone marrow cellularity of the mouse. *Gerontology.* 16:25.
19. Chen, M. G. 1971. Age-related changes in hematopoietic stem cell populations of a long-lived hybrid mouse. *J. Cell. Physiol.* 78:225.
20. Ogden, D. A., and H. S. Miklem. 1976. The fate of serially transplanted bone marrow cell population from young and old donors. *Transplantation.* 22:287.

21. Harrison, D. E., C. M. Astle, and J. W. Doubleday. 1977. Stem cell lines from old immunodeficient donors give responses in young recipients. *J. Immunol.* 118:1223.
22. Ross, E. A. M., N. Anderson, and H. S. Micklem. 1982. Serial depletion and regeneration of the murine hematopoietic system. *J. Exp. Med.* 155:432.
23. Schofield, R., T. M. Dexter, B. I. Lord, and N. G. Tests. 1986. Comparison of haemopoiesis in young and old mice. *Mech. Ageing Dev.* 34:1.
24. Chen, M. G. 1974. Impaired Elkind recovery in hematopoietic colony-forming cells of aged mice. *Proc. Soc. Exp. Biol. Med.* 145:1181.
25. Albright, J. W., and T. Makinodan. 1976. Decline in the growth potential of spleen-colonizing bone marrow stem cells of long-lived aging mice. *J. Exp. Med.* 144:1204.
26. Lipschitz, D. A., and K. B. Udupa. 1984. Effect of donor age on long-term culture of bone marrow in vitro. *Mech. Ageing Dev.* 24:119.
27. Harrison, D. E., C. M. Astle, and J. A. Delaittre. 1978. Loss of proliferative capacity in immunohemopoietic stem cells caused by serial transplantation rather than aging. *J. Exp. Med.* 147:1526.
28. Tyan, M. L. 1977. Age-related decrease in mouse T cell progenitors. *J. Immunol.* 118:846.
29. Kay, M. M. B. 1984. Immunological aspects of aging: Early changes in thymic activity. *Mech. Ageing Dev.* 28:193.
30. Twomey, J. J., R. J. Luchi, and N. M. Kouttab. 1982. Null cell senescence and its potential significance to the immunobiology of aging. *J. Clin. Invest.* 70:201.
31. Gorcyzynski, R. M., and M.-P. Chang. 1984. Peripheral (somatic) expansion of the murine cytotoxic T lymphocyte repertoire. II. Comparison of diversity in recognition repertoire of alloreactive T cells in spleen and thymus of young or aged DBA/2J mice transplanted with bone marrow cells from young or aged donors. *J. Immunol.* 133:2381.
32. Wolf, N. S., and R. K. Arora. 1982. Depletion of reserve in the hemopoietic system: I. Self-replication by stromal cells related to chronological age. *Mech. Ageing Dev.* 20:127.
33. Mauch, P., L. E. Botwinick, E. L. Hannon, J. Obbagy, and S. Hellman. 1982. Decline in bone marrow proliferative capacity as a function of age. *Blood.* 60:245.
34. Astle, C. M., and D. E. Harrison. 1984. Effects of marrow donor and recipient age on immune responses. *J. Immunol.* 132:673.
35. Mathews, K. I., and D. A. Crouse. 1981. An in vitro investigation of the hematopoietic microenvironment in young and aged mice. *Mech. Ageing Dev.* 17:289.
36. Hirokawa, K. 1977. The thymus in aging. *In* Immunology and Aging. T. Makinodan and E. Yunis, editors. Plenum Press, New York. 51–72.
37. Pyke, K. W., and J. F. Bach. 1979. The in vitro migration of murine fetal liver cells to thymic rudiments. *Eur. J. Immunol.* 9:317.
38. Trainin, N., M. Small, T. Zipori, T. Umiel, A. I. Kook, and V. Rotter. 1975.

Characteristics of THF, a thymic hormone. *In* The Biological Activity of Thymic Hormones. D. W. Van Bekkum, editor. Kooyker Scientific Publications, Rotterdam. 261–264.

39. Schlesinger, D. H., and G. Goldstein. 1975. The amino acid sequence of thymopoietin II. *Cell.* 5:361.
40. Goldstein, A. L., T. L. K. Low, M. McAdoo, J. McClure, G. B. Thurman, J. Rossio, C.-Y. Lai, D. Chang, S.-S. Wang, C. Harvey, A. H. Ramel, and J. Meienhofer. 1977. Thymosin α_1: Isolation and sequence analysis of an immunologically active thymic polypeptide. *Proc. Natl. Acad. Sci. USA.* 74:725.
41. Dardenne, M., J. M. Pleau, N. K. Man, and J. F. Bach. 1977. Structural study of circulating thymic factor, a peptide isolated from pig serum. I. Isolation and purification. *J. Biol Chem.* 252:8040.
42. Hirokawa, K., J. E. McClure, and A. L. Goldstein. 1982. Age-related changes in localization of thymosin in the human thymus. *Thymus.* 4:19.
43. Haynes, B. F., M. Robert-Guroff, R. S. Metzgar, G. Franchini, V. S. Kalyanaraman, T. J. Palker, and R. C. Gallo. 1983. Monoclonal antibody against human T cell leukemia virus p19 defines a human thymic epithelial antigen acquired during ontogeny. *J. Exp. Med.* 157:907.
44. Boyd, E. 1932. The weight of the thymus gland in health and in disease. *Am. J. Dis. Child.* 43:1162.
45. Santisteban, G. A. 1960. The growth and involution of lymphatic tissue and its interrelationships to aging and to the growth of the adrenal glands and sex organs in CBA mice. *Anat. Rec.* 136:117.
46. Hirokawa, K., and T. Makinodan. 1975. Thymic involution: Effect on T cell differentiation. *J. Immunol.* 114:1659.
47. Hirokawa, K., and T. Sado. 1978. Early decline of thymic effect on T cell differentiation. *Mech. Ageing Dev.* 7:89.
48. Hirokawa, K., K. Sato, and T. Makinodan. 1982. Influence of age of thymic grafts on the differentiation of T cells in nude mice. *Clin. Immunol. Immunopathol.* 24:251.
49. Bach, M.-A., and G. Beaurain. 1979. Respective influence of extrinsic and intrinsic factors on the age-related decrease of thymic secretion. *J. Immunol.* 122:2505.
50. Sato, K., M.-P. Chang, and T. Makinodan. 1984. Influence of age on the ability of thymic adherent cells to produce factors in vitro which modulate immune responses of thymocytes. *Cell. Immunol.* 87:473.
51. Makinodan, T., and M. M. B. Kay. 1980. Age influence on the immune system. *Adv. Immunol.* 29:287.
52. Stutman, O. 1974. Cell-mediated immunity and aging. *Fed. Proc.* 33:2028.
53. Kay, M. M. B., J. Mendoza, J. Diven, T. Denton, N. Union, and M. Lajiness. 1979. Age-related changes in the immune system of mice of 8 medium and long-lived strains and hybrids. I. Organ, cellular and activity changes. *Mech. Ageing Dev.* 11:295.
54. Krogsrud, R. L., and E. H. Perkins. 1977. Age-related changes in T cell function. *J. Immunol.* 118:1607.

55. Callard, R. E., and A. Basten. 1978. Immune function in aged mice. IV. Loss of T cell and B cell function in thymus-dependent antibody response. *Eur. J. Immunol.* 8:552.
56. Sohnle, P. G., S. E. Larson, C. Collins-Lech, and A. R. Guansing. 1980. Failure of lymphokine-producing lymphocytes from aged humans to undergo activation by recall antigens. *J. Immunol.* 124:2169.
57. Gillis, S., R. Kozak, M. Durante, and M. E. Weksler. 1981. Immunological studies of aging. Decreased production of and response to T cell growth factor by lymphocytes from aged humans. *J. Clin. Invest.* 67:937.
58. Miller, R. A., and O. Stutman. 1981. Decline, in aging mice, of the *anti*-2,4,6-trinitrophenyl (TNP) cytotoxic T cell response attributable in loss of Lyt-2$^-$, interleukin 2-producing helper cell function. *Eur. J. Immunol.* 11:751.
59. Thoman, M. L., and W. O. Weigle. 1982. Cell-mediated immunity in aged mice: An underlying lesion in IL-2 synthesis. *J. Immunol.* 128:2358.
60. Gilman, S. C., J. S. Rosenberg, and J. D. Feldman. 1982. T lymphocytes of young and aged rats. II. Functional defects and the role of interleukin-2. *J. Immunol.* 128:644.
61. Chang, M.-P., T. Makinodan, W. J. Peterson, and B. L. Strehler. 1982. Role of T cells and adherent cells in age-related decline in murine interleukin 2 production. *J. Immunol.* 129:2426.
62. Goidl, E. A., J. B. Innes, and M. E. Weksler. 1976. Immunological studies of aging. II. Loss of IgG and high avidity plaque-forming cells and increased suppressor cell activity in aging mice. *J. Exp. Med.* 144:1037.
63. Segre, D., and M. Segre. 1976. Humoral immunity in aged mice. II. Increased suppressor T cell activity in immunologically deficient old mice. *J. Immunol.* 116:735.
64. Makinodan, T., J. W. Albright, P. I. Good, C. P. Peter, and M. L. Heidrick. 1976. Reduced humoral immune activity in long-lived old mice: An approach to elucidating its mechanisms. *Immunology.* 31:903.
65. Roder, J. C., D. A. Bell, and S. K. Singhal. 1977. Regulation of the immune response in autoimmune NZB/BZW F_1 mice. I. The spontaneous generation of splenic suppressor cells. *Cell. Immunol.* 29:272.
66. Doria, G., C. Mancini, and L. Adorini. 1982. Immunoregulation in senescence: Increased inducibility of antigen-specific suppressor T cells and loss of cell sensitivity to immunosuppression in aging mice. *Proc. Natl. Acad. Sci. USA.* 79:3803.
67. Barthold, D. R., S. Kysela, and A. D. Steinberg. 1974. Decline in suppressor T cell function with age in female NZB mice. *J. Immunol.* 112:9.
68. Krakauer, R. S., T. A. Waldmann, and W. Strober. 1976. Loss of suppressor T cells in adult NZB/BZW mice. *J. Exp. Med.* 144:663.
69. Thoman, M. L., and W. O. Weigle. 1983. Deficiency in suppressor T cell activity in aged animals. *J. Exp. Med.* 157:2184.
70. Hallgren, H., and E. Yunis. 1977. Suppressor lymphocytes in young and aged humans. *J. Immunol.* 118:2004.
71. Antel, J. P., and B. G. W. Arnason. 1979. Suppressor cell function in man:

Evidence for altered sensitivity of responder cells with age. *Clin. Immunol. Immunopathol.* 13:119.
72. Abe, T., C. Morimoto, T. Toguchi, M. Kiyotaki, and M. Homma. 1981. Evidence of aberration of T-cell subsets in aged individuals. *Scand. J. Immunol.* 13:151.
73. Gupta, S., and R. A. Good. 1979. Subpopulations of human T lymphocytes. X. Alterations in T, B, third population cells, and T cells with receptors for immunoglobulin M (T_μ) or G (T_γ) in aging humans. *J. Immunol.* 122:1214.
74. Goodwin, J. S., and R. P. Messner. 1979. Sensitivity of lymphocytes to prostaglandin E_2 increases in subjects over age 70. *J. Clin. Invest.* 64:434.
75. Shocken, D. D., and G. S. Roth. 1977. Reduced β-adrenergic receptor concentrations in ageing man. *Nature.* 267:856.
76. Petrovic, J. S., and R. Z. Markovic. 1975. Changes in cortisol binding to soluble receptor proteins in rat liver and thymus during development and ageing. *Dev. Biol.* 45:176.
77. Abrass, I. B., and P. J. Scarpace. 1981. Human lymphocyte β-adrenergic receptors are unaltered with age. *J. Gerontol.* 36:298.
78. Landmann, R., H. Bittiger, and F. R. Buhler. 1981. High affinity β-2-adrenergic receptors in mononuclear leucocytes: Similar density in young and old normal subjects. *Life Sci.* 29:1761.
79. Abrass, I. B., and P. J. Scarpace. 1982. Catalytic unit of adenylate cyclase: Reduced activity in aged-human lymphocytes. *J. Clin. Endocrinol. Metab.* 55:1026.
80. Callard, R. E., A. Basten, and R. V. Blanden. 1979. Loss of immune competence with age may be due to a qualitative abnormality in lymphocyte membranes. *Nature.* 281:218.
81. Noronha, A. B. C., J. P. Antel, R. P. Roos, and B. G. W. Arnason. 1980. Changes in concanavalin A capping of human lymphocytes with age. *Mech. Ageing Dev.* 12:331.
82. Biro, J., and E. Beregi. 1979. Electron microscopical and immunoelectron microscopical examination of the lymphocytes of young and old people after influenza vaccination. *Acta Gerontol.* 9:235.
83. Kennes, B., C. Hubert, D. Brohee, and P. Neve. 1981. Early biochemical events associated with lymphocyte activation in ageing. *Immunology.* 42: 119.
84. Lichtman, A. H., G. B. Segel, and M. A. Lichtman. 1983. The role of calcium in lymphocyte proliferation (an interpretive review). *Blood.* 61: 413.
85. Tam, C. F., and R. L. Walford. 1978. Cyclic nucleotide levels in resting and mitogen-stimulated spleen cell suspensions from young and old mice. *Mech. Ageing Dev.* 7:309.
86. Tam, C. F., and R. L. Walford. 1980. Alterations in cyclic nucleotides and cyclase-specific activities in T lymphocytes of aging normal and patients with Down's syndrome. *J. Immunol.* 125:1665.
87. Mark, D. H., and M. E. Weksler. 1982. Immunologic studies of aging. VIII.

No change in cyclic nucleotide concentration in T lymphocytes from old humans despite their depressed proliferative response. *J. Immunol.* 129: 2323.

88. Chapman, M. L., M. R. Zaun, and R. W. Gracy. 1983. Changes in NAD levels in human lymphocytes and fibroblasts during aging and in premature aging syndromes. *Mech. Ageing Dev.* 21:157.
89. Jacobs, P. A., W. M. Court Brown, and R. Doll. 1961. Distribution of human chromosome counts in relation to age. *Nature.* 191:1178.
90. Awa, A. A. 1975. Chromosome aberrations in somatic cells. *J. Rad. Res.* 16 (suppl.):122.
91. Buys, C. H. C. M., J. Osinga, and G. J. P. A. Anders. 1979. Age-dependent variability of ribosomal RNA–gene activity in man as determined from frequencies of silver staining nucleolus organizing regions on metaphase chromosomes of lymphocytes and fibroblasts. *Mech. Ageing Dev.* 11:55.
92. Denton, T. E., S. L. Liem, K. M. Cheng, and J. V. Barett. 1981. The relationship between aging and ribosomal gene activity in humans as evidenced by silver staining. *Mech. Ageing Dev.* 15:1.
93. Zakharov, A. F., A. Z. Davudov, V. A. Benjush, and N. A. Egolina. 1982. Polymorphisms of Ag-stained nucleolar organizer regions in man. *Hum. Genet.* 60:334.
94. Johnson, R., C. Chrisp, and B. L. Strehler. 1972. Selective loss of ribosomal RNA genes during the aging of postmitotic tissues. *Mech. Ageing Dev.* 1:183.
95. Strehler, B. L., M.-P. Chang, and L. K. Johnson. 1979. Loss of hybridizable ribosomal DNA from human postmitotic tissues during aging. I. Age-dependent loss in human myocardium. *Mech. Ageing Dev.* 11:371.
96. Strehler, B. L., and M.-P. Chang. 1979. Loss of hybridizable ribosomal DNA from human postmitotic tissues during aging. II. Age-dependent loss in human cortex–hippocampal and somatosensory cortex comparison. *Mech. Ageing Dev.* 11:379.
97. Preumont, A. M., P. Van Gansen, and J. Brachet. 1978. Cytochemical study of human lymphocytes stimulated by PHA in function of donor age. *Mech. Ageing Dev.* 7:25.
98. Norman, A., S. Cochran, D. Bass, and D. Roe. 1984. Effects of age, sex, and medical x-rays on chromosome damage. *Int. J. Radiat. Biol.* 46:317.
99. Barton, R. W., and W.-K. Yang. 1975. Low molecular weight DNA polymerase: Decreased activity in spleens of old BALB/c mice. *Mech. Ageing Dev.* 4:123.
100. Shmookler-Reis, R. J., C. K. Lumpkin, Jr., J. R. McGill, K. T. Riabowol, and S. Goldstein. 1983. Extrachromosomal circular copies of an inter-Alu unstable sequence in human DNA are amplified during in vitro and in vivo ageing. *Nature.* 301:394.
101. Scholar, E. M., M. Rashidian, and M. L. Heidrick. 1980. Adenosine deaminase and purine nucleoside phosphorylase activity in spleen cells of aged mice. *Mech. Ageing Dev.* 12:323.
102. Gutowski, J. K., J. Innes, M. E. Weksler, and S. Cohen. 1984. Induction

of DNA synthesis in isolated nuclei by cytoplasmic factors. II. Normal generation of cytoplasmic stimulatory factors by lymphocytes from aged humans with depressed proliferative responses. *J. Immunol.* 132:559.

103. Vijayalaxmi, and H. J. Evans. 1984. Measurement of spontaneous and x-irradiation-induced 6-thioguanine-resistant human blood lymphocytes using a T-cell cloning technique. *Mutat. Res.* 125:87.
104. Trainor, J. J., D. J. Wigmore, A. Chrysostomou, J. L. Dempsey, R. Seshardri, and A. A. Morley. 1984. Mutation frequency in human lymphocytes increases with age. *Mech. Ageing Dev.* 27:83.
105. Inamizu, T., and T. Makinodan. 1984. Influence of age on the frequency of 6-thioguanine (6-TG) resistant murine T cells. *Fed. Proc.* 43:1822.
106. Chu, E. H.-Y. 1974. Induction and analysis of gene mutations in cultured mammalian somatic cells. *Genetics.* 74:115.
107. Alberts, B., D. Bray, J. Lewis, M. Raff, K. Roberts, and J. D. Watson. 1983. Molecular Biology of the Cells. Garland, New York.

3

Infection and Immunity in Relation to Aging

Rita B. Effros and Roy L. Walford

University of California at Los Angeles School of Medicine
Los Angeles, California

I. INTRODUCTION

Infectious diseases are a major cause of morbidity and mortality in the elderly population (1). As examples, respiratory infections, particularly influenza and pneumonia, are the fourth leading cause of death in the elderly (2); gram-negative sepsis in the aged population may exceed 50% (3); infectious endocarditis displays a mortality of 40–70% in patients over the age of 60 (4); urinary tract infections occur in 15% of all elderly patients (5); tuberculosis occurs with the greatest frequency and highest death rate in the aged (6); and in the United States the highest incidence of tetanus, with a mortality rate of 80%, is in persons older than 65 years (7).

Undoubtedly multiple factors contribute to the statistics above. Socioeconomic conditions, senescent changes in digestive and absorptive capacities, alterations in major organs such as the lungs, chronic degenerative diseases, and increased hospitalizations may place the geriatric population at greater risk to infections. However, a major cause of the increased susceptibility to infections in the elderly may also be the well-documented decline of the aged immune system.

The first section of this chapter summarizes some of the experimental evidence demonstrating the effects of age on the immune response to infectious agents in humans and rodents. We then review experimental influenza in mice as a model system for studying immunity to infection in relation to aging, emphasizing our own work in this area. Finally, we discuss possible mechanisms that may underlie some of the age-related defective immune responses to infections.

II. INFECTION AND IMMUNITY IN HUMANS

Epidemiological studies have established that children with congenital immunodeficiencies (8), foreign graft recipients subjected to immunosuppressive therapy (9), and patients with acquired immunodeficiency syndrome (10) are all highly vulnerable to infection. It is therefore assumed that the decrement in immune function associated with aging plays a role in the increased susceptibility of the elderly population to infections. However, much of the literature regarding infections in aged humans is clinically oriented, with an emphasis on improved diagnosis and descriptive case presentations (11,12) rather than experimental evidence showing the actual contribution of the immune deficit to infection. Nevertheless, several reports do address specific immunological functions with respect to the response to infectious agents. For example, in a 3-year influenza vaccination study, Howells et al. (13) found that elderly patients had lower hemagglutination-inhibiting antibody levels and a poorer serological response to vaccination than young persons in the same city. In another study the binding of T cells to cholera toxin was measured in old and young human volunteers (14). Using a fluorescence-activated cell sorter, the investigators found that the number of cells capable of binding high concentrations of the toxin was significantly lower in the old subjects. Monocyte and polymorphonuclear function, which contributes to defense against infectious agents, has also been studied. Testing 55 aged subjects, Antonaci et al. (15) reported that the peripheral blood monocytes showed decreased phagocytosis and chemotaxis to leukocyte-derived chemotactic factor. Diminished intracellular killing of *Candida* and reduced chemiluminescence (a marker of intracellular killing) have also been reported (16).

The possibility of external manipulation to compensate for the senescence associated immunological decline is suggested in two reports. Joris and Girard (17) showed that the weak skin reaction of aged subjects to tuberculin PPD (purified protein derivative) can be "reactivated" to the level seen in young subjects by using higher doses of antigen and prolonged stimulation. Study of influenza vaccination showed no difference in mortality rates between elderly vaccinated and unvaccinated cohorts until the third year of observation, when the vaccinated group enjoyed significantly lower mortality and a lower incidence of bronchopneumonia (13). This finding justifies the use of the vaccine in the older age group and suggests that more highly immunogenic preparations of antigen may be capable of accelerating the development of immunity in the elderly.

III. DOWN'S SYNDROME

Down's syndrome (DS) is recognized as being probably the best available model of accelerated aging in humans (18,19). Life span is clearly diminished in DS—fewer than 10% of DS subjects survive beyond 40 years of age (20,21). By 40 years, pathological changes characteristic of Alzheimer's disease are almost universally observed in DS (22-26). Early involutional changes, even in newborns, are seen in the thymus in DS (27,28), and a significantly lower activity of a thymus-dependent serum factor is reported (29). At the cellular level, DS also shows similarities to normal aging. There is a decreased in vitro replicative capacity of fibroblasts from subjects with DS (30) and an increased susceptibility to transformation by SV-40 virus (31,32).

The majority of studies on immune function in DS subjects show a substantial decline compared to age-matched controls. Abnormally low levels of "natural" antibodies against tetanus toxoid, ϕX175 phage, and influenza, a delayed initiation of primary antibody responses, and a decreased skin reaction to mumps antigen and PPD have all been reported for DS subjects (21,33,34). A decreased yield of neutrophils was found in blood drawn from DS patients, and neutrophil half-life was reduced by 50% of the control values (35). Neutrophil chemotaxis to endotoxin-activated serum was defective in DS individuals. Numerous reports show a decline in the T-cell response to mitogens (36-39), and preliminary work by Medici (cited in Ref. 19) indicates that this defect may be due primarily to suboptimal monocyte function. Finally, the normal augmentation of natural killer (NK) cell activity by interferon has been found to be deficient in DS persons (40).

Unfortunately the data on incidence of infections in DS subjects is very sparse. However, there is some indication that these individuals may be at risk in combating infections. The frequency of death from respiratory infection is 125 times and from other infectious diseases is 52 times higher in DS than in normals (41). In addition, hepatitis B surface antigen was found in 20% of institutionalized DS and in only 6% of the age-matched controls from the same institution (42). The occurrence of antibody to hepatitis B surface antigen was significantly greater in DS individuals than in staff controls (19). Thus, the few studies that have been reported suggest a relationship between DS, declining immunity, and increased incidence of infection.

IV. INFECTION AND IMMUNITY OF ANIMAL MODELS

A. *Listeria monocytogenes*

One of the most carefully studied models of an age-associated decline in antimicrobial immunity is the murine listeriosis system. This model has the advantage of analyzing an acute infection that runs its course in less than 2 weeks, making it unlikely that the immune system of the host will age during the course of the experiment. Furthermore, the immunobiology of the disease has been extensively studied and is known to involve two major classes of protective cells: T cells and macrophages. Patel (43) has demonstrated that in response to a sublethal infection with *Listeria monocytogenes*, aged mice show a smaller than normal increase in spleen weight, spleen cellularity, and splenic T cells. Dose-response analyses of adoptively transferred protective T cells revealed that senescent mice generated 10-fold fewer protective T cells and that these cells were 100-fold less efficient than cells from young mice. In contrast to the antigen-specific immune decline displayed by the aged T cells, the innate mechanisms of antibacterial resistance do not seem to show any reduction in their capacity to control the growth of *Listeria* within the spleen.

B. *Toxoplasma gondii*

The studies of Gardner and Remington (44,45) on another intracellular parasite, *Toxoplasma gondii*, demonstrate the age-related decline of several components of the immune system. When compared with young mice, old mice showed a significant decrease in antibody titers both at the peak of the acute infection, and also during the chronic phase of the infection. Evaluation of the presence of *Toxoplasma* cysts, a measure of latent infection, revealed a sixfold increase in brain cyst number in the aged mice. This larger number of cysts together with the observed increased susceptibility of old mice to *T. gondii* suggests that the age-related decrease in the early antibody response allows the increased multiplication of the organism in vivo, leading to increased cyst numbers and/or death. Another major difference between the age groups was seen in the macrophage activation during the chronic phase of the disease. Populations of macrophages from very young and very old (> 25 months) mice infected with the *T. gondii* showed a marked decrease in activation compared to adult mice. Although T lymphocytes have been shown to be important in macrophage activation, no difference was seen in antigen-specific transformation between young adult and very old mice.

C. Oncogenic Viruses

The immune reaction to oncogenic viruses is an important area of gerontology that has received only minimal attention. The increased incidence of tumors with increasing age is well documented, but the focus of such research is often on immune surveillance and the nonspecific NK response. The relationship between a causative virus and the specific immune response to the viral infection may be equally important here. Pazmino and Yuhas (46) have shown that the senescent loss of resistance to the murine (Malony) sarcoma virus (MSV-M) is correlated with the increased incidence of tumor growth. Sensitivity to the oncogenic effects of MSV-M is maximal at birth, declines rapidly as the mouse approaches young adulthood, and reappears in old age. The sensitivity of the various age groups to tumor appearance is increasingly related to their ability to synthesize antibodies that can specifically neutralize MSV-M.

D. Nonspecific Immune Mechanisms

Evidence for a decline with age in *nonspecific* immune mechanisms suggests that these, too, contribute to the increase in infections in the elderly. A study on the mouse-specific parasite *Trypanosoma musculi* found that aged mice of several different strains developed more severe infections than did young adults (47). An analysis of the antibody-dependent cellular cytotoxicity reactions against *T. musculi* revealed no difference between the age groups. However, assays measuring the binding of NK cells to appropriate targets showed a marked decline in the older mice. This occurred even though at maximal stimulation with *T. musculi*, no difference was measured in the frequency of NK cells between young and old spleen populations. The authors conclude that the functional efficiency of NK cells is impaired with age. They find this defect to be amplified by a second defect: the production of macrophage interferon. In another study, Louria et al. (48) report that *Staphylococcus aureus* infection, which is dealt with primarily by the polymorphonuclear system, is much worse in older than younger mice.

E. Multiple Infections

The analysis of the effect of the declining immune system on the resistance to infection in the aged population can be confounded by the simultaneous occurrence of several infections. Studies that have experimentally simulated this situation show interesting results. For example, an increased susceptibility to influenza infection by intranasal inoculation was noted in aged CBA/CA and A/J mice (49), and such virus infection also impaired the lymphoblastogenic response to mitogens, but (surprisingly), the virus infection in aged animals was less lethal after a subsequent infection with a small inoculum of *Listeria*. In another study, Janev et al. (50) demonstrate that in the progerialike syndrome of Selye in rats, considered to be experimentally induced accelerated aging, repeated inoculation with *Brucella abortus* and *Diplococcus pneumoniae* improve the activity of the reticuloendothelial system.

F. Effect of Dosage

A second factor that may affect the outcome of experimental infections is the dosage of the infectious agent. Esposito and Pennington (51) used both *S. aureus* and *Klebsiella pneumoniae* to show that at different concentrations of inocula, comparison between young adult and senescent mice yielded different results. At higher inocula, senescent mice showed enhanced pulmonary clearance mechanisms. At lower doses, the young mice cleared viable bacteria more rapidly than the aged animals. This finding is reminiscent of the PPD skin reaction studies in humans mentioned above (17).

G. Viral Infection and Autoimmunity

A potential link between infection and autoimmunity has been suggested by several investigators (52,53). However, the question of why there is an increased incidence of autoantibodies in the aged population has not been resolved. It is possible that a certain percentage of viral infections lead to autoimmunity, and the elderly, by virtue of their longer lifetime, have simply had more opportunity for viral infections. However, it may also be true that the diminished or distorted immune response to infection seen in the elderly is a crucial factor leading to virus-associated autoimmunity. A report by Kay (54) suggests that this may indeed be the case. Following an outbreak of Sendai infection in a mouse colony, it was shown that the old, but not the young adult, mice exhibited numerous autoimmune phenomena, including antiglomerular basement membrane antibodies, membranous glomerular nephritis, and appearance of Coombs positivity. The report also showed that the decline of certain T-cell functions preceded the autoimmune disease.

In another virus system, the link between autoimmunity and infection was demonstrated at the level of individual B-cell clones. Tardieu et al. (55) infected mice with reovirus types 1 and 3 and showed that during the in vivo immune response to the virus, autoantibodies were generated that reacted to a wide variety of normal tissues. They next demonstrated that monoclonal antibodies derived from these mice could identify numerous antigenic structures shared between viral determinants and normal tissues. The key question is, of course, whether the incidence of these parameters increases with age. This question may pertain to exposure to viral antigens during vaccination as well.

H. Occasional Advantage of Declining Immunity

When either high-titered antibody or strong specific cellular immunity confers protection to the host, the aged population may be at risk of infection. However, when the immune response itself contributes to the pathology of the disease, senescent subjects may have an advantage. For example, in lymphocytic choriomeningitis (LCM), the cytotoxic T lymphocytes (CTL) that are activated against infected targets proceed to kill the infected cells of the central nervous system. The stronger the CTL response, the greater the deleterious immunopathological effects. Doherty (56) has shown that in senescent mice the capacity to generate LCM-specific CTL is greatly diminished. This finding provides a possible explanation for an earlier observation by Anderlik et al. (57) that the clinical course and the histological picture of LCM infection were significantly milder in aged mice. A similar correlation was reported for human subjects with systemic lupus erythematosus (SLE) (58). In this case, nonspecific cell-mediated immune functions were tested in young and old patients and showed an inverse correlation with the severity of SLE symptoms.

V. INFLUENZA AS A MODEL SYSTEM IN MICE

Although influenza as a disease has been essentially unvarying in the typical patient during the past 400 years, it continues to defy control by artificial immunization. Research on influenza prophylaxis suggests that the elderly population does benefit from vaccination, although the beneficial effect may not be evident for several years (13). At a recent workshop on influenza, it was recommended that increased efforts be made to evaluate T-cell immunity following vaccination and to aim vaccine preparations at stimulating T cells (59). This was suggested because T cells are cross-reactive for all A-strain viruses and might therefore confer more long-lasting immunity than B cells, which are exquisitely specific for the immunizing strain. In addition, since influenza-specific antibody titer does not always correlate with protection from death, cellular immunity may be a more critical factor.

The murine influenza model for studying the effect of aging on the immune response to infection has the advantage of allowing large numbers of genetically identical subjects to be studied. Genetic homogeneity is crucial in aging studies, since old subjects show an increased variability in most parameters when compared to young subjects. Also, the divergence in T- and B-cell specifities for the virus that has been shown in humans (60,61) occurs in mice as well (62,63). Our own studies have focused on the T-cell response to the virus for several reasons. First, it is this aspect of immunity that is the most severely compromised in the aged population. Second, it has been shown for several virus systems, including influenza, that high in vitro CTL activity correlates with protection from death (64). In the influenza model there is also a positive correlation between the peak of CTL activity and a decrease in pulmonary viral titer (65). These events occur well before the peak of the antibody response.

A. Primary Response

We first examined the CTL response of individual old and young mice following in vivo inoculation with influenza. Previous studies had demonstrated that in young adult mice the peak of this activity, as manifested in a ^{51}Cr release assay, occurs at day 5 (66). However, at this timepoint, the response of all the old mice was usually absent, or at best, minimal. A kinetic study of the old mice demonstrated that their peak CTL response was somewhat delayed, occurring on days

7-9 after immunization. However, even at peak response, the magnitude of the CTL activity among old mice was significantly less than that of the young mice (67). Analysis of the specificity of the T-cell response in the aged animals showed the same extensive cross-reactivity to a serologically distinct influenza A virus, thereby eliminating one potential cause of the diminished response.

B. Secondary Response

Since most infections of the elderly human population involve memory responses, we next compared the secondary CTL response in young and old mice (68). Here too, the mean response of the aged cohort was significantly less than the young group. Table 1 illustrates that 12 of 16 old mice tested showed diminished responses, while 4 animals displayed CTL function comparable to the young mice.

To dissect the possible factors contributing to the diminished response, we utilized an in vitro microculture system so that replicate cultures could be monitored sequentially for several different parameters. Spleen cells from old and young mice previously immunized with PR8 were restimulated with PR8 and then cultured for 5 days. On days 1, 3, 4, and 5 cultures were pulsed with tritiated thymidine for 6 h to measure proliferation. As shown in Figure 1, the kinetics of the two age groups were similar, with the peak of proliferation occurring on day 4. However, the old cultures showed only about 40% of the proliferation seen in the young cultures. The production of interleukin 2 (IL-2) by old cultures was also significantly diminished, in agreement with several other reports measuring production of this lymphokine following various methods of stimulation (69,70). Addition of exogenous IL-2 to the microcultures at day 0 resulted in the augmentation of the CTL activity, but never to the level observed

Table 1 Kinetics of Secondary in vivo CTL Response[a]

Age (months)	Days after A/HK	% cytotoxicity on: Infected MC57G	Normal MC57G
3	3	39	0
3	4	55	0
25	3	6, 15, 15, 5	0
25	4	12, 39, 40, 20	0
25	5	3, 60, 18, 20	0
25	6	16, 38, 15, 22	0

[a]All mice received a primary immunization with A/PR8 6 weeks before ^{51}Cr release assay. On the days indicated, a secondary inoculation with A/HK was administered. Results are shown for individual spleens of old mice at an effector-target ratio of 100:1.
Source: Ref. 68.

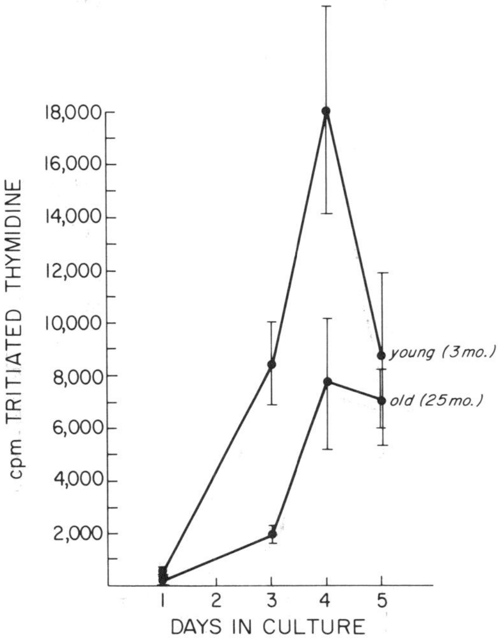

Figure 1 Kinetics of proliferation following secondary in vitro stimulation.

in the cultures from young animals (67). The IL-2-related defect was presumably operative in the primary in vivo response, indicating that the addition of the factor during secondary stimulation could only partially correct the problem.

C. Precursor Frequency Analysis

One of the possible causes of a decrease in the CTL response is a diminished frequency of CTL precursors (pCTL) in the old mice. We therefore used the limit dilution technique to compare the precursor frequencies for influenza-modified self in old and young mice (71). The unexpected finding that emerged from these experiments was that the age of the mice used to prepare the *antigen-presenting cells* (APC) was the critical factor in determining the precursor frequency. Thus, when old and young responders were both cultured with young APC, there was no difference in the pCTL frequency. This apparent "change" in precursor frequency can be seen in Figure 2, where responder cells from five individual old mice were stimulated with old and young APC. Cell mixing experiments showed no evidence of suppression in the old APC—these cells merely seem to function suboptimally in antigen presentation. The effect of this

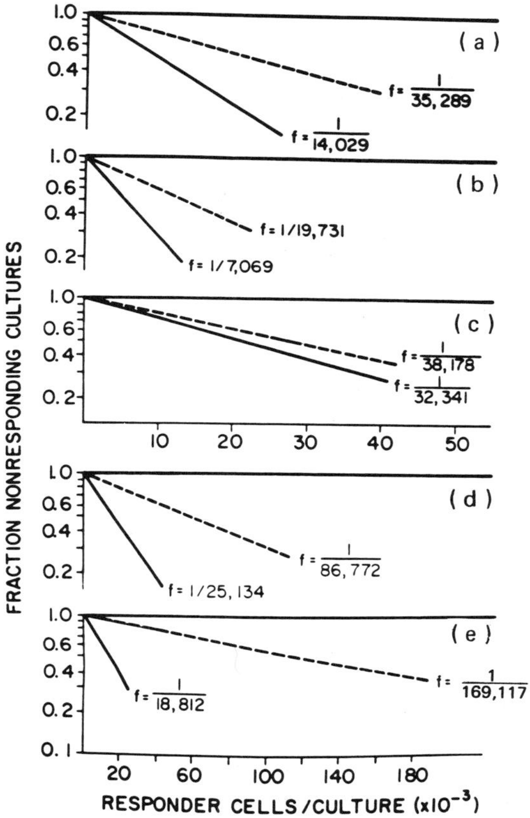

Figure 2 The improved CTL precursor frequency for individual "old" spleens cultured with young (–) vs. old (- - -) APC. The same pool of old or young APC was used for all these analyses.

diminished AP function was also seen when old APC were cultured with *young* responder populations. Thus, we have suggested that some aspect of AP function–processing and/or presenting of antigen–is diminished in aged animals.

To analyze the precise nature of this defect, we have been comparing splenic adherent cells (SAC) from young and old mice for several different functions. Preliminary data on IL-1 production demonstrates a decreased production of this lymphokine in old mice following influenza inoculation, even though before infection both age groups produced equivalent amounts (Figure 3). Influenza-infected SAC were also compared for their ability to stimulate purified memory T cells to develop virus-specific cytotoxicity. As shown in Figure 4, the

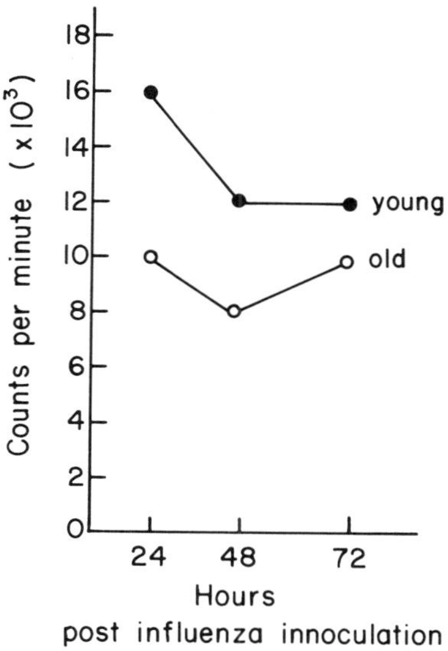

Figure 3 Interleukin-1 production.

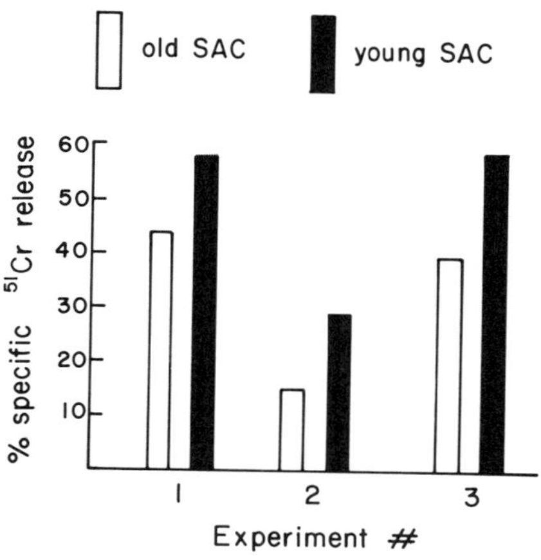

Figure 4 Specific cytotoxicity generated in vitro by culturing memory T cells with old or young SAC.

CTL activity generated from identical populations of memory T cells is significantly lower when they were stimulated with old versus young SAC.

Thus, our experiments have led to the conclusion that for the influenza virus system, the age-related defects in IL-2 production, proliferation, and cytotoxicity that we have reported previously can be traced, at least in part, to diminished APC function by macrophages. The precise nature of the particular event in the complex series of steps leading to antigen presentation that may be at fault has yet to be defined. Nevertheless, the finding of a possible defect in antigen-presenting function in aging subjects has broad implications for influenza prophylactic programs directed at the elderly. It may be, for example, that certain viral preparations will be more difficult for the immune systems of the elderly to process and/or present. This problem may not be evident in antibody titration assays and may require the additional testing of specific T-cell functions. The importance of aiming vaccine research at the T-cell response has been emphasized by others (59), mainly because antibody titers do not always correlate with protection from death. Our own work gives an additional rationale for utilizing T-cell assays to evaluate vaccine preparations. Since the vaccine protection is most important in the elderly population, it may be crucial to assess the ability of a senescent immune system to present particular antigenic preparations effectively.

VI. POSSIBLE MECHANISMS FOR IMMUNOLOGICALLY RELATED INCREASE IN INFECTION WITH AGE

A. Thymic Involution

The one change that appears to be a universal feature of aging in all species studied thus far is the involution of the thymus. The process, which begins at puberty, has been shown in humans to be accompanied by a decline in the serum concentration of thymic hormones (72). It has been suggested that all the age-associated changes that have been shown to occur in the immune response are dependent on this basic change in the thymus (73). Certainly T-cell maturation and function, which is critical in the response to infectious agents, is highly dependent on the thymus. The key question that remains unanswered is whether the process of thymic atrophy is the *primary* cause of immunological decline, or whether the atrophy itself is the result of more basic changes, such as modulation in the neuroendocrine system or even intrinsic, genetically programmed cellular aging. In any case, a link between aging, infections, and thymic function was suggested in a study by Pandolfi et al. (74), who noted a significant reduction in infections in a group of elderly hospital patients following a 3-month treatment with thymic extract.

B. Decrease in Modified-Self Reactivity with Age

One of the effects of a decline in thymic function might be a deficiency in the ability of T cells to recognize self-MHC (major histocompatibility complex) antigens. It is well established that one of the conditions requisite for all aspects of T-cell function, from early activation through the final effector phase, is the recognition of MHC-coded antigens. Any interference with either the expression or the recognition of these antigens will result in a compromised immune response. This phenomenon has been repeatedly demonstrated in vitro in antibody blocking experiments (75). The relevance of the problem to the aging immune system is suggested very clearly in a set of elegant experiments performed by Gershon et al. (76). The goal was to examine the role of the aged environment in supporting the development of anti–modified-self reactivity. Radiation chimeras were produced by reconstituting lethally irradiated 18-month-old BDF1 mice with anti-Thy-1 plus complement-treated bone marrow cells from BCF1 mice 6–8 weeks old. When the hosts reached age 24–28 months they were tested for their ability to respond to self antigen modified by trinitrophenyl (TNP). This ability declines with age, as attested by the marked decrease in anti-TNP reactivity in the aged intact BDF1 mice. The same lack of modified-self-reactivity was also demonstrated in the BCF1→BDF1 chimeras constructed in aged hosts. Since the BCF1 bone marrow from young donors was the same as that used to establish the BCF1→BDF1 chimeras in young hosts that have a normal response, the problem could not be related to the bone marrow cells or to the chimeric state itself. It appears that the aged environment prevents a potentially competent T-cell precursor in the bone marrow from reaching full cytolytic reactivity to modified-self determinants. The same conclusion was reached by Zharhary and Klinman in a completely different system (77). An analysis of the aged B-cell reactivity patterns to PR8 influenza virus showed no decrease in the repertoire diversity. It was therefore suggested that the observed reduction in repertoire diversity in serum antibody of old mice may be due to factors in the aged environment.

C. The "Aged Environment"

The term "aged environment" is, of necessity, a vague description, given the minimal amount of data defining the types of change that may constitute this milieu. An intriguing possibility is suggested in a study by Field (78), who noted certain morphological similarities between the slow virus disease "scrapie" and the aging process in normal animals. It was found that with advancing age, new antigens either identical with or similar to those occurring with scrapie make their appearance in both mice and humans. These antigens are detected by immunizing normal guinea pigs with old tissues. The appearance of these new antigens is greatly increased by thymectomy and can be retarded by implantation of neonatal thymus tissue. It is suggested that the "new antigen" may depend on molecular rearrangement of existing membrane structures. The notion of steric rearrangement or altered antigen display of cell surface antigen is reinforced by the experiments of Callard et al. (79) showing mutual mixed lymphocyte reactivity between spleens of syngeneic old and young mice, but not in age-matched cultures. Also, the work of Licastro et al. (80), showing profoundly reduced autologous mixed lymphocyte reactivity in aged human subjects who even had normal alloreactivity suggests a defect in self-recognition. The alterations may be related to the well-documented aging-associated changes in membrane viscosity. In addition, there is evidence that lateral mobility of protein molecules is retarded in aging cells. Vetvicka et al. (81) studied the binding of six different lectins as well as anti-H-2 and anti-Ia antisera to the surface of mouse peritoneal macrophages. In all cases, old macrophage membranes exhibited lower mobility, as measured by patch and cap formation. A similar finding was reported by Naeim and Walford (82), studying receptors of concanavalin A (Con A) on T cells from old donors and patients with Down's syndrome (which is believed to mimic normal senescence).

D. Chronic Viral Infections

There are several other possible explanations for the probable association of immune defects of the elderly and the observed high incidence of infections. In their study of mice infected with Sendai virus, Kay et al. (83) showed that chronic viral infection in aged animals can accelerate the immunological changes associated with aging. In this regard, Oyeyinka has posed the possibility that lymphoid failure itself accelerates senescence by predisposing individuals to infection and degenerative diseases (84). A genetic component is favored by B'atory et al. (85) in a study of T-cell reactivity of HLA-typed young and old subjects. These investigators found that a genetic factor, segregating with the MHC, correlates with the impaired or preserved T-lymphocyte reactivity in old subjects. A similar relation with the H-2 system has been reported in mice (86). This finding is reminiscent of the numerous HLA–disease associations, some of which putatively involve infectious agents, such as the HLA B-27/*Klebsiella*/ ankylosing spondylitis model (87).

E. Effect of Endotoxins

Many of the observed senescent immunological changes do not correlate with the status of thymic function (88). Horan and Fox (89) have therefore suggested that these immunological changes can be induced by endotoxins from the cell walls of gram-negative bacteria. The colon is a large repository for these organisms, and bacterial breakdown products are found in portal venous blood. Spillover into the peripheral circulation may be caused by the senescence-associated waning function of Kupffer cells, thereby leading to many of the immunological changes previously attributed to aging.

F. Nutritional Inadequacy in Old Age

Although we are one of the richest nations of the world, the average 3000-calorie diet of many Americans shows widespread nutritional deficiency. Protein, vitamin C, and various B vitamins have been found to be the nutrients most frequently lacking. Malnutrition is even more common among the elderly than among the "average" citizen. In a study of 200 elderly persons, almost 50% were found to have inadequate diets, with approximately similar rates of inadequacy among institutionalized and noninstitutionalized subjects (90). In another study, 50% of the elderly subjects were found to consume less than two-thirds of the recommended daily allowance for zinc (91). Deficiencies in iron and chromium have also been reported for elderly subjects (92). Since nutritional modulation of life span in mice has always resulted in improved immune function, it is clear that malnutrition is a potential factor contributing to the declining immune function of the elderly. The one nutrient that has been rather extensively analyzed in this regard is zinc. It has been shown that zinc deficiency is associated with the impaired capacity of T cells to respond to lectins (93), to provide helper function (94), and to generate cytotoxic cells (95). Furthermore, serum thymic factor activity has been reported to be dependent on zinc (96). Most recently, Winchurch et al. (97) have shown that the depressed antibody responses of aged mice can be augmented significantly by the in vitro addition of zinc to the cultures. It has also been shown that lithium and potassium ions have an enhancing effect on lectin-induced proliferation in both elderly and DS subjects (98). Thus, from the few available reports, one can hypothesize that borderline malnutrition is a potential contributory factor to a faulty immune response to infection in the elderly.

VII. CONCLUDING REMARKS

The increased risk of the elderly population to infectious disease is a major medical problem. Since immunosenescence is well documented for aged subjects, it may be possible to selectively manipulate certain components of the immune system or to target prophylactic regimens to the particular needs of the aged immune system. This type of intervention will be possible only when a more complete definition of the precise nature of the immune defects has been reached.

ACKNOWLEDGMENTS

This work was supported by U.S. Public Health Service grants AG03524 (a New Investigator Research Award to R.B.E.) and AG00424.

REFERENCES

1. Kohn, R. P. 1982. Cause of death in very old people. *JAMA*. 247:2793.
2. Verghese, A., and S. L. Berk. 1983. Bacterial pneumonia in the elderly. *Medicine* (Baltimore). 62:271.
3. Hodgin, V. G., and J. P. Sanford. 1965. Gram-negative rod bacteremia. *Am. J. Med.* 39:952.
4. Cantrell, M., and T. T. Yoshikawa. 1983. Aging and infective endocarditis. *J. Am. Geriatr. Soc.* 31:216.
5. Yoshikawa, T. T., and L. B. Guze. 1982. UTI: special problems in the elderly. *Geriatrics.* 37:109.
6. Nagami, P. H., and T. T. Yoskikawa. 1983. Tuberculosis in the geriatric patient. *J. Am. Geriatr. Soc.* 31:356.
7. Schneider, E. L. 1983. Infectious diseases in the elderly. *Ann. Intern. Med.* 98:395.
8. Fudenberg, H. H., R. A. Good, H. C. Goodman, W. Hitzig, H. G. Kunkel, I. M. Roitt, F. S. Rosen, D. S. Rowe, M. Seligman, and J. R. Soothill. 1971. *Bull. WHO.* 45:125.
9. Pazmino, N. H., and J. M. Yuhas. 1973. Senescent loss of resistance to murine sarcoma virus (Maloney) in the mouse. *Cancer Res.* 33:2668.
10. Masur, H. 1983. *Disease a Month.* 30:5.
11. Bentley, D. W. 1984. Bacterial pneumonia in the elderly: Clinical features, diagnosis, etiology and treatment. *Gerontology.* 30:297.
12. Andrews, J., P. Chandraseekaran, and D. McSwiggan. 1984. Lower respiratory tract infections in an acute geriatric male ward: A one-year prospective surveillance. *Gerontology.* 30:290.
13. Howells, C. H. L., C. K. Vesselinova-Jenkins, A. D. Evans, and J. James. 1975. Influenza vaccination and mortality from bronchopneumonia in the elderly. *Lancet.* 1:381.
14. Tsuru, S., Y. Zinnaka, and K. Nomoto. 1981. Decrease in cholera toxin-binding T cells in aged mice and human volunteers. *Int. Arch. Allergy Appl. Immunol.* 64:217.
15. Antonaci, S., E. Jirillo, M. T. Ventura, A. R. Garofalo, and L. Bonomo. 1984. Non-specific immunity in aging: Deficiency of monocyte and polymorphnuclear cell-mediated functions. *Mech. Ageing Dev.* 24:367.
16. Van Epps, D. E., J. S. Goodwin, and S. Murphey. 1978. Age-dependent variations in polymorphonuclear leukocyte chemiluminescence. *Infect. Immun.* 22:57.
17. Joris, F., and J. P. Girard. 1975. Immune response in aged and young subjects, following administration of large doses of tuberculin. *Int. Arch. Allergy Appl. Immunol.* 48:584.
18. Martin, G. M. 1978. *In* Genetic Effects on Aging. D. Bergsma and D. E. Harrison, editors. Alan R. Liss, New York. 5.
19. Walford, R. L., T. G. Gossett, F. Naeim, C. F. Tam, J. L. Van Lancker, E. V. Barnett, D. Chia, R. S. Sparks, J. L. Fahey, C. Spina, R. A. Gatti, M. A. Medici, H. Grossman, H. Hibrawi, and M. Motda. 1981. Immuno-

logical and biochemical studies of Down's syndrome as a model of accelerated aging. *In* Immunological Aspects of Aging. D. Segre and L. Smith, editors. Marcel Dekker, New York. 479–532.

20. Berg, W. R. 1975. *In* Endocrine and Genetic Diseases of Childhood. L. I. Gardner, editor. W. B. Saunders Co., Philadelphia. p. 730.
21. Smith, G. F., and J. M. Berg. 1976. Down's Anomaly. Churchill-Livingston, Edinburgh.
22. Jervis, G. A. 1970. Premature senility in Down's syndrome. *Ann. N.Y. Acad. Sci.* 171:559.
23. Owens, D., J. C. Dawson, and S. Losin. 1971. Alzheimer's disease in Down's syndrome. *Am. J. Ment. Defic.* 75:606.
24. Burger, P. C., and F. S. Vogel. 1973. The development of the pathological changes of Alzheimer's disease and senile dementia in patients with Down's syndrome. *Am. J. Pathol.* 73:457.
25. Ellis, W. G., J. R. McCulloch, and C. L. Corley. 1974. Presenile dementia in Down's syndrome. *Neurology.* 24:101.
26. Mehne, P., and P. Grunwald. 1975. *10th Int. Cong. Gerontol. Jerusalem.* 74.
27. Rigas, D. A., P. Elsasser, and F. Hecht. 1970. Impaired in vitro response of circulating lymphocytes to phytohemagglutinin in Down's syndrome: Dose- and time-response curves and relation to cellular immunity. *Int. Arch. Allergy Appl. Immunol.* 39:587.
28. Levin, S., M. Schlesinger, Z. Handzel, T. Hahn, Y. Altman, R. Czernobilsky, and J. Boss. 1979. Thymic deficiency in Down's syndrome. *Pediatrics.* 63:80.
29. Duse, M., M. A. Brugo, A. Martins, C. Tassi, C. Ferrario, and A. G. Ugazio. 1980. Immunodeficiency in Down's syndrome: Low levels of serum thymic factor in trisomic children. *Thymus.* 2:127.
30. Schneider, E. L., and C. J. Epstein. 1972. Replication rate and life span of cultured fibroblasts in Down's syndrome. *Proc. Soc. Exp. Biol. Med.* 141:1092.
31. Todaro, G. J., and G. M. Martin. 1967. Increased susceptibility of Down's syndrome fibroblasts to transformation by SV40. *Proc. Soc. Exp. Biol. Med.* 124:1232.
32. Trosko, J. E., and C. C. Chang. 1976. *In* Aging, Carcinogenesis and Radiation Biology. K. C. Smith, editor. Plenum Press, New York. 399.
33. Burgio, G. R., and A. G. Ugazio. 1978a. Editorial: Das Down-Syndrom als Immunmangel-Modell (Down's syndrome as a model of immunodeficiency. Facts and speculations). *Helv. Paediatr. Acta.* 33:5.
34. Sutnick, A. I., T. London, B. S. Blumberg, and B. J. S. Gertsley. 1971. Susceptibility to leukemia: Immunologic factors in Down's syndrome. *J. Natl. Cancer Inst.* 47:923.
35. Raab, S. O., W. J. Mellman, F. A. Oski, and D. Baker. 1966. Abnormal leukocyte kinetics: An explanation for the enzyme abnormalities observed in trisomy-21 (Down's syndrome). *J. Pediatr.* 69:952.

36. Franceschi, D., F. Licastro, P. Paolucci, M. Masi, S. Cavicci, and M. Zannotti. 1978. T and B lymphocyte subpopulation in Down's syndrome. A study on non-institutionalised subjects. *J. Ment. Defic. Res.* 22:179.
37. Blumberg, B. S., B. J. S. Gerstley, A. T. Sutnick, I. Millman, and W. T. London. 1970. Australia antigen, hepatitis virus, and Down's syndrome. *Ann. N.Y. Acad. Sci.* 171:486.
38. Mellman, W. J., L. H. Younkin, and D. Baker. 1970. Abnormal lymphocyte function in trisomy 21. *Ann. N.Y. Acad. Sci.* 171:537.
39. Gershwin, M. E., F. M. Grinella, J. J. Castles, and J. K. T. Trent. 1977. Immunologic characteristics of Down's syndrome. *J. Ment. Defic. Res.* 21: 237.
40. Nurmki, T., K. Huttunen, O. Lassila, M. Hentonen, A. Sakkinen, S. Linna, and A. Tiilikainen. 1982. Natural killer cell function in trisomy-21 (Down's syndrome). *Clin. Exp. Immunol.* 47:735.
41. Oster, J., M. Mikkelson, and A. Nielson. 1964. *Proc. Int. Copenhagen Cong. Sci. Study Ment. Retard.* 1:231.
42. Burgio, G. R., and A. G. Ugazio. 1978b. Immunity in Down's syndrome. *Eur. J. Pediatr.* 127:293.
43. Patel, P. J. 1981. Aging and antimicrobial immunity. Impaired production of mediator T cells as a basis for the decreased resistance of senescent mice to listeriosis. *J. Exp. Med.* 154:821.
44. Gardner, I. D., and J. S. Remington. 1978. Aging and the immune response. I. Antibody formation and chronic infection in *Toxoplasma gondii*-infected mice. *J. Immunol.* 120:939.
45. Gardner, I. D., and J. S. Remington. 1977. Age-related decline in the resistance of mice to infection with intracellular pathogens. *Infect. Immun.* 16:593.
46. Pazmino, N. H., and J. M. Yuhas. 1973. Senescent loss of resistance to murine sarcoma virus (Maloney) in the mouse. *Cancer Res.* 33:2668.
47. Albright, J. W., and J. F. Albright. 1982. The decline of immunological resistance of aging mice to *Trypanosoma musculi*. *Mech. Ageing Dev.* 20:315.
48. Louria, D. B., P. Sen, and M. Buse. 1982. Age-dependent differences in outcome of infections, with special reference to experiments in mice. *J. Am. Geriatr. Soc.* 30:769.
49. Ahlstedt, S., and A. Sohl-Akerlund. 1981. Protective effect of sublethal intraperitoneal *Listeria* infection secondary to intranasal influenza infection in aged immunodeficient mice. *Int. Arch. Allergy Appl. Immunol.* 66:350.
50. Janev, E., L. Kostowa, and H. Taskov. 1976. Cellular immunity against bacteria (intracellular and extracellular parasites) in experimentally aged rats [translation]. *ZFA Dresden.* 31:53.
51. Esposito, A. L., and J. E. Pennington. 1983. Effects of aging on antibacterial mechanisms in experimental pneumonia. *Am. Rev. Respir. Dis.* 128:662.
52. Williams, R. C. Jr. 1977. *In* Autoimmunity. Genetic, Immunologic, Virologic and Clinical Aspects. N. Talal, editor. Academic Press, Orlando, Fla. 457.

53. Hirsch, R. S., and M. R. Profit. 1975. *In* Viral Immunology and Immunopathology. A. L. Notkins, editor. Academic Press, Orlando, Fla. 419.
54. Kay, M. M. B. 1979. Parainfluenza infection of aged mice results in autoimmune disease. *Clin. Immunol. Immunopathol.* 12:301.
55. Tardieu, M., M. L. Powers, D. A. Hafler, S. L. Hauser, and H. L. Weiner. 1984. Autoimmunity following viral infection: Demonstration of monoclonal antibodies against normal tissue following infection of mice with reovirus and demonstration of shared antigenicity between virus and lymphocytes. *Eur. J. Immunol.* 14:561.
56. Doherty, P. C. 1977. Diminished T cell surveillance function in old mice infected with lymphocyte choriomeningitis virus. *Immunology.* 32:751.
57. Anderlik, P., I. Szeri, S. B'anos, and B. Radnai. 1975. Course of lymphocytic choriomeningitis virus infection in young and aged mice. *Acta Microbiol. Acad. Sci. Hung.* 22:27.
58. Foad, B. S., S. Khullar, E. H. Freimer, A. B. Kirsner, and R. P. Sheon. 1975. Cell-mediated immunity in systemic lupus erythematosus: Alterations with advancing age. *J. Lab. Clin. Med.* 85:132.
59. McMichael, A. J., B. A. Askonas, R. G. Webster, and W. G. Laver. 1982. Vaccination against influenza: B-cell or T-cell immunity? *Immunol. Today.* 3:255.
60. McMichael, A. J., and B. A. Askonas. 1978. Influenza virus-specific cytotoxic T cells in man; induction and properties of the cytotoxic cell. *Eur. J. Immunol.* 8:705.
61. Biddison, W. E., S. Shaw, and D. L. Nelson. 1979. Virus specificity of human influenza virus immune cytotoxic T cells. *J. Immunol.* 122:660.
62. Effros, R. B., P. C. Doherty, W. Gerhard, and J. Bennink. 1977. Generation of both cross-reactive and virus-specific T-cell populations after immunization with serologically distinct influenza A viruses. *J. Exp. Med.* 145:557.
63. Zweerink, H. J., B. A. Askonas, D. M. Millican, S. Courtneige, and J. Skehel. 1977. Cytotoxic T cells to type A influenza virus; viral hemagglutinin induces A-strain specificity while infected cells confer cross-reactive cytotoxicity. *Eur. J. Immunol.* 7:630.
64. Lu, L. Y., and B. A. Askonas. 1980. Cross-reactivity for different type A influenza viruses of a clone T-killer cell line. *Nature.* 288:164.
65. Yap, K. L., and G. L. Ada. 1978. The recovery of mice from influenza virus infection: Adoptive transfer of immunity with immune T lymphocytes. *Scand. J. Immunol.* 7:389.
66. Doherty, P. C., R. B. Effros, and J. Bennink. 1977. Heterogeneity of the cytotoxic response of thymus-derived lymphocytes after immunization with influenza viruses. *Proc. Natl. Acad. Sci. USA.* 74:1209.
67. Effros, R. B., and R. L. Walford. 1983. Diminished T cell response to influenza virus in aged mice. *Immunology.* 49:387.
68. Effros, R. B., and R. L. Walford. 1983. The immune response of aged mice to influenza: Diminished T cell proliferation, IL-2 production and cytotoxicity. *Cell. Immunol.* 81:298.
69. Thoman, M. L., and W. O. Weigle. 1982. Cell-mediated immunity in aged mice: An underlying lesion in IL-2 synthesis. *J. Immunol.* 128:2358.

70. Miller, R. A., and O. Stutman. 1981. Decline, in aging mice, of the anti-2,4,6-trinitrophenyl (TNP) cytotoxic T cell response attributable to loss of Lyt-2⁻, interleukin 2-producing helper cell function. *Eur. J. Immunol.* 11:751.
71. Effros, R. B., and R. L. Walford. 1984. The effect of age on macrophage antigen presentation. *Cell. Immunol.* 88:531.
72. Lewis, V. M., J. J. Twomey, P. Bealmear, G. Goldstein, and R. A. Good. 1978. Age, thymic involution and circulating thymic hormone activity. *J. Clin. Endocrinol. Metab.* 47:145.
73. Wecksler, M. 1981. The senescence of the immune system. *Hosp. Prac.* Oct:53.
74. Pandolfi, F., I. Quint, F. Montella, M. C. Voci, A. Schipani, G. Urasia, and F. Aiuti. 1983. T-dependent immunity in aged humans. II. Clinical and immunological evaluation after three months of administering thymic extract. *Thymus.* 5:235.
75. Burakoff, S. J., R. N. Germain, H. E. Dorf, and B. Benacerraf. 1976. Inhibition of cell-mediated cytolysis of trinitrophenyl-derivatized target cells by alloantisera to the products of the K and D loci of the H-2 complex. *Proc. Natl. Acad. Sci. USA.* 73:625.
76. Gershon, H. E., E. C. Lattime, and O. Stutman. 1980. Host age and H-2 tolerance in chimeric mice: Mixed lymphocyte reactivity, cell-mediated lympholysis and responses to hapten-modified self. *Mech. Ageing Dev.* 13:253.
77. Zharhary, D., and N. R. Klinman. 1984. B cell repertoire diversity to PR8 influenza virus does not decrease with age. *J. Immunol.* 133:2285.
78. Field, E. J. 1978. Immunological assessment of ageing: Emergence of scrapie-like antigens. *Ageing.* 7:28.
79. Callard, E. R., A. Basten, and B. V. Blanden. 1979. Loss of immune competence with age may be due to a qualitative abnormality in lymphocyte membranes. *Nature.* 281:218.
80. Licastro, F., P. L. Tabacchi, M. Chiricolo, R. Parente, M. Cenci, F. Barboni, and C. Franceschi. 1983. Defective self-recognition in subjects of far-advanced age. *Gerontology.* 29:64.
81. Vetvicka, V., L. Fornusek, H. Tlaskalov'a-Hogenov'a, and B. Rihov'a. 1982. Changes in some properties and functions of plasma membranes of macrophages from young, adult and aged mice. *Dev. Comp. Immunol.* 6:755.
82. Naeim, F., and R. L. Walford. 1980. Disturbance of redistribution of surface membrane receptors on peripheral mononuclear cells of patients with Down's syndrome and of aged individuals. *J. Gerontol.* 35:650.
83. Kay, M. M., J. Mendoza, S. Hausman, and B. Dorsey. 1979. Age-related changes in the immune system of mice of eight medium and long-lived strains and hybrids. II. Short- and long-term effects of natural infection with parainfluenza type 1 virus (Sendai). *Mech. Ageing Dev.* 11:347.
84. Oyeyinka, G. O. 1984. Age and sex differences in immunocompetence. *Gerontology.* 30:128–95.

85. B'atory, G., C. Onody, E. Gy'odi, J. Nemesk'eri, and G. G. Petr'anyi. 1983. HLA and T-lymphocyte function in old age. *Hum. Immunol.* 7:187.
86. Meredith, P., and R. L. Walford. 1977. Effect of age on response to T and B cell mitogens in mice congenic at the H-2 locus. *Immunogenetics.* 5:109.
87. Avakian, H., J. Welch, A. Ebringer, and C. C. Entwistle. 1980. Ankylosing spondylitis, HLA-B27 and *Klebsiella.* II. Cross-reactivity studies with human tissue typing sera. *Br. J. Exp. Pathol.* 61:91.
88. Makinodan, T., S. J. James, T. Inamizu, and M. P. Chang. 1984. Immunologic basis for susceptibility to infection in the aged. *Gerontology.* 30:279.
89. Horan, M. A., and R. A. Fox. 1984. Ageing and the immune response—A unifying hypothesis. *Mech. Ageing Dev.* 26:165.
90. Clark, M., and L. M. Wakefield. 1975. Food choices of institutionalized vs. independent living elderly. *J. Am. Diet. Assocn.* 66:600.
91. Hsu, J. M. 1979. Current knowledge on zinc, copper and chromium in aging. *World Rev. Nutr. Diet.* 33:42.
92. Nordstrum, J. W. 1982. Trace mineral nutrition in the elderly. *Am. J. Clin. Nutr.* 36:788.
93. Carlomagno, M. A., and D. N. McMurray. 1983. Chronic zinc deficiency in rats: Its influence on some parameters of humoral and cell-mediated immunity. *Nutr. Res.* 3:69.
94. Fernandes, G., M. Nair, K. Onoe, T. Tanaka, R. Floyd, and R. A. Good. 1979. Impairment of cell-mediated immunity functions by dietary zinc deficiency in mice. *Proc. Natl. Acad. Sci. USA.* 76:457.
95. Frost, P., P. Rabbani, J. Smith, and A. Prasad. 1981. Cell-mediated cytotoxicity and tumor growth in zinc deficient mice. *Proc. Soc. Exp. Biol. Med.* 167:333.
96. Iwata, T., G. S. Incenfy, T. Tanaka, G. Fernandes, C. J. Menedez-Botet, K. Pih, and R. A. Good. 1979. Circulating thymic hormone levels in zinc deficiency. *Cell. Immunol.* 47:100.
97. Winchurch, R. A., D. J. Thomas, W. H. Adler, and T. J. Lindsay. 1984. Supplemental zinc restores antibody formation in cultures of aged and spleen cells. *J. Immunol.* 133:561.
98. Licastro, F., M. Chiricolo, P. Tabacchi, F. Barboni, M. Zanotti, and C. Franceschi. 1983. Enhancing effect of lithium and potassium ions on lectin-induced lymphocyte proliferation in aging and Down's syndrome subjects. *Cell. Immunol.* 15:111.

4

Cell Biology of the Impaired Proliferation of T Cells from Elderly Humans

Risë Schwab and Marc E. Weksler

Cornell University Medical College
New York, New York

I. INTRODUCTION

The impaired proliferation of T cells from elderly humans following mitogen stimulation, in particular the response to plant lectins such as phytohemagglutinin (PHA) and concanavalin A (Con A), is a well-established characteristic of immune senescence (1,2). Many T-cell responses, including proliferation induced by mitogens, require accessory cell help. Although age-associated changes in accessory cell function for mitogen-induced T-cell proliferation have been reported, they do not explain the impaired proliferative response of T cells from elderly humans. The primary defect resides within the T-cell population and cannot be reversed by mixing T cells from elderly humans with accessory cells from young persons (3).

T-cell mitogenesis can be divided into two stages. The first stage is mitogen dependent and involves events that induce T cells to become activated, that is, to leave the quiescent G_0 phase of the cell cycle and to enter the G_1 phase. The binding of a mitogen to its receptor on the T-cell surface induces, under the appropriate conditions, a number of metabolic changes leading to an increase in cell volume and the expression of new cell surface determinants, many of which are receptors for growth factors. The second stage is mitogen independent and involves events that stimulate T cells to leave G_1 and to progress through the S phase and ultimately to divide. While the second stage of T-cell mitogenesis is mitogen independent, it does depend on the interactions of growth factors such as interleukin 2 (IL-2) and transferrin with their cell surface receptors. These growth factor-receptor interactions are essential signals for T cells to complete the S, G_2, and M phases of the cell cycle. In the absence of appropriate growth factors, T cells can be activated (G_0-G_1 shift) but will fail to proliferate.

The impaired proliferative response of T cells from elderly humans usually has been documented by measuring tritiated thymidine (^{3}H-Tdr) incorporation. However, ^{3}H-Tdr incorporation is a relatively late event in the cell cycle, occurring during the S phase or DNA replicative phase and first observed after 30–36 h in culture. To understand the mechanism of the impaired proliferation of T cells from elderly humans, it is essential to explore the steps that precede and lead to DNA replication and to consider the changes in the distribution of T cells in peripheral blood that accompany aging. A combination of techniques has provided an increasingly complete picture of the events associated with T-cell mitogenesis. Thus our understanding of T-cell senescence has been increased by cell cycle analysis using flow cytometric techniques, changes in the expression of cell surface determinants, measurement of the production of and response to growth factors, and an examination of the transcription of specific genes, as well as ^{3}H-Tdr incorporation.

II. QUANTITATIVE DIFFERENCES IN T-CELL SUBSETS WITH AGE

The age-associated decrease in T-cell proliferation is not due to a decreased number of T cells in peripheral blood of old humans. Most investigators have found that the relative and absolute numbers of T cells are comparable in young and old human subjects, despite thymic involution (1,4,5). This is probably explained by the long life span of human T cells. Some reports have described a decline in the relative or absolute number of T cells with age (6–8). We have found that the number of lymphocytes expressing the CD3 determinant, present on mature T cells, is comparable in healthy old and young human subjects (9).

Peripheral blood T cells are composed of a population of helper-inducer cells, which express the CD4 determinant, and a population of cytotoxic-suppressor cells, which express the CD8 determinant. Although the total number of T cells is unchanged with age, there are significant shifts in the distribution of the CD4- and CD8-bearing T-cell subsets in the peripheral blood of old humans (8,10). We found the number of OKT4-positive T cells to be significantly greater, while the number of OKT8-positive T cells is significantly lower (Table 1). This altered ratio of CD4- and CD8-bearing T cells, however, does not explain the proliferative defect, since there was no correlation between the ratio of the CD4 to CD8 T-cell subsets and ^{3}H-Tdr incorporation by peripheral blood T cells stimulated by PHA or Con A. Furthermore, the proliferative response of isolated CD4-bearing T cells is impaired in the elderly compared to the young (R. Schwab, unpublished observations).

Table 1 T-Cell Subpopulations in Young and Old Individuals

Age of donor (years)	Subpopulations[a]	
	CD4	CD8
19–31	60.2 ±1.8	38.7 ±2.3
65–84	73.4 ±3.3	28.6 ±3.0

[a]Data are given as mean percentages of OKT3-positive population (T cells) ± standard error. The number of OKT3-positive cells in peripheral blood of young donors was comparable to that from old donors.
Source: Ref. 9.

III. DECREASED PROLIFERATIVE RESPONSE OF T CELLS FROM OLD HUMANS TO PHYTOHEMAGGLUTININ

T cells from old humans cultured with plant lectins such as PHA incorporate less ^{3}H-Tdr than do T cells from young humans (1,2,11,12). This age-associated decreased response to PHA does not result from a reduced number of peripheral blood T cells in old individuals or from a defect in the capacity of T cells from old humans to interact with lectins. The number and the affinity of PHA receptors on lymphocytes from old and young humans are comparable (13). However, fewer T cells from elderly subjects are capable of responding to PHA. In peripheral blood of old humans, there are less than half as many T cells as in peripheral blood of young humans that enter the G_1 phase of the cell cycle when cultured with PHA (12). Furthermore, the T cells that are activated by PHA do not undergo as many divisions in culture as do T cells from young. There is no difference in the lag time for cycle entry (G_0-G_1 shift) or in the time it takes to pass through each phase of the cell cycle in T-cell cultures from old and young subjects.

IV. THE IMPAIRED RESPONSE TO ANTI-CD3 MONOCLONAL ANTIBODIES

The CD3 determinant, originally identified by the OKT3 monoclonal antibody, is expressed on mature human T cells and is associated with the T-cell receptor for antigen (14). The CD3 determinant is a tripeptide complex that is noncovalently associated with the antigen receptor heterodimer. Monoclonal antibodies recognizing CD3, as well as those recognizing the antigen receptor, induce proliferation of T cells in the presence of adherent accessory cells (14–16). In addition, anti-CD3 antibodies block the proliferative response of T cells induced by soluble antigens and allogeneic cells, as well as target cell lysis by cytotoxic T cells. Anti-CD3 antibodies recognize a surface determinant that probably acts as

Table 2 ^{3}H-Tdr Incorporation by T Cells from Young and Old Individuals Stimulated by OKT3 and PHA

	Incorporation (mean cpm × 10^{-3} ± SE) from:	
Mitogen	Young donors	Old donors
OKT3	34.1 ±4.2	14.6 ±2.0
PHA	89.0 ±7.1	77.7 ±9.3

Source: Ref. 3.

the activation signal transducer following the interaction of antigen with its receptor on the T cell. For this reason, the response of T cells to anti-CD3 antibodies is a good model of the activation of T cells by antigen in vivo, and probably is better than the response of T cells to plant lectins.

We have found that the response of T cells from elderly donors to OKT3 is significantly less, as measured by ^{3}H-Tdr incorporation, than that of T cells from young donors in paired comparisons (Table 2). We found this to be true of 95% of the elderly tested. In contrast, the response to PHA was impaired in only 60% of the elderly in the paired comparisons. Thus, the response to OKT3 appears to be more sensitive to the age of the T-cell donor than is the response to PHA. This has been proved by showing that T cells from old donors whose response to PHA is comparable to that of young donors are significantly impaired in their response to OKT3.

Mitogenesis induced by anti-CD3 antibodies is dependent on adherent accessory cells (Table 3). Thus, the incorporation of ^{3}H-Tdr is reduced by approximately 90% when accessory cells are depleted. The addition of autologous or allogeneic accessory cells to purified T cells restores the response, and the age-

Table 3 Effect of Allogeneic Monocytes on T-Cell Response to OKT3

Donors	Cell preparation	^{3}H-Tdr incorporation (cpm × 10^{-3} ± SE)
Young	T cells alone	4.5 ±1.2
	T + autologous monocytes	32.9 ±6.5
	T + allogeneic monocytes, young	26.0 ±4.5
	T + allogeneic monocytes, old	33.1 ±4.5
Old	T cells alone	4.7 ±1.4
	T + autologous monocytes	19.5 ±4.8
	T + allogeneic monocytes, old	16.4 ±3.3
	T + allogeneic monocytes, young	16.6 ±4.5

Source: Ref. 3.

associated defect is observed. Although the response to antigen is restricted by the major histocompatibility complex (MHC), these studies showed that the response of T cells to OKT3 is not. Furthermore, we found that accessory cells from old or young donors are equal in their capacity to restore the response of T cells from young donors. T cells from old donors show the age-associated defect in the presence of accessory cells from either old or young donors. No evidence was found that the function of accessory cells from old donors is impaired with respect to facilitating T-cell proliferation by anti-CD3. Thus, the age-associated defect in the response to anti-CD3 rests not in the accessory cells but in the T cells.

V. CELL CYCLE ANALYSIS OF THE IMPAIRED MITOGENESIS OF T CELLS FROM ELDERLY HUMANS

The age-associated proliferative defect has been defined by the reduced incorporation of ^{3}H-Tdr by T cells from elderly humans. As noted previously, however, ^{3}H-Tdr incorporation is a late event, occurring during the S phase or DNA replicative phase of the cell cycle. In addition, ^{3}H-Tdr incorporation itself may bias the proliferative response (17). T cells from elderly donors are more sensitive to the radiobiological effects of ^{3}H-Tdr incorporation and show increased levels of chromosomal damage and cell cycle arrest (18,19).

Flow cytometric techniques can be used, in the absence of a radioactive probe, to measure the activation and proliferation of T cells through the cell cycle (20). Multiparameter flow cytometric analysis allows each cell to be placed into a particular compartment of the cell cycle (G_0, G_{1a}, G_{1b}, S, G_2, M) based on its RNA and DNA contents. The metachromatic dye acridine orange differentially stains DNA and RNA and can be used to determine cell cycle distribution.

We have found that more than 99% of peripheral blood T cells from both old and young donors are in the G_0 or resting phase of the cell cycle when placed in culture (21). G_0 phase is characterized by a diploid content of DNA and relatively low content of RNA. Cells that are activated and enter G_1 can then be identified by their increased content of RNA. After 24 h with PHA, a significantly lower percentage of cells from old donors (22%) than from young donors (34%) were in G_1. After 48 h in culture, the number of cells in G_1 had increased in cultures from both old and young donors, but the percentage of cells in G_1 was still lower in the old (50%) than in the young (66%). Similar results were obtained using OKT3 as a mitogen.

The S phase is characterized by a significant increase in the cellular content of RNA and DNA. The percentage of T cells with twice diploid DNA content was compared. Fewer T cells from old donors pass through G_1 into S phase.

While these cells continued through G_2 and M, fewer T cells from old donors reenter G_1 and continue to cycle. This is not due to a slower passage of activated T cells from old donors through the cell cycle. In fact, the length of the cell cycle is comparable in proliferating T cells from old and young donors.

VI. EARLY EVENTS IN T-CELL ACTIVATION

Activation of T cells is initiated by the binding of a ligand to its receptor followed by the aggregation of these receptors. Most mitogenic ligands cross-link their receptors. The activation of T cells by the bivalent monoclonal antibody OKT3 requires accessory cells, probably because only in this way can the CD3-OKT3 complexes be sufficiently cross-linked. Thus, changes in the fluidity of the plasma membrane may impair aggregation of membrane receptors and thereby the activation of T cells. Changes in the mobility of cell surface receptors with age have been reported. The percentage of Con A capping on lymphocytes from old humans is decreased (22). Increased membrane microviscosity with age strongly correlates with a decreased proliferative response to Con A (23).

The binding and cross-linking of a mitogen rapidly induces membrane depolarization and changes in potassium and sodium ion fluxes and in Na^+/K^+ ATPase activity. These electrolyte shifts appear to be unchanged with age (24). Within minutes, the level of intracellular Ca^{2+} increases. Calcium ion plays a major role in a cascade of metabolic pathways that ultimately lead to DNA synthesis. Lymphocytes from old humans are more sensitive than young to Ca^{2+} chelators and require more Ca^{2+} supplements to restore proliferation following such inhibition (25). Activation of membrane methyltransferases, methylation of phospholipids, induction of ornithine decarboxylase, phosphatidylinositol turnover, and changes in arachidonic metabolism also occur within minutes. Whether these early events are comparable in activated T cells from old and young donors is not known. While cells in G_0 do carry on a low level of RNA and protein synthesis, activated T cells accelerate the levels of protein and RNA synthesis and increase the number of active ribosomes.

T cells that have been activated express new surface determinants in a sequential manner (26,27). Some are first detected early in G_1 and increase in density during cell cycle progression, while others are not detected until S, G_2, or M. The expression of G_1 markers appears to be important in regulating entry into S phase. Two of these G_1 markers have been identified as receptors for growth factors—the receptor for interleukin 2 and the receptor for transferrin. The impaired sequential expression of receptors for growth factors could contribute to the defect in the proliferation of T cells from old donors.

VII. IL 2 PRODUCTION, IL 2 RECEPTOR EXPRESSION AND T CELL PROLIFERATION

Activated T cells produce interleukin 2 and express receptors for this growth factor in early G_1. Entry of activated T cells into the S phase and subsequent proliferation are directly dependent on the interaction of IL-2 with its receptor (28–31). Monoclonal antibodies directed against IL-2 or its receptor block T-cell proliferation (32,33). Removal of IL-2 from actively cycling cells results in a decrease in the number of cells in S phase and an increase in the number of cells in early G_1 (i.e., G_{1a}). Addition of IL-2 to these cultures allows these cells to pass through G_1 (G_{1a}-G_{1b} progression) and enter S phase.

Recently, it has been reported that there are high- and low-affinity receptors for IL-2 (34). Both high- and low-affinity receptors for IL-2 bind the anti-Tac monoclonal antibody, which has been extensively used to characterize the receptor. The high-affinity IL-2 receptors are associated with proliferation, but the function of the low-affinity receptors is unknown, although activated T cells express 8–20 times as many low-affinity receptors as high-affinity receptors. Thus, an impaired expression of high-affinity IL-2 receptors may contribute to the decreased proliferative response of T cells from old humans.

Activated T cells from old humans have a decreased capacity to produce and respond to IL-2 (35). Activated T cells from old donors absorb less IL-2 than do T cells from young donors. Addition of exogenous IL-2 to T-cell cultures from old donors enhances T-cell proliferation, but to a lesser degree than that of T cells from young donors. Thus, both impaired production of IL-2 and altered expression of functional high-affinity IL-2 receptors probably contribute to the age-associated impaired proliferative response of T cells.

The expression of the IL-2 receptor on activated T cells is followed by expression of the transferrin receptor during late G_1. Antibodies to the IL-2 receptor block ^{3}H-Tdr incorporation if added to culture before expression of the transferrin receptor (26). Antibodies to transferrin or to the transferrin receptor also block T-cell proliferation. Interaction of IL-2 with its receptor leads to transferrin receptor expression before entry into S phase. Interaction of transferrin with its receptor, therefore, is a critical step following the interaction of IL-2 with its receptor in regulating the progression of T cells into the S phase of the cell cycle. This may be another step that is impaired in the proliferative response of T cells from old donors.

The proliferation of human T cells is suppressed by monocyte-produced prostaglandin E2 (PGE2) (36–38). T cells from old donors are more sensitive to inhibition by endogenously produced PGE2 than are T cells from young donors. PGE2 may exert its immunosuppressive effects by interfering with two distinct and essential pathways in T-cell activation. PGE2 inhibits IL-2 production but does not appear to affect IL-2 receptor expression, and PGE2 may inhibit expression of the transferrin receptor (39). The addition of indomethacin, a cyclooxygenase inhibitor that blocks PGE2 production, results in an augmented proliferation of activated T cells. We found that T cells from both old and young donors cultured with mitogens in the presence of indomethacin show an enhanced response (3). However, the response of T cells from old donors still remains lower than the response of T cells from young donors. Thus, the increased sensitivity of T cells from old donors to PGE2 can only partly explain the age-associated defect in T-cell proliferation.

VIII. CYTOPLASMIC STIMULATORY FACTORS FOR DNA SYNTHESIS

Cell division requires a coordinated series of metabolic events, some in the cytoplasm leading to cell growth and others in the nucleus leading to DNA replication. Cytoplasmic extracts from proliferating cell lines and from mitogenic hormone-stimulated cells have been shown to induce DNA synthesis in quiescent frog nuclei (40,41). Gutowski et al. (42,43) have identified a cytoplasmic factor, ADR (activator of DNA replication), produced by PHA-activated lymphocytes, that induces DNA synthesis in quiescent nuclei isolated from frog splenocytes. ADR is not released from cells, has no effect on intact cells, and cannot be detected in the cytoplasm of unstimulated cells. Comparable levels of ADR are found in cytoplasmic extracts of PHA-activated lymphocytes from young and old donors, although the PHA-induced proliferative response of lymphocytes from old donors is significantly impaired (Table 4). In PHA-activated lympho-

Table 4 Cytoplasmic Stimulatory Activity in PHA-Activated Lymphocytes from Young and Old Donors

Culture[a]	Experiment A	Experiment B
	^{3}H-Tdr incorporation (mean cpm × 10^{-3} ±SD)[b]	
Young PBL + PHA	34.4 ±0.6	65.8 ±2.1
Old PBL + PHA	6.8 ±0.8	42.9 ±6.1
	^{3}H[TTP] incorporation (mean cpm × 10^{-3} ±SD)[c]	
Nuclei alone	1.3 ±0.4	2.6 ±0.3
Nuclei + young ADR	10.1 ±1.1	6.1 ±0.6
Nuclei + old ADR	11.2 ±3.2	5.9 ±0.6

[a]Peripheral blood lymphocytes (PBL) from young and old donors were cultured with PHA for 66 h. Cytoplasmic extracts were isolated and incubated with isolated frog spleen nuclei.
[b]Isotope incorporation by PBL in response to PHA.
[c]Isotope (tritiated thymidine-5′-triphosphate) incorporation by isolated frog spleen nuclei.
Source: Ref. 43.

cytes from young donors, proliferation correlated with the amount of ADR detectable in cytoplasmic extracts. Activated lymphocytes from old donors failed to show the same correlation. These data suggest that the impaired proliferative response of T cells from old donors may be the result of an impairment at the level of the nucleus. However, while ADR may be an important signal to induce DNA replication, it may not be sufficient to signal the nuclear commitment to DNA replication in T cells from old donors. This is supported by preliminary data examining the response of isolated nuclei of lymphocytes from old and young donors (44). Nuclei of cells from old donors are impaired in their response to a standard preparation of ADR (cytoplasmic extract from a T-lymphoma line) compared to nuclei of cells from young donors.

IX. NUCLEAR ACTIVATION IN T-CELL MITOGENESIS

Cell cycle progression depends not only on the sequential expression of receptors for growth factors and the production of growth factors, but also on the expression of intranuclear regulatory proteins such as the DNA-binding, c-myc-encoded products (45,46). The c-myc proto-oncogene protein product appears to be involved in nuclear activation that accompanies the transition of T cells from G_0 to G_1. Activation of the c-myc oncogene is induced by T-cell mitogens and is associated with the shift from quiescence. The steady-state level of c-myc mRNA is detectable at low levels in resting T cells, but increases 5- to 10-fold within 2–3 h following exposure to an activation signal. Therefore, c-myc activation may be associated with the proliferative capacity of activated T cells.

Increased transcription of the genes for IL-2 and the IL-2 receptor are, like transcription of the c-myc oncogene, rapidly induced following activation of human T cells. Transcription of c-myc, IL-2, and IL-2 receptor genes are independent of de novo protein synthesis and are not dependent on each other (47). Transcription of the transferrin receptor gene, however, occurs later in T-cell activation and is dependent on de novo protein synthesis. The age-associated impairment in T-cell proliferation, therefore, may be due to an impairment in nuclear activation, perhaps in the transcription of c-myc or of other genes. Preliminary studies at the Cornell University Medical College support this hypothesis.

X. CYTOPLASM VERSUS NUCLEUS IN CELLULAR SENESCENCE

Somatic cell hybridization has been used extensively to analyze the contributions of the nucleus and the cytoplasm to cellular senescence. Both the nucleus and the cytoplasm have been shown to play a role in the decreased replicative ability of late-passage fibroblasts. The senescent phenotype (loss of DNA replicative capacity) has been shown to be dominant in fusions between senescent and young human diploid fibroblasts.

Normal human diploid lung fibroblasts have a defined and well-characterized life span. The fusion of senescent nonreplicative human lung fibroblasts with replicative young fibroblasts produced heterodikaryons in which the young nuclei were inhibited from entering DNA S phase (48). Thus, senescent fibroblasts appear to contain an inhibitor of DNA synthesis. This is supported by experiments in which cytoplasts (enucleated cells) from senescent fibroblasts were fused with young fibroblasts. This fusion resulted in greater than 40% inhibition of DNA synthesis in the fusion products (49). Coculture of senescent late-passage fibroblasts with early-passage fibroblasts had no inhibitory effect on the proliferative capacity of the early passage cells. Further experiments fusing isolated nuclei with cytoplasts demonstrate that the nucleus also contributes to the characteristic life span of these cells. The fusion product of a young nucleus with an old cytoplast replicated only a few times, again demonstrating the contribution of the cytoplasm to cellular aging. However, fusion of a nucleus from an aged cell with the cytoplast of a young cell had no effect on the old nucleus. The old nucleus did not replicate. Therefore, both the nucleus and the cytoplasm contribute to the defined life span of these fibroblasts.

An inhibitor of DNA synthesis in human T cells has not yet been identified. A cytoplasmic activator of DNA synthesis, ADR, has been identified and shown to be produced comparably in activated T cells from old and young donors. However, nuclei from T cells of old donors are impaired in their response to ADR. Other cytoplasmic signals for replication, such as interaction of IL-2 with its receptor, may also be impaired, contributing to immune senescence. Thus, the impaired replicative capacity of T cells from old humans results partly from defects in the response of the nucleus to cytoplasmic signals. It is not clear at this time whether the cytoplasm of T cells from old donors also contains proteins that inhibit nuclear activation.

XI. CONCLUSIONS

The impaired proliferative capacity of T cells from old humans is the result of a number of factors. With age, fewer T cells initially respond to mitogens, although the total number of T cells is comparable to young, and fewer activated cells progress through the cell cycle. In addition, there are fewer cells that after completing one cell cycle, reenter G_1 and continue to proliferate. Since progression through the cell cycle is the result of a complex of signals. there are many points at which the appropriate signal may be missing, leading to cell cycle arrest and the subsequent failure to proliferate.

The age-associated reduction in the proliferative response to mitogens is associated with the failure of activated T cells from old donors to produce and respond to IL-2. A critical level of IL-2 production and IL-2 receptor expression are required for continued progression of T cells through the cell cycle. The subsequent expression of the transferrin receptor and its interaction with the growth factor transferrin then allows these cells to enter S phase, during which DNA is replicated. Thus, an age-associated decrease in the amount of IL-2 produced and an impairment in the expression of biologically active IL-2 receptors would inhibit the repeated replication of T cells in culture. Evidence suggests that other stimulators of DNA replication, such as ADR, may also provide essential signals for the nuclear commitment to DNA replication.

In the absence of the appropriate signals, T cells can be blocked at any stage of the cell cycle. DNA replication and T-cell proliferation (S-M progression) can be dissociated from T-cell activation (G_0-G_1 shift). To understand T-cell senescence it is, therefore, essential to examine the steps that precede and lead to DNA replication. The early activation events may be the most decisive in determining the fate of activated T cells. For this reason, future studies of the proliferation of T cells from elderly donors must examine these early events.

REFERENCES

1. Weksler, M. E., and T. H. Hutteroth. 1974. Impaired lymphocyte function in aged humans. *J. Clin. Invest.* 53:99.
2. Makinodan, T., and M. B. Kay. 1980. Age influence on the immune system. *Adv. Immunol.* 29:287.
3. Schwab, R., P. B. Hausman, E. Rinnooy-Kan, and M. E. Weksler. 1985. Immunological studies of aging. X. Impaired T lymphocytes and normal monocyte response from elderly humans to the mitogenic antibodies OKT3 and Leu 4. *Immunology.* 55:677.
4. Hallgren, H. M., J. H. Kersey, D. P. Dubey, and E. J. Yunis. 1978. Lymphocyte subsets and integrated immune function in aging humans. *Clin. Immunol. Immunopathol.* 10:65.
5. Gupta, S., and R. A. Good. 1979. Subpopulations of human T lymphocytes. X. Alterations in T, B, third population cells, and T cells with receptors for immunoglobulin M or G in aging humans. *J. Immunol.* 122:1214.
6. Davey, F. R., and S. Huntington. 1977. Age-related variation in lymphocyte subpopulations. *Gerontology.* 23:381.
7. Reddy, M. M., and K. Goh. 1979. B and T lymphocytes in man. IV. Circulating B, T, and "null" lymphocytes in aging population. *J. Gerontol.* 34:5.
8. Nagel, J. E., F. J. Chrest, and W. H. Adler. 1981. Enumeration of T lymphocyte subsets by monoclonal antibodies in young and aged humans. *J. Immunol.* 127:2086.
9. Schwab, R., L. Staiano-Coico, and M. E. Weksler. 1983. Immunological studies of aging. IX. Quantitative differences in T lymphocyte subsets in young and old individuals. *Diagn. Immunol.* 1:195.
10. Moody, C. E., J. B. Innes, L. Staiano-Coico, G. S. Incefy, H. T. Thaler, and

M. E. Weksler. 1981. Lymphocyte transformation induced by autologous cells. XI. The effect of age on the autologous mixed lymphocyte reaction. *Immunology*. 44:431.

11. Inkeles, B., J. B. Innes, M. M. Kuntz, A. S. Kadish, and M. E. Weksler. 1977. Immunological studies of aging. III. Cytokinetic basis for the impaired response of lymphocytes from aged humans to plant lectins. *J. Exp. Med.* 145:1176.
12. Hefton, J. M., G. J. Darlington, B. A. Casazza, and M. E. Weksler. 1980. Immunologic studies of aging. V. Impaired proliferation of PHA-responsive human lymphocytes in culture. *J. Immunol.* 125:1007.
13. Antel, J., J. J. F. Oger, E. Dropcho, D. P. Richman, H. H. Kuo, and B. G. Arnason. 1980. Reduced T lymphocyte cell reactivity as a function of human aging. *Cell. Immunol.* 54:184.
14. Reinherz, E. L., S. Meuer, K. A. Fitzgerald, R. E. Hussey, H. Levine, and S. F. Schlossman. 1982. Antigen recognition by human T lymphocytes is linked to surface expression of the T3 molecular complex. *Cell.* 30:735.
15. VanWauwe, J., and J. Goossens. 1981. Mitogenic actions of orthoclone OKT3 on human peripheral blood lymphocytes: Effects of monocytes and serum components. *Int. J. Immunopharmacol.* 3:203.
16. Landegren, U., J. Anderson, and H. Wigzell. 1984. Mechanism of T lymphocyte activation by OKT3 antibodies: A general model for T cell induction. *Eur. J. Immunol.* 14:138.
17. Pollack, A., C. B. Bagwell, and G. L. Irvin III. 1979. Radiation from ^{3}H-Tdr perturbs the cell cycle progression of stimulated lymphocytes. *Science.* 203:1025.
18. Staiano-Coico, L., Z. Darzynkiewicz, J. M. Hefton, R. Dutkowski, G. J. Darlington, and M. E. Weksler. 1983. Increased sensitivity of lymphocytes from people over 65 to cell cycle arrest and chromosomal damage. *Science.* 219:1335.
19. Dutkowski, R. T., R. Lesh, L. Staiano-Coico, H. Thaler, G. J. Darlington, and M. E. Weksler. 1985. Increased chromosomal instability in lymphocytes from elderly humans. *Mutat. Res.* 149:505.
20. Melamed, M. R., and R. Mullaney. 1979. Flow Cytometry and Sorting. John Wiley, New York.
21. Staiano-Coico, L., Z. Darzynkiewicz, M. R. Melamed, and M. E. Weksler. 1984. Immunological studies of aging. IX. Impaired proliferation of T lymphocytes detected in elderly humans by flow cytometry. *J. Immunol.* 132:1788.
22. Avertano, B., C. Noronha, J. P. Antel, R. P. Roos, and B. G. Arnason. 1980. Changes in concanavalin A capping of human lymphocytes with age. *Mech. Ageing Dev.* 12:331.
23. Rivnay, B., S. Bergman, M. Shinitzky, and A. Globerson. 1980. Correlations between membrane viscosity, serum cholesterol, lymphocyte activation and aging in man. *Mech. Ageing Devel.* 12:119.
24. Kennes, B. J., P. F. Moest, and P. E. Neve. 1982. Biochemical events associated with lymphocyte activation in aging: K^+ transport and sensitivity of the Na^+–K^+ pump to digoxine. *Exp. Gerontol.* 17:245.

25. Kennes, B., C. Hubert, D. Brohee, and P. Neve. 1981. Early biochemical events associated with lymphocyte activation in aging. I. Evidence that Ca^{2+}-dependent processes induced by PHA are impaired. *Immunology*. 42:119.
26. Neckers, L. M., and J. Cossman. 1983. Transferrin receptor induction in mitogen-stimulated human T lymphocytes is required for DNA synthesis and cell division and is regulated by interleukin 2. *Proc. Natl. Acad. Sci. USA*. 80:3494.
27. Cotner, T., J. M. Williams, L. Christenson, H. M. Shapiro, T. B. Strom, and J. Strominger. 1983. Simultaneous flow cytometric analysis of human T cell activation antigen expression and DNA content. *J. Exp. Med.* 157:461.
28. Cantrell, D. A., and K. A. Smith. 1983. Transient expression of interleukin 2 receptors: Consequences for T cell growth. *J. Exp. Med.* 158:1985.
29. Cantrell, D. A., and K. A. Smith. 1984. The interleukin 2–T cell system: A new cell growth model. *Science*. 224:1312.
30. Smith, K. A., and D. A. Cantrell. 1985. Interleukin 2 regulates its own receptors. *Proc. Natl. Acad. Sci. USA*. 82:864.
31. Bettens, F., F. Kristensen, C. Walker, G. D. Bonnard, and A. L. deWeck. 1984. Lymphokine regulation of human lymphocyte proliferation: Formation of resting G_0 cells by removal of interleukin 2 in cultures of proliferating T lymphocytes. *Cell. Immunol.* 86:337.
32. Leonard, W. J., J. M. Depper, T. Uchiyama, K. A. Smith, T. A. Waldmann, and W. C. Greene. 1982. A monoclonal antibody that appears to recognize the receptor for human T-cell growth factor: Partial characterization of the receptor. *Nature*. 300:267.
33. Depper, J. M., W. J. Leonard, R. J. Robb, T. A. Waldmann, and W. C. Greene. 1983. Blockade of the interleukin 2 receptor by anti-Tac antibody: Inhibition of human lymphocyte activation. *J. Immunol.* 131: 690.
34. Robb, R. J., W. C. Greene, and C. M. Rusk. 1984. Low and high affinity cellular receptors for interleukin 2: Implications for the level of Tac antigen. *J. Exp. Med.* 160:1126.
35. Gillis, S., R. Kozak, M. Durante, and M. E. Weksler. 1981. Immunologic studies of aging. Decreased production of and response to T cell growth factor by lymphocytes from aged humans. *J. Clin. Invest.* 67:937.
36. Goodwin, J. S., and R. P. Messner. 1979. Sensitivity of lymphocytes to prostaglandin E2 increases in subjects over 70. *J. Clin. Invest.* 64:424.
37. Goodwin, J. S. 1982. Changes in lymphocyte sensitivity to prostaglandin E, histamine, hydrocortisone and x-irradiation with age: Studies in a healthy elderly population. *Clin. Immunol. Immunopathol.* 25:243.
38. Goodwin, J. S., and J. Ceuppens. 1983. Regulation of the immune response by prostaglandins. *J. Clin. Immunol.* 3:295.
39. Chouib, S., K. Welte, R. Mertelsmann, and B. Dupont. 1985. Prostaglandin E2 acts at two distinct pathways of T lymphocyte activation: Inhibition of interleukin 2 production and down-regulation of transferrin receptor expression. *J. Immunol.* 135:1172.
40. Jazwinski, S. M., J. L. Wang, and G. M. Edelman. 1976. Initiation of repli-

cation in chromosomal DNA induced by extracts from proliferating cells. *Proc. Natl. Acad. Sci. USA.* 73:2231.

41. Das, M. 1980. Mitogenic hormone-induced intracellular message: Assay and partial characterization of an activator of DNA replication induced by epidermal growth factor. *Proc. Natl. Acad. Sci. USA.* 77:112.
42. Gutowski, J. K., and S. Cohen. 1983. Induction of DNA synthesis in isolated nuclei by cytoplasmic factors from spontaneously proliferating and mitogen-activated lymphoid cells. *Cell. Immunol.* 75:300.
43. Gutowski, J. K., J. Innes, M. E. Weksler, and S. Cohen. 1984. Induction of DNA synthesis in isolated nuclei by cytoplasmic factors. II. Normal generation of cytoplasmic stimulatory factors by lymphocytes from aged humans with depressed proliferative responses. *J. Immunol.* 132:559.
44. Gutowski, J. K., J. Innes, S. Cohen, and M. E. Weksler. 1984. Immunological studies of aging. X. Impaired incorporation of ^{3}H-thymidine in isolated lymphoid nuclei from old humans induced by cytoplasmic factors. *In* Lymphoid Cell Functions in Aging. A. L. deWeck, editor. Eurage, Rijswijk, The Netherlands. 275.
45. Kelly, K., B. Cochran, C. D. Stiles, and P. Leder. 1983. Cell-specific regulation of the c-myc gene by lymphocyte mitogens and platelet-derived growth factor. *Cell.* 35:603.
46. Kaczmarek, L., J. K. Hyland, R. Watt, M. Rosenberg, and R. Baserga. 1985. Microinjected c-myc as a competence factor. *Science.* 228:1313.
47. Kronke, M., W. J. Leonard, J. M. Depper, and W. C. Greene. 1985. Sequential expression of genes involved in human T lymphocyte growth and differentiation. *J. Exp. Med.* 161:1593.
48. Yanishevsky, R. M., and G. H. Stein. 1980. Ongoing DNA synthesis continues in young human diploid cells (HDC) fused to senescent HDC, but entry into S phase is inhibited. *Exp. Cell Res.* 126:469.
49. Drescher-Lincoln, C. K., and J. R. Smith. 1983. Inhibition of DNA synthesis in proliferating human diploid fibroblasts by fusion with senescent cytoplasts. *Exp. Cell Res.* 144:455.

5

The Effects of Aging on Murine B-Cell Responsiveness

Dorith Zharhary* and Norman R. Klinman

Scripps Clinic and Research Foundation
La Jolla, California

I. INTRODUCTION

As detailed in several chapters of this book, aging is accompanied by marked changes in immune responsiveness. In general, these changes are evidenced by a decrease in both cellular and humoral immunity (1-7). While the decrease in humoral immunity can be attributed, in part, to diminished helper T-cell function (5-7), it is now clear that B-cell responsiveness, per se, is also markedly altered in aged individuals (8-12).

Our laboratory at the Scripps Clinic has conducted an extensive analysis of B-cell responses in aged mice at the level of single precursor cells (10-13). The results of these studies indicate that aging exerts a pleitropic affect on the B-cell compartment. Although the capacity of the bone marrow of aged individuals to generate B cells, as well as the functional capabilities of mature responding B cells in aged individuals, appear to be similar to those of young individuals (11), several important differences between aged and young animals have been identified. The most pronounced of these differences are: (a) aged mice appear to have accumulated a high level of anti-idiotypic suppression that probably dampens the responsiveness of available B cells (10) and may, in addition, contribute to a decreased frequency of mature B cells responsive to various antigens; (b) while the frequency of newly generated bone marrow B

**Current affiliation*: Weizmann Institute of Science, Rehovot, Israel

cells specific for several antigens is normal in aged mice, the frequency of mature splenic precursor cells responsive to these antigens is decreased more than two-fold on a per-B-cell basis (11,12); and (c) the frequency of B cells responsive to at least one antigen, phosphorylcholine (PC), is increased in the splenic B-cell population of aged individuals (13). In BALB/c mice, this increase is found in the populations of PC-responsive B cells that do and do not bear the usually dominant TEPC-15 (T15) idiotype (13–17). The increased frequency of splenic PC-responsive B cells is apparently reflective of a marked increase in the frequency of newly generated PC-responsive B cells in the bone marrow. It is likely that this increase in the generation of PC-responsive B cells reflects age-associated changes in the expression of immunoglobulin variable region genes.

It is clear that these disparities between the B-cell responsiveness of aged versus young individuals could account for much of the altered humoral responsiveness of aged individuals. It is also likely that the three aforementioned alterations could be interrelated. This chapter describes each of the parameters of B-cell responsiveness in aged individuals as determined by analyses of responses at the clonal level and attempts to relate these parameters to the alterations in humoral responsiveness of aged individuals noted by our laboratory and others. Finally, we attempt to interrelate the various alterations of immune function associated with aging in an effort to elucidate the physiology of the immune system, per se, and as it relates to physiological aging.

II. MATURE, RESPONSIVE B CELLS ARE NORMAL IN AGED MICE

Most of the changes in the responsiveness of splenic B cells of aged mice seem to be quantitative rather than qualitative. While the frequency of antigen-responsive B cells specific for some antigens is reduced in spleens of aged mice (11,12), B cells that are triggered respond normally (11). The average amount of antibody produced by clones of cells producing anti-2,4-dinitrophenyl (DNP) antibody is similar whether responsive spleen cells are derived from old or young mice. To the extent that the amount of antibody per clone is a reflection of the extent of cell division after antigenic stimulation and the amount of antibody secreted by the cells in a clone, these functions would appear to be normal in responsive B cells from aged mice (11). Multiple isotypes are produced by splenic B cells from aged mice, but, while a high proportion of B cells from young mice tend to switch immunoglobulin classes from IgM to IgG (18–20), more clones derived from aged mice tend to produce solely IgM (11). As seen in Table 1, only 35% of the clones from aged mice produce IgG as compared with 71% of the clones derived from young spleens. This reduction in IgG production, which has been previously found in intact mice (6), was thought to be solely a result of T-cell defects in the aged mice, but our findings suggest that this might be a B-cell defect as well.

Table 1 Relative Affinity and Immunoglobulin Isotype Composition of DNP-Specific Monoclonal Antibodies Derived from Splenic B Cells of BALB/c Mice

Immuno-globulin	Clones producing isotype (%)		Relative affinity (I-50)[a]	
	Old[b]	Young[c]	Old[b]	Young[c]
IgM	71	89	16.0×10^{-4} M	19.1×10^{-4} M
IgG	*35*	71	76.1×10^{-6} M	76.6×10^{-6} M
IgA	44	47	23.3×10^{-6} M	40.3×10^{-6} M

[a]Relative affinity was determined using a radioimmunoassay by hapten inhibition of antibody binding to plates coated with DNP-BSA and expressed as hapten concentration causing 50% inhibition of antibody binding.
[b]Old mice were 24 months old.
[c]Young mice were 3 months old.
Source: Abstracted from Ref. 11.

The observation that the frequency of B cells specific for some antigens is reduced in spleens of aged mice while normal in the bone marrow implies that mature B cells remain functional for less time in aged mice than in young mice and may indicate that B cells are eliminated in the aged environment. Moreover, the evidence that increased auto-anti-idiotypic suppression operates in aged mice (10,21-23) raises a question regarding the selectivity of this presumptive elimination. Studies from several laboratories have shown restricted heterogeneity of the antibodies produced in immunized aged mice (6,21), as well as a reduction in the average affinity of these antibodies (6,24). To account for such findings, Kishimoto et al. suggested that aging is associated with a decrease in frequency of high-affinity B cells (9). We find that clones derived from splenic B cells of aged mice produce antibodies with relative affinities that are comparable to antibodies produced by B cells derived from young mice (Table 1) (11). Since these results demonstrate that high-affinity antibodies can be produced by B cells obtained from aged mice, the reduced average affinity of serum antibodies produced after in vivo immunization is probably a consequence of post-immunization environmental regulatory effects in the aged mice (6,7).

To further study whether the reduced frequency of responsive B cells in spleens of aged mice is selective, we determined the fine-specificity repertoire of antibodies produced by BALB/c splenic B cells against the hemagglutinin molecule of PR8-influenza virus (PR8-HA) and against the hapten (4-hydroxy,3-nitrophenyl)acetyl (NP) (12,25). In both antigenic systems, not only was the diversity of the repertoire similar in splenic B cells derived from aged versus young mice, but also the representations of various reactivity patterns were similar. In contrast, Goidl et al. found that the repertoire of trinitrophenyl (TNP)-specific idiotypes produced in aged mice in response to TNP-Ficoll, differed from that in young mice (22). They suggested that this difference in the repertoire between young and aged mice may be a consequence of an increased anti-idiotypic regulation that operates upon antigenic stimulation in the aged mice. Our own studies, however, while indicating subtle differences in repertoire expression (see below), generally indicate no substantial differences in the expressed primary B-cell repertoire. Thus, it seems that despite ample evidence for the existence of an enhanced level of idiotypic regulation in aged versus young mice, the reduction in the frequency of antigen-responsive primary B cells in aged mice is not selective and affects equally most specificities. In aged mice, splenic B cells that are capable of responding to antigenic stimulation represent a diverse array of specificities and affinities and respond to this stimulation as efficiently as B cells from young mice (11,12,25). Thus, any selective effects of anti-idiotypic regulation that might lead to apparent repertoire differences in aged versus young mice are likely to occur after in vivo antigenic stimulation (see below).

III. ANTI-IDIOTYPIC SUPPRESSION IS INCREASED IN AGED MICE

It is generally accepted that the immune system of an individual has the capacity to recognize its own idiotypic determinants and that this recognition may lead to regulation of the immune response (26-30). However, it is not clear whether such idiotypic regulation is normally present in the absence of antigenic stimulation, in young individuals (29,31). We have shown that with increasing age, anti-idiotypic recognition may accumulate in the absence of any overt antigenic stimulation and may down-regulate primary immune responses of aged mice (10). This was shown by the demonstration that upon transfer of B cells from young mice to an aged, irradiated, carrier-primed recipient, anti-DNP monoclonal responses were suppressed. This suppression occurred only when the young donors and aged recipient mice were syngeneic at the Igh locus. The observation that normal responses were obtained in aged recipients when donor B cells were obtained from young mice differing from the aged recipients in the Ig heavy-chain allotype-idiotype locus suggested that the observed down-regulation was not due to the "aged environment" per se. Rather, the down-regulation appeared to result from an Igh-specific (idiotypic?) cellular recognition. This was further demonstrated by the fact that this specific suppression could be transferred to carrier-primed, irradiated young individuals by the injection of high numbers of spleen cells from naive aged donors (10). The cell responsible for this down-regulation is thought to be a T cell, since anti-Thy-1.2 plus complement treatment eliminates this effect.

It appears that T cells from nonantigenically stimulated aged mice can down-regulate the responsiveness of the primary B-cell repertoire in nonimmune mice as well (32). This type of regulation was evident in studies of monoclonal B-cell responses in chimeric mice constructed by the transfer of bone marrow cells from young mice along with T cells from spleens of aged versus young mice to irradiated young syngeneic hosts (32). The frequency of antigen-specific B cells in the spleen of these chimeric mice was determined 7-15 days later using the fragment culture technique. We found that the frequency of DNP-specific B cells in the spleen of chimeric mice that received T cells from aged mice was significantly lower than in control chimeric mice constructed with T cells from young mice.

Additional support for the postulate that T cells of aged mice may regulate the expression of the primary B-cell repertoire comes from our recent studies on aged nude mice (32). In these studies we found that the frequency of DNP^-, (4-hydroxy-3,5-dinitrophenyl) acetyl $(NNP)^-$, and NP-specific B cells in spleens of aged and young (22 vs. 3 months) athymic BALB/c nu/nu mice was the same. Thus, it appears that the B-cell repertoire of aged mice is greatly affected by the presence of T cells. However, this T-cell regulation of B-cell expression appears to be panspecific, affecting all B cells irrespective of clonotype since, as has already been discussed, the primary B-cell repertoire retains its diversity in aged mice.

The existence of an anti-idiotypic regulation subsequent to immunization is well established (29). In aged mice, however, anti-idiotypic regulation occurring post-antigenic stimulation seems to be elevated (6,21,22). In agreement with this conclusion, we have observed that 4 weeks after immunization of young versus aged B10.D2 mice with NP-Bovine serum albumin (BSA), the frequency of secondary NP-specific B cells was significantly lower in aged versus young mice. Although both primary and secondary B cells specific for DNP are two- to threefold lower in spleens of aged versus young mice, it can be seen in Table 2 that the frequency of secondary λ-bearing B cells specific for NP is unusually low in immunized aged B10.D2 mice. This finding suggests that a specific suppression of λ-bearing, NP-specific B cells occurs in the aged mice after in vivo immunization. The NP response in B10.D2 mice (Igh^b) is known to

Table 2 Frequency of Secondary B Cells in Aged and Young Mice

	Average frequency per 10^6 cells injected[a]		
Response	Old	Young	Young/old
DNP	7.6	22.1	2.9
NP	1.22	6.9	5.65
κ-bearing antibody response	0.69	2.1	3.04
λ-bearing antibody response	0.5	4.7	9.4

[a]The frequency of secondary splenic B cells was determined in fragment cultures 4 weeks after intraperitoneal injection of 100 μg of either DNP-BSA or NP-BSA in complete Freund's adjuvant.

be relatively restricted and to bear a common idiotype (NP^b) (33,34), and this may indicate that this particular clonotype family may be disproportionately disfavored by idiotype-specific suppression following immunization of B10.D2 aged mice.

IV. THE FREQUENCY OF NEWLY GENERATED AND MATURE B CELLS IN AGED MICE

The most readily identified disparity in the B-cell compartment of aged versus young animals is the marked difference in the frequency of splenic B cells responsive to certain antigens. In Table 3, it can be seen that the frequency of B cells responsive to DNP, NNP, and NP is substantially reduced, on a per-B-cell basis, in the splenic B-cell populations of aged mice. Since these antigens are recognized by a relatively high frequency of primary B cells and represent a broad sampling of the primary B-cell repertoire, we have concluded that in general, the frequency of responsive mature B cells in aged animals is lower than that of young animals. This finding is consistent with those of other laboratories using different approaches. Kishimoto and Yamamura have injected limiting numbers of cells to an irradiated host and assessed the number of foci specific to the immunized antigen-SRBC in the recipient spleen and have concluded that the number of antibody-forming precursors is diminished in spleens of aged mice (8). Using limiting dilution assays as well, Price and Makinodan have also concluded that the number of reactive B-cell precursors is reduced in spleens of aged mice (1). They found a reduction of 3.5-fold in the frequency of responding B cells in aged versus young mice, which is quite similar to what we find (2.5-3-

Table 3 Antigen-Specific Precursor Cell Frequencies Determined in Fragment Cultures

Frequency	Antigen	Mouse strain	Spleen		sIg^- bone marrow	
			Old[a]	Young[b]	Old[a]	Young[b]
Reduced	DNP	BALB/c	1.1	2.3	0.4	0.57
	NP	BALB/c	0.28	0.54	0.13	0.15
		B10.D2	0.39	0.75	–	–
	NNP	B10.D2	0.7	1.78	–	–
Normal	PR8	BALB/c	0.57	0.56	–	–
	PR8-HA	BALB/c	0.23	0.22	–	–
Elevated	PC	BALB/c	0.97	0.57	0.25	0.04

[a]Old mice were 24 months old.
[b]Young mice were 3 months old.
Source: Abstracted from Refs. 11–14.

fold). It is interesting to note that the frequency of secondary B cells is reduced 3-fold as well in spleens of aged mice (Table 2). This may imply that secondary B cells are the progeny of primary cells or that secondary B cells in aged mice are down-regulated in the same manner as primary B cells.

The reduction in the frequency of responsive splenic B cells in aged animals is not true for all antigens, however. It can also be seen in Table 3 that the frequency of splenic B cells responsive to the antigens of the influenza virus PR8 is approximately the same as the frequency in young animals on a per-B-cell basis. Interestingly, the frequency of PC-responsive B cells is significantly higher in splenic B cells of aged individuals (13). Thus it remains a possibility that the decreased frequency of splenic B cells to certain antigens may reflect a skewing of the repertoire in aged mice rather than a decreased responsiveness.

Both the decreased frequency of B cells responsive to some antigens and the increased frequency of responsive B cells for other antigens could be a reflection of any number of underlying environmental influences on the B-cell repertoire. Considerably greater insight into the processes that may be responsible for disparities in the frequency of responsive B cells to various antigens of aged versus young mice may be gained by the analysis of the surface-immunoglobulin-negative (sIg^-) bone marrow B-cell population (11,17,35). This laboratory has conducted an extensive analysis of the antibody repertoire as expressed in sIg^- cells obtained by the analysis of cells remaining after removal of all surface-immunoglobulin-positive (sIg^+) cells from murine bone marrow cell populations. The intent of these studies has been to evaluate the antibody repertoire in a B-cell population that should closely represent the purely genetic contributions to repertoire expression. Additionally, by comparing the repertoire expressed in these immature B-cell populations with that expressed in the mature splenic B-cell populations, it has been possible to evaluate the impact of various environmental influences on the expression of the mature primary B-cell repertoire. The bona fides of the sIg^- B-cell population, as obtained by rosetting all sIg^+ cells from bone marrow cell populations, has been demonstrated in several ways (11, 17,35,36). First, the precursor cells that remain in this population not only are sIg^- but also represent the population of bone marrow B cells that is tolerance susceptible (38). In addition, stimulated sIg^- B cells give rise to clones that produce IgM or IgA but not IgG antibodies (11,17,35). Both these properties are characteristic of the most immature of responsive B cells (20). Furthermore, in several systems it has been possible to identify specificities that exist in the sIg^- pool of B cells that do not exist in mature bone marrow or splenic B cells (17). Finally, in animals that have been rendered profoundly tolerant with DNP-DGL, DNP-specific precursor cells persist only in the sIg^- cell population (36). Similarly, in mice treated from birth with anti-T15 idiotypic antibody, whose mature B-cell populations show few, if any, $T15^+$ PC-reactive precursors, $T15^+$ precursors exist in normal numbers in the sIg^- bone marrow population (17).

Thus, the sIg⁻ bone marrow cell pool apparently represents a population of newly generated cells that have the capacity to generate receptors and to respond in fragment culture. However, at the time of isolation, these cells have not yet expressed their sIg receptors, and therefore, have not interfaced with the environment through these receptors.

The frequency of sIg^- cells of various specificities present in the bone marrow of aged BALB/c mice is shown in Table 3. It can be seen that for the antigens DNP and NP, the frequency of newly generated sIg^- precursor cells is similar to that in young animals. Indeed, for DNP, the frequency of both sIg^- and sIg^+ bone marrow precursor cells is similar in aged and young BALB/c mice. Thus, aged individuals do not appear to have a deficiency in their capacity to generate antigen-responsive B cells. Rather, the efficiency with which these cells emerge from the bone marrow to the spleen is low, for any of several possible reasons. For example, these cells may be inactivated by environmental (such as anti-idiotypic) influences. Alternatively, B cells of aged mice may inherently have a shorter functional half-life than those generated in young mice, or emerging B cells may home to peripheral organs differently in aged and young individuals.

The most striking finding is the extraordinarily high frequency of newly generated PC-responsive B cells in the sIg^- pool of aged animals (13). This increase is particularly notable in the population of PC-responsive B cells that do not bear the T15 idiotype. That the antibody products of these cells are indeed PC specific has been demonstrated by the capacity of soluble phosphorylcholine to inhibit their binding to plates coated with PC-BSA. Indeed, even though the frequency of PC-responsive B cells in the splenic B-cell population of aged BALB/c mice is higher than that of young BALB/c mice, the proportion of newly generated B cells that emerge to the splenic B-cell population is, if anything, lower than the proportion of newly generated DNP- and NNP-specific B cells. Thus, a diminution in the proportion of newly generated bone marrow B cells that achieve the status of mature primary splenic B cells appears to be a consistent finding for all tested B-cell specificities in aged versus young individuals. Thus, the effects of any changes in environmental influences in aged mice, such as antigenic or anti-idiotypic regulation, are likely to be panspecific and do not disproportionately affect B cells of certain idiotypes relative to others. This finding is borne out by an analysis of NP-specific B cells wherein the representation of λ- and κ-bearing B cells, whose antibody products display various reactivity patterns, is essentially the same in the sIg^- pool as in the splenic B-cell pool (12).

As mentioned above, the most intriguing aspect of these findings is the increase in frequency of newly generated PC-specific B cells in the bone marrow of aged versus young BALB/c mice. In previous studies, we have demonstrated that the frequency of sIg^- B cells of both $T15^+$ and $T15^-$ types is directly proportional to the frequency of occurrence of newly generated clones within the sIg$^-$ bone marrow populations (17). Thus, the sixfold increase in newly generated T15$^-$ PC-specific B cells in the sIg$^-$ pool of aged mice presumably reflects an increase in the frequency with which appropriate heavy- and/or light-chain variable region genes are expressed in the stem cell pool of these individuals.

If true, this conclusion has many important ramifications. Studies from this and other laboratories have clearly documented the reproducible sequential expression of various antigen-responsive B cells during neonatal development (37-39). These findings have recently been given a molecular basis by the finding that certain V_H genes are expressed at a much higher frequency in fetal and early neonatal cells than are others (40,41). The increase in PC-responsive sIg$^-$ B cells in aged individuals may indicate that such time-ordered control of V_H expression is not restricted to the neonatal period. In addition, since the overall size of the sIg$^-$ pool does not appear to increase with age, it is likely that an increase in the generation of certain specificities would be accompanied by a decrease in the generation of other specificities. Clearly the experiments carried out to date are insufficient to even begin to document such changes. However, the studies of other laboratories mentioned above have indicated that the idiotypic repertoire of aged individuals may differ from that of young individuals (6,21,22). These findings present the possibility that such differences in idiotypic representation may reflect true differences in V_H gene expression. Finally, as we and others have shown, changes in the environment of animals throughout their lifetime, such as the absence of T cells in nu/nu individuals or long-term caloric restriction (42), can markedly diminish the changes in immune responsiveness associated with aging. It will be of considerable interest to determine whether such changes also influence the changes observed in the repertoire of sIg$^-$ cells that accompany aging. In this sense, the changes in V_H expression could be viewed as a potential marker for the aging process and the influence of various environmental factors on this process might be assessed.

V. CONCLUSION

The studies discussed above demonstrate several parameters in which the B-cell responsiveness of aged mice differs from that of young mice. Overall, there appears to be a decreased frequency of mature, antigen-responsive splenic B cells in aged mice. While for some antigens equivalent or even higher levels of responsiveness may be present in the spleen, the most telling difference may be the finding that in proportion to the frequency of newly generated cells in the bone marrow, the frequency of mature, responsive splenic B cells is substantially reduced for all antigens. Thus, while the generation of B cells from the bone marrow stem cell pool appears to be unaffected with aging, the emergence from the bone marrow of these cells and their establishment within the mature splenic

B-cell repertoire is clearly inhibited in aged individuals. Thus, either the ultimate anatomical distribution of newly generated cells in aged versus young animals differs or the functional half-life of newly generated cells in aged animals is shortened. The latter could be an intrinsic property of the newly generated B cells in aged mice or the product of down-regulatory mechanisms present in the environment of aged individuals.

In addition to the well-established decrease in T-cell helper function associated with aging, many of the findings cited above demonstrate an important role for T-cell-mediated down-regulation in the diminution of B-cell responsiveness associated with aging. These findings take two forms. First, there appears to be a marked increase in T-cell-dependent, anti-idiotypic down-regulation of primary B-cell stimulation in aged individuals. Additionally, we have presented findings from both repopulation studies and studies of athymic nude mice that T cells present in the aged environment are, at least in part, responsible for the aforementioned decrease in frequency of responsive mature primary B cells in spleens of aged mice. Although it is tempting to speculate that this latter effect is a consequence of the increased anti-idiotypic regulation associated with T cells of aged animals, this association has not been demonstrated experimentally.

Perhaps the most surprising finding from our studies of precursor cells in aged individuals is the increased frequency of PC-responsive cells emanating from bone marrow stem cells in aged individuals. This finding clearly reflects a change in the expression of immunoglobulin variable regions at the molecular level associated with aging. It will be of considerable interest to evaluate the extent of this change with respect to a broader spectrum of antibody specificities. In addition, this change in repertoire expression associated with aging may serve as a marker for aging and as a means by which various experimental manipulations that appear to affect aging related changes in the immune response may be evaluated. Finally, the relationship of changes in the newly generated B-cell specificity repertoire associated with aging and the increased autoimmunity in aged individuals should be evaluated.

REFERENCES

1. Price, G. B., and T. Makinodan. 1972. Immunologic deficiencies in senescence. I. Characterization of intrinsic deficiencies. *J. Immunol.* 108:403.
2. Nordin, A. A., and T. Makinodan. 1974. Humoral immunity in aging. *Fed. Proc.* 33:2033.
3. Makinodan, T. 1972. Age-related changes in antibody forming capacity. *In* Tolerance, Autoimmunity and Aging. M. Sigel and R. Good, editors. Charles C Thomas, Springfield, Ill. 3–17.
4. Callard, R. E., A. Basten, and L. K. Waters. 1977. Immune function in aged mice. II. B cell function. *Cell. Immunol.* 31:26.

5. Krosgrud, R. L., and E. H. Perkins. 1977. Age-related changes in T-cell function. *J. Immunol.* 118:1607.
6. Goidl, E. A., J. B. Innes, and M. E. Weksler. 1976. Immunological studies of aging. II. Loss of IgG and high avidity plaque-forming cells and increased suppressor cell activity in aging mice. *J. Exp. Med.* 144:1037.
7. Segre, D., and M. Segre. 1976. Humoral immunity in aged mice. II. Increased suppressor T cell activity in immunologically deficient old mice. *J. Immunol.* 116:735.
8. Kishimoto, S., and Y. Yamamura. 1971. Immune responses in aged mice: Changes of antibody-forming cell precursors and antigen-reactive cells with aging. *Clin. Exp. Immunol.* 8:957.
9. Kishimoto, S., T. Takahana, and H. Mizumachi. 1976. In vitro immune responses to the 2,4,6-trinitrophenyl determinant in aged C57BL/6J mice: Changes in the humoral immune response to, avididity for the TNP determinant and responsiveness to LPS effect with aging. *J. Immunol.* 116: 294.
10. Klinman, N. R. 1981. Antibody-specific immunoregulation and the immunodeficiency of aging. *J. Exp. Med.* 154:547.
11. Zharhary, D., and N. R. Klinman. 1983. Antigen responsiveness of the mature and generative B cell population of aged mice. *J. Exp. Med.* 157: 1300.
12. Zharhary, D., and N. R. Klinman. 1986. The frequency and fine specificity of B cells responsive to 4-hydroxy-3-nitrophenyl acetyl (NP) in aged mice. *Cell Immunol.* (in press).
13. Zharhary, D., and N. R. Klinman. 1986. A selective increase in the generation of phosphorylcholine specific B cells associated with aging. *J. Immunol.* 136:368.
14. Lieberman, R., M. Potter, W. Mushinski, W. Humphrey, Jr., and S. Rudikoff. 1974. Genetics of a new IgV_H (T15 idiotype) marker in the mouse regulating natural antibody to phosphorylcholine. *J. Exp. Med.* 139:983.
15. Gearhart, P. J., N. Sigal, and N. R. Klinman. 1975. Heterogeneity of the BALB/c anti-phosphorylcholine antibody response at the precursor cell level. *J. Exp. Med.* 141:56.
16. Cerny, J., R. Cronkhite, and C. Heussen. 1983. Antibody response of mice following neonatal treatment with a monoclonal anti-receptor antibody. Evidence for B cell tolerance and T suppressor cells specific for different idiotypic determinants. *Eur. J. Immunol.* 13:244.
17. Klinman, N. R., and M. R. Stone. 1983. The role of variable region gene expression and environmental selection in determining the anti-phosphorylcholine B cell repertoire. *J. Exp. Med.* 158:1948.
18. Klinman, N. R., J. P. Press, and G. Segal. 1973. Overlap stimulation of primary and secondary B cells by cross-reacting determinants. *J. Exp. Med.* 138:1276.
19. Gearhart, P. J., N. H. Sigal, and N. R. Klinman. 1975. Production of antibodies of identical idiotype but diverse immunoglobulin classes by cells derived from a single stimulated B cell. *Proc. Natl. Acad. Sci. USA.* 72:1707.

20. Teale, J. M., D. Lafrenz, N. R. Klinman, and S. Strober. 1981. Immunoglobulin class commitment exhibited by B lymphocytes separated according to surface isotype. *J. Immunol.* 126:1952.
21. Szewczuk, M. R., and R. J. Campbell. 1980. Loss of immune competence with age may be due to auto-anti-idiotypic antibody regulation. *Nature.* 286:164.
22. Goidl, E. A., G. J. Thorbecke, M. E. Weksler, and G. W. Siskind. 1980. Production of auto-anti-idiotypic antibody during the normal immune response: Changes in the auto-anti-idiotypic antibody response and the idiotype repertoire associated with aging. *Proc. Natl. Acad. Sci. USA.* 77:6788.
23. Goidl, E. A., J. W. Choy, J. J. Gibbons, M. E. Weksler, G. J. Thorbecke, and G. W. Siskind. 1984. Production of auto-anti-idiotypic antibody during the normal immune response. VII. Analysis of the cellular basis for the increased auto-anti-idiotype antibody production by aged mice. *J. Exp. Med.* 157:1635.
24. Doria, G., G. D'Agostaro, and A. Porette. 1978. Age dependent variations of antibody avidity. *Immunology.* 35:601.
25. Zharhary, D., and N. R. Klinman. 1984. B cell repertoire diversity to PR8-influenza virus does not decrease with age. *J. Immunol.* 133:2285.
26. Rodkey, L. S. 1974. Studies of idiotypic antibodies. Production and characterization of auto-anti-idiotypic antisera. *J. Exp. Med.* 139:712.
27. Eichmann, K. 1978. Expression and function of idiotypes on lymphocytes. *Adv. Immunol.* 26:195.
28. Kohler, H. 1975. The response to phosphorylcholine: Dissecting an immune response. *Transplant. Rev.* 27:24.
29. Pierce, S. K., and N. R. Klinman. 1977. Antibody specific immunoregulation. *J. Exp. Med.* 146:509.
30. Accolla, R. S., P. J. Gearhart, N. H. Sigal, M. P. Cancro, and N. R. Klinman. 1977. Idiotype-specific neonatal suppression of phosphorylcholine-responsive B cells. *Eur. J. Immunol.* 7:876.
31. Zharhary, D., R. L. Riley, B. G. Froscher, and N. R. Klinman. 1983. Genetic and environmental control of B cell idiotype expression. *In* The Biology of Idiotypes. M. Greene and A. Nisonoff, editors. Plenum Press, New York. 249.
32. Zharhary, D. 1985. T cell involvement in the decrease of antigen-responsive B cells in aged mice. *Fed. Proc.* 44:1716 (abstr. 7635).
33. Makela, O., and K. Karajalainen. 1977. Inherited immunoglobulin idiotypes of the mouse. *Immunol. Rev.* 34:119.
34. Nishikawa, S., T. Toshitada, and K. Rajewsky. 1983. The expression of a set of antibody variable regions in lipopolysaccharide-reactive B cells at various stages of ontogeny and its control by anti-idiotypic antibody. *Eur. J. Immunol.* 13:318.
35. Riley, R. L., D. E. Wylie, and N. R. Klinman. 1983. B cell repertoire diversification precedes immunoglobulin receptor expression. *J. Exp. Med.* 158:1733.

36. Klinman, N. R., A. F. Schrater, and D. H. Katz. 1981. Immature B cells as the target for in vitro tolerance induction. *J. Immunol.* 126:1970.
37. Press, J. L., and N. R. Klinman. 1973. Enumeration and analysis of antibody-forming cell precursors in the neonatal mouse. *J. Immunol.* 111:829.
38. Klinman, N. R., and J. L. Press. 1975. The characterization of the B cell repertoire specific for the DNP and TNP determinants in neonatal BALB/c mice. *J. Exp. Med.* 141:1133.
39. Cancro, M. P., D. E. Wylie, W. Gerhard, and N. R. Klinman. 1979. Patterned acquisition of the antibody repertoire. *Proc. Natl. Acad. Sci. USA.* 76:6577.
40. Yancopoulis, G. D., S. D. Desiderio, M. Paskind, J. F. Kearney, D. Baltimore, and F. Alt. 1984. Preferential utilization of the most J_H-proximal V_H gene segments in pre-B cell lines. *Nature.* 311:727.
41. Perlmutter, R. M., J. F. Kearney, S. P. Chang, and L. E. Hood. 1985. Developmentally controlled expression of immunoglobulin V_H genes. *Science.* 227:1597.
42. Fernandes, G., R. A. Good, and E. J. Yunis. 1977. Attempts to correct age-related immunodeficiency and autoimmunity by cellular and dietary manipulation in inbred mice. *In* Immunology and Aging. T. Makinodan, and E. Yunis, editors. Plenum Press, New York. 111.

6

Changes in the Mucosal-Associated B-Cell Response with Age

Andrew W. Wade and Myron R. Szewczuk

Queen's University
Kingston, Ontario, Canada

I. INTRODUCTION

A significant portion of aging research has focused on changes in the immune system, first because genetic analysis of aging patterns has yielded speculation that aging itself may be linked to genes controlling the immune system (1), and second because aged individuals become increasingly vulnerable to life-threatening infections and cancer (2–7). The mechanisms are undoubtedly complex, but aged individuals are more susceptible to death from pneumonia (2), influenza (8), tuberculosis (9), infective endocarditis (10), and urinary tract (11) and intra-abdominal (12) infections. Causal relationships between these conditions (or cancer) and the age-associated decline in immune reactivity have yet to be definitely established. However, (a) Hirokawa et al. have recently described a relationship between declining T-cell-dependent immunological responses, susceptibility to malignant tumors (lymphoma), and the length of life span in two strains of mice (13), and (b) numerous reports have linked the increase of infectious disease in the elderly to their reduced immunological vigor (14–16).

In support of these contentions, numerous studies have reported a reduction in most T-cell-dependent immune responses in aged mice, rats, and humans (reviewed in Refs. 17–19, and 20). With few exceptions, this work has focused on describing the age-associated alterations in immune reactivity of tissues representative of the systemic immune system: peripheral blood, spleen, and peripheral lymph nodes (PLN). While this work is clearly important, information on the changes in immune reactivity in the mucosal immune system would be clearly relevant for elucidating the mechanisms of disease establishment in the elderly. The potential importance of this information is underscored by accumulating evidence that microorganisms entering the host encounter a functionally compartmentalized and distinct lymphoid area underlying the mucosal surfaces of the lung, genital tract, and intestine. This lymphoid area is recognized to be distinct because of its unique cell populations, cell trafficking/homing patterns, and immune responsiveness (reviewed in Refs. 17 and 21-23).

This chapter reviews and presents work performed recently in the Department of Microbiology and Immunology at Queen's University with (a) a description of the age-associated change to T-cell-dependent and -independent immune responses in systemic and mucosal-associated tissues, (b) a discussion of the concurrent regulatory changes, and (c) a review of evidence for our working hypothesis that the mucosal lymphoid system may be exempt from the age-associated influences down-regulating the systemic immune system.

II. CHANGES TO SYSTEMIC AND MUCOSAL B-CELL RESPONSES WITH AGE

A. Primary Responses

The focus of previous aging work has been to examine the role of the involuting thymus and thymus-derived cells on the decline in immune reactivity of old mice (reviewed in Refs. 17 and 20). This has mostly been accomplished through studies of T-cell-dependent responses ranging from mitogenic proliferation (24-26), the generation of cytotoxic T lymphocytes (27-29), and T-cell-dependent antibody formation (30-34). In similar studies, we have shown that when C57BL/6J male mice are immunized intraperitoneally (I.P.) with trinitrophenylated bovine γ-globulin (TNP-BGG), IgM, IgG, and IgA anti-TNP plaque-forming cell (PFC) responses of the spleen (35-37) and peripheral lymph nodes (37,38) decline with increasing age. However, if PFC responses were concomitantly measured in the mucosal-associated [mediastinal (BLN) and mesenteric (MLN)] lymph nodes, it was found that IgM, IgG, and IgA PFC responses did not decline, but instead remained elevated over the age span (36).

Goidl et al. (34), examining the nature of the age-related PFC response decline, observed that the avidity of indirect PFC produced in response to TNP-BGG became significantly less heterogeneous in the spleen of old mice, with a specific loss of high-avidity PFC. Using a slightly different method of measurement, Kishimoto et al. (39) found a 33-fold reduction in the avidity of direct PFC in the spleen of old mice after in vitro stimulation with trinitrophenylated sheep red blood cells (TNP-SRBC). In parallel studies, we have examined the avidity of PFC produced during the primary response to TNP-BGG by assessing the degree of PFC inhibition induced by various concentrations of free TNP-ϵ-amino-*n*-caproic acid (EACA) (40). When tissues representative of the systemic immune system were examined (spleen and PLN), it was found that the avidity of IgM, IgG, and IgA PFC became restricted in heterogeneity by 8 months of age, with specific losses of high-avidity PFC (40). The avidity of the PFC response in the MLN and BLN of the same animals remained heterogeneous over the age span, with some reduction in the avidity of IgG and IgA PFC at 24 months (40).

These results indicated that the systemic and mucosal-associated immune systems do not demonstrate parallel age-associated defects in T-cell-dependent antibody formation. Instead, any changes in responsiveness of the MLN and BLN are manifested later in life or not at all. The restricted avidity of the PFC response in the spleen of old mice resembles the avidity determined in the spleen of T-cell-deficient, B-cell-reconstituted, radiation-chimeric mice used in a study to evaluate the influence of T cells on antibody affinity (41). Consequently, a deficit in T-cell help [a common finding in many aging studies (32,33)] would account for the results seen here. If this were the case, our findings might indicate that T helper (Th) cells remain unimpaired in mucosal tissues of old mice. Alternatively, it could be argued that because lyt-2^- cells recirculate preferentially to MLN and Peyer's patches (PP) (42), the inferred normal Th cell activity in the MLN of old mice (relative to that in the spleen), might simply be a result of an age-associated accumulation of these cells within the gut. We addressed this question by examining changes in the number of Thy 1.2^+, lyt-1^+, and lyt-2^+ cells in the spleen, bone marrow (BM), thymus (thy), MLN, BLN, PP, and PLN (axillary, brachial, caudal, inguinal, and lumbar) of variously aged C57BL/6J mice (Wade and Szewczuk, in preparation). It was found that significant increases of Thy 1.2^+ and lyt-1^+ cells occurred in the spleen after 2 months of age, while lyt-2^+ cell numbers in this tissue remained essentially unaffected over the age span. Age-associated shifts of these cell populations in the PP, MLN, and BLN showed remarkable similarity, with significant reductions in Thy 1.2^+, lyt-1^+, and lyt-2^+ cells when compared with the young age group. Although these results indicated that our initial supposition was incorrect, we next examined changes in these three cell populations within the same seven tissues of aged mice after first priming (I.P.) the mice with a T-dependent antigen, trinitrophenylated keyhole limpet hemocyanin (TNP-KLH). Using such a protocol we found that 14 days after immunization, Thy 1.2^+ and lyt-1^+ cell numbers in the spleen of aged mice were little changed from the levels determined for nonimmune mice; however lyt-2^+ cells did decline significantly after 12 months of age. The age-associated reduction of these three cell populations in the PP, MLN, and BLN of nonimmune animals appeared to have been completely restored in these tissues 14 days after immunization. Specifically, we could identify no change with age in numbers of Thy 1.2^+, lyt-1^+, or lyt-2^+ cells derived from mucosal tissues of

TNP-KLH immune mice. The results therefore, do not support the idea that lyt-1^+ cells accumulate within the gut of older animals, but they do illustrate the remarkable uniformity of mucosal T-cell subpopulation changes with age. The data show that T-cell populations within systemic tissues of aged animals are minimally influenced by acute immunization, whereas complete recovery of cell numbers to levels found in young mice occurs in mucosal tissue of old mice immunized intraperitonally with a T-dependent antigen.

B. Secondary Responses

To further characterize the age-related PFC response dichotomy between systemic and mucosal tissue, various aged C57BL/6J male mice were immunized intraperitoneally with 500 μg of TNP-BGG in complete Freund's adjuvant (CFA), boosted 3 weeks later, and assayed for anti-TNP PFC responses after a further 7 days. Table 1 shows the geometric mean of the IgM, IgG, and IgA PFC responses obtained in the spleen, MLN, and BLN. It can be seen that the splenic response increased in all three isotypes up to 8 months of age, but declined gradually thereafter. The number of IgG PFC at 20 months was significantly reduced from levels determined for 8-month-old mice ($p < .05$). However, PFC responses in the MLN and BLN were less influenced by senescence and did not significantly change after 8 months of age. It is apparent therefore that the primary and secondary mucosal-associated lymph node response remains essentially unaffected by age, whereas PFC responses in the spleen of aged mice become compromised in both, with a less marked effect seen in the secondary response.

C. Intragastric Immunization

We were interested in determining whether the enhanced mucosal immune response of old mice could also be observed if antigen was directly applied to mucosal surfaces. Consequently, we immunized various aged animals intragastrically (I.G.) with 500 μg of TNP-BGG in CFA and measured PFC responses after 14 days. Table 2 shows that direct stimulation of mucosal tissue results in an IgM, IgG, and IgA PFC response in the spleen and MLN that remains elevated, or peaks at the oldest age group examined. From studies of lymphocyte trafficking and homing (43–45), it is apparent that mucosal lymphocytes comprise a unique population of cells: they not only bear specialized high endothelial venule binding structures on their surface (45,46), but upon antigen priming in situ, the cells demonstrate the ability to home back to the site of antigen priming (44) after a round of systemic migration (47). The enhanced PFC response in the MLN of old mice primed intragastrically (Table 2) may therefore represent the activation, trafficking, and subsequent seeding of gut tissue by cells previously demonstrated to be only slightly affected by age (36; Table 1).

Table 1 Effect of Age on the Secondary Response in the Spleen, Mesenteric Lymph Node, and Mediastinal Lymph Node Following Intraperitoneal Immunization with TNP-BGG[a]

Tissue	Age (months)	Number of animals	Anti-TNP PFC/10^8 cells[b]		
			IgM	IgG	IgA
Spleen	2	9	3,415 (±1.0)	3,433 (±0.93)	1,430 (±0.75)
	4	11	3,744 (±0.87)	13,899 (±0.65)	1,922 (±1.03)
	8	14	9,568 (±1.04)	21,751 (±0.80)	5,790 (±1.26)
	14	7	5,248 (±0.87)	9,834 (±0.82)[c,d]	3,073 (±1.43)
	20	8	5,379 (±1.31)	10,815 (±1.57)	2,355 (±1.35)
MLN	2	9	2,249 (±0.38)	4,228 (±1.23)	1,690 (±0.82)
	4	8	1,849 (±1.19)	10,240 (±0.98)	1,565 (±0.73)
	8	11	6,536 (±0.52)	33,388 (±0.78)	8,033 (±0.91)
	14	7	4,582 (±1.59)	21,927 (±2.57)	5,218 (±2.35)
	20	6	5,556 (±1.31)	22,149 (±1.43)	9,685 (±1.11)
BLN	2	9	4,535 (±0.99)	7,758 (±0.93)	1,430 (±0.75)
	4	8	4,497 (±1.19)	13,886 (±1.53)	1,815 (±1.03)
	8	11	7,846 (±1.19)	35,137 (±0.97)	4,707 (±0.84)
	14	7	11,438 (±2.00)	18,989 (±2.33)	9,212 (±2.61)
	20	7	19,177 (±1.66)	33,935 (±1.45)	12,982 (±1.37)[e]

[a]Various aged C57BL/6J male mice were immunized intraperitoneally with 500 μg of TNP-BGG in complete Freund's adjuvant (CFA), boosted with 500 μg of TNP-BGG in phosphate-buffered saline 21 days later, and assayed for IgM, IgG, and IgA PFC responses in the spleen, mesenteric lymph node (MLN), and mediastinal lymph node (BLN) after a further 7 days by methods described elsewhere (36).
[b]The geometric mean of the PFC response of individually assayed animals from at least three independent experiments is presented.
[c]The statistical significance of the response was evaluated with the two-tailed t test by comparing PFC numbers from aged animals with those of 8-month-old animals. Unless specified, any change in the PFC response with age was not significant.
[d]The response was significantly reduced at this age: $p < .05$.
[e]The response was significantly elevated at this age: $p < .05$.

Table 2 Effect of Age on the Primary Response in the Spleen and Mesenteric Lymph Node Following Intragastric Immunization with TNP-BGG[a]

Tissue	Age (months)	Number of animals	Anti-TNP PFC/10^8 cells[b]		
			IgM	IgG	IgA
Spleen	2	18	465 (±0.59)	152 (±1.06)	271 (±0.94)
	4	16	605 (±0.67)	65 (±1.12)	142 (±0.91)
	8	13	636 (±0.68)	161 (±0.41)[c,d]	226 (±0.82)
	11	13	502 (±1.72)	223 (±1.57)[e]	238 (±1.24)
	20	9	668 (±0.60)	663 (±0.71)[f]	998 (±1.11)[f]
MLN	2	18	1243 (±0.71)	1093 (±0.84)	864 (±1.03)
	4	15	601 (±1.28)	644 (±1.35)	985 (±0.81)
	8	7	1243 (±0.84)	1325 (±0.87)	1345 (±0.76)
	11	9	584 (±0.69)	432 (±1.45)	1071 (±1.99)
	20	8	1053 (±0.95)	3479 (±1.76)[g]	5006 (±2.36)[g]

[a]Various aged C57BL/6J male mice were immunized intragastrically with 500 μg of TNP-BGG in CFA, and assayed 14 days later as outlined in note a to Table 1.

[b]The geometric mean of the PFC responses of individually assayed animals from at least three independent experiments are presented.

[c]The statistical significance of the response was evaluated with the two-tailed t test by comparing PFC numbers from aged animals with those of 4-month-old animals. Unless specified, any change in the PFC response with age was not significant.

[d]The response was significantly elevated at this age: $p < .02$.

[e]The response was significantly elevated at this age: $p < .025$.

[f]The response was significantly elevated at this age: $p < .001$.

[g]The response was significantly elevated at this age: $p < .05$.

Homing to mucosal areas after systemic migration by these mucosally stimulated cells is evidently not complete, since the PFC response of the spleen also did not decline with age (although the response remained below that of the MLN).

Pierce and Gowans (48) have shown that the optimal mucosal response to cholera toxoid in rats could be generated by a combined immunization protocol involving initial intraperitoneal administration of antigen, followed by a boost intraduodenally. We therefore intraperitoneally immunized a series of animals with TNP-BGG, intragastrically boosted them after 3 weeks, and examined anti-TNP PFC in the spleen, BLN, and MLN 7 days later. Unexpectedly, this immunization regime induced marginally depressed PFC responses in the spleen by old age (Table 3) and unimpaired responses through 20 months of age in the MLN and BLN (with the exception of IgM PFC responses in the MLN). An explanation for the age-associated response pattern in these animals is not immediately apparent, but it is clear that this mixed immunization protocol does not maximally stimulate MLN cells even at a young age (see Table 1). The results (with those of Table 2) do indicate that PFC responses remain elevated in the mucosa of aged animals after using an alternative form of antigen presentation.

D. Primary Response to T-Independent Antigens

As a measure of the functional B-cell status in aged animals, several investigators have used the approach of stimulating animals with T-cell-independent antigens (28,49,50). Although their strict T-independent status has been questioned in vitro (51,52), it is evident that the IgM antibody response produced after in vivo immunization with a T-independent type 2 antigen (TI-2) is still highly T independent (51). Examination of in vitro responses to T-independent type 1 (TI-1) antigens under a variety of conditions demonstrates that they can be considered "more" T independent than TI-2 antigens (51,53,54). Since we were interested in evaluating the status of systemic and mucosal B cells in aged mice (independently of major requirements for T-cell help), we immunized various aged mice with optimum concentrations of TNP-Ficoll (TI-2), TNP-Dextran (TI-2), or TNP-*Brucella abortus* (BA) (TI-1) and evaluated PFC responses after a predetermined optimal period. Initial experiments employing the intravenous (I.V.) route of immunization demonstrated that IgM, IgG, and IgA anti-TNP PFC responses to all three TI antigens declined with age after 8–16 months in the spleen and MLN (Wade and Szewczuk, unpublished results). Preliminary results from a study employing the I.P. route of immunization have shown that PFC responses to TNP-Ficoll and TNP-Dextran decline with age in the spleen of old animals, while responses of the MLN increased over the age span. Although the latter experiments have not been repeated with TNP-BA, the results, as they stand, indicate that I.P., but not I.V. immunization, of aged mice with TI antigens reveals an relatively unimpaired mucosal B-cell (lyb-5^{+}?) population. From

Table 3 Effect of Age on the Secondary Response in the Spleen, Mesenteric Lymph Node, and Mediastinal Lymph Node Following Intraperitoneal and Intragastric Immunization with TNP-BGG[a]

Tissue	Age (months)	Number of animals	Anti-TNP PFC/10^8 cells[b] IgM	IgG	IgA
Spleen	2	4	1204 (±1.33)	1070 (±0.90)	689 (±1.26)
	4	8	1132 (±0.59)	2365 (±0.89)	638 (±1.35)
	8	15	481 (±1.15)	1602 (±1.13)	524 (±1.25)
	14	8	989 (±0.80)	2373 (±0.81)	875 (±1.08)
	20	7	1033 (±0.93)	736 (±0.34)[c,d]	409 (±0.60)
MLN	2	4	2041 (±1.05)	1415 (±0.67)	1896 (±0.88)
	4	6	720 (±1.27)	1581 (±0.75)	1688 (±1.62)
	8	13	462 (±0.99)	2719 (±0.48)	456 (±1.02)[e]
	14	7	2637 (±1.49)	2719 (±2.48)	2001 (±2.28)
	20	7	1844 (±1.65)	3025 (±1.49)	6622 (±2.18)
BLN	2	4	1682 (±0.75)	1421 (±1.10)	935 (±0.64)
	4	6	1993 (±1.53)	2520 (±1.04)	1844 (±1.46)
	8	11	1535 (±1.69)	2841 (±1.20)	2111 (±0.99)
	14	7	3567 (±1.15)	4534 (±1.08)	3933 (±1.65)
	20	5	5343 (±1.04)	5611 (±0.97)	4457 (±1.29)

[a]Variously aged C57BL/6J male mice were immunized intraperitoneally with 500 μg of TNP-BGG in CFA, boosted intragastrically 21 days later with 500 μg of TNP-BGG in phosphate-buffered saline, and assayed after a further 7 days as outlined in note a to Table 1.
[b]The geometric mean of the PFC responses of individually assayed animals from at least two independent experiments are presented.
[c]The statistical significance of the response was evaluated with the two-tailed t test by comparing PFC numbers from aged animals with those of 4-month-old animals. Unless specified, any change in the PFC response with age was not significant.
[d]The response was significantly reduced at this age: $p < .05$.
[e]The response was significantly reduced at this age: $p < .01$.

the experiments employing I.V. immunization, it is speculated that either (a) antigen entering the mucosa from the blood is incapable of properly activating the mucosal B cells in old mice or (b) blood-borne antigen does not effectively reach mucosal areas in aged animals.

III. CHANGES TO SYSTEMIC AND MUCOSAL IDIOTYPE REGULATION WITH AGE

Previous work from this laboratory has demonstrated that aged C57BL/6J male mice, immunized with TNP-BGG, responded with higher PFC levels in the presence of low concentrations of TNP-EACA. [Hapten-augmentation (HA) of PFC responses has been correlated with the reversible binding of auto-anti-idiotypic antibody to the surface of B cells (35,37,55-58).] These HA-PFC are produced in the spleen of young animals during a normal immune response (55, 57,59), but they increase in number by old age in response to both T-dependent (60) and T-independent (60-62) antigens. Since effector cell blockade by anti-idiotypic antibody has been shown to suppress antibody secretion (63,64), it was hypothesized that this could be one additional mechanism for the diminished immune responsiveness of old animals (35,61).

We examined this phenomenon in adoptive transfer experiments involving the transfer of isolated splenic B and T cells from young or old mice into irradiated young recipients (65). It was found that only the combination of B cells (old) with T cells (old) would result in the generation of HA-PFC after immunization with TNP-BGG. Further studies analyzing their appearance in various mouse strains demonstrated that the ability to generate HA-PFC in the spleen by 6-11 months of age was linked to the Igh-C, and another undetermined locus (58).

If C57BL/6J male mice of various ages were immunized intraperitoneally with TNP-BGG and their PFC responses examined in the spleen, MLN, and BLN 14 days later, the high levels of IgM, IgG, and IgA HA-PFC in the spleen of old animals were not identified in the mucosal-associated lymph nodes (37). In this study, Szewczuk and Campbell (37) have shown that TNP-specific B cells are recognized, bound, and reversibly inhibited by anti-idiotypic antibody on their surface, whereas no such antibody could be demonstrated on the surface of mucosal lymphocytes of the same animals. An analysis of this phenomenon in nine mouse strains demonstrated that some strains (C57BL/6J, DBA/2J, and C3H/HeJ) that develop high levels of HA-PFC in their spleens (58) by old age do not have HA-PFC in their MLN or BLN at any age (66). In contrast, strains (129/J, AKR/J, and C57L/J) that lose HA-PFC numbers with age maintain high levels in their MLN and BLN over the age span examined. CBA/J and SJL/J mice, respectively, maintained high and low levels of HA-PFC in their spleens, MLN, and BLN at 2 and 7-11 months of age. NZB/BinJ mice produced low levels of HA-PFC in their spleens and high levels in their MLN and BLN at 2 and 6 months of age (66). Except for the latter three mouse strains, the results indicate that mice produce comparable amounts of HA-PFC in their spleen and mucosal-associated lymph nodes when young; as they age, splenic but not mucosal levels undergo a change. In the context of work performed by Goidl et al. (61), suggesting that the idiotype repertoire of cells changes with age in the spleen, these results indicate that at a young age the anti-TNP idiotype repertoire of cells within the mucosal-associated lymph nodes is similar to that in the spleen, but as the animal ages, any changes in the spleen are not mirrored in the mucosa of these mice. The methods employed here do not demonstrate any change in the idiotype repertoire of PFC in the spleen and MLN of CBA/J or SJL/J mice over the age span. In contrast, the anti-TNP idiotype repertoires expressed in the spleen and MLN of NZB/BinJ mice are demonstrably different at both young and old ages (66).

To evaluate the hypothesis that the anti-TNP idiotype repertoire in the spleen and MLN of C57BL/6J mice becomes nonoverlapping by old age, we collected serum from young and old C57BL/6J mice previously immunized with TNP-BGG and tested its ability to reversibly inhibit the PFC response of spleen and MLN cells from young and old mice. Since reversible suppression in this system is thought to be mediated by circulating anti-idiotypic antibody (37,55,59), we would predict that only PFC from the spleen (not the MLN) of old mice would be inhibited in this protocol. In accord with previous findings (35), serum from old immune mice was more inhibitory than serum from young animals in the PFC cell responses of young and old animals (Table 4). Similarly the greater inhibition of splenic PFC responses from old mice (vs. young) by serum from old immune animals agrees with work performed by Goidl et al. (61), suggesting that the idiotype repertoire stimulated by TNP-Ficoll undergoes a change with age. Our results show that immune serum from old mice (a) inhibits PFC from the spleen of both young and old mice to a greater degree than does serum from young immune animals and (b) has little effect on PFC from the MLN of either young or old animals (Table 4). It must be emphasized that we have not identified the serum component responsible for the selective inhibition in this study, but previous work has implicated serum auto-anti-idiotypic antibody in this suppression (37). The results, therefore, support the hypothesis that the idiotype repertoire produced in response to TNP-BGG is not the same on B cells in the spleen and MLN of old mice.

In a final series of experiments, we examined the ability of TNP-EACA to augment the PFC response of animals of various ages previously immunized intragastrically with TNP-BGG in CFA. Table 5 demonstrates that I.G. immunization induced high levels of HA-PFC in young, but not old, mice. Taken with the results in Table 2, the data demonstrate that direct mucosal stimulation allows not only for an elevated systemic and mucosal PFC response in aged

Table 4 Effect of Sera from Young and Old C57BL/6J Mice Immunized with TNP-BGG on the Splenic and Mesenteric Lymph Node PFC Response of Young and Old TNP-BGG Immune Mice[a]

			% of NMS-incubated response ($\bar{x}$ = SEM)[d]		
Tissue	Immune cells[b]	Serum[c]	IgM PFC	IgG PFC	IgA PFC
Spleen	4 month	Young	104 ±27.54	134 ±21.81	104 ±25.41
		Old	60 ±9.77	98 ±22.88	86 ±18.76
	20 month	Young	105 ±24.25	172 ±65.05	134 ±27.83
		Old	63 ±9.77	56 ±10.67	33 ±11.02
MLN	4 month	Young	92 ±24.98	123 ±34.83	98 ±43.60
		Old	123 ±10.21	84 ±19.29	115 ±30.62
	20 month	Young	212 ±83.00	73 ±25.95	115 ±38.66
		Old	108 ±50.90	96 ±28.3	136 ±34.71

[a]Young and old C57BL/6J male mice were immunized with TNP-BGG in CFA and assayed for anti-TNP PFC 7 days later. Immune cell suspensions were initially incubated with 10^{-8} M TNP-EACA to remove bound anti-idiotypic antibody as described by Goidl et al. (55). A standard cell concentration from the MLN and spleen was then incubated with serum from young or old TNP-BGG-immunized mice or nonimmune animals (NMS) for 10 min on ice. After one wash, the cells were assayed for IgM, IgG, and IgA anti-TNP PFC as previously described (11). Any inhibition was reversible, since incubation of the cells in 10^{-9}–10^{-5} M TNP-EACA allowed recovery of the response.

[b]Cells from the spleen and MLN were pooled from two or three animals immunized with 500 μg of TNP-BGG 14 days before assay.

[c]Serum was collected and pooled from 4–6 and 20-month-old C57BL/6J male mice 14 days after immunization with 500 μg of TNP-BGG. The anti-TNP antibody was removed by (2×) batch absorption with TNP-BGG-Sepharose (15 min, 4°C). The titer of anti-TNP antibody remaining after absorption was undetectable by passive hemagglutination with TNP-conjugated sheep red blood cells.

[d]The results are presented as the arithmetic mean (= SEM) from six independent experiments. The percentage of NMS-incubated response was determined by the following formula: 100 × number of PFC (test serum) / number of PFC (NMS). The NMS was derived from old mice (8–10 months), which accounts for the augmentation occasionally seen.

Table 5 Effect of Age on the Appearance of Anti-Idiotype Blocked, Hapten-Augmentable IgG PFC During the Primary Immune Response to TNP-BGG Administered Intragastrically to C57BL/6J Male Mice[a]

Tissue	Age (months)	IgG PFC/10^8 cells[b]		Incidence of >20% augmentation (%)	% Augmentation GM (± SD)[c]
		Without TNP-EACA	With TNP-EACA		
Spleen	2	152	187	11/18 (61%)	23 (± 2.20)
	4	65	221	8/8 (100%)	240 (± 1.11)
	8	161	275	9/10 (90%)	71 (± 1.58)
	11	223	236	5/13 (38%)	6 (± 2.46)
	20	663	769	4/9 (44%)	16 (± 1.82)
MLN	2	1093	1126	6/18 (33%)	3 (± 1.84)
	4	644	1326	4/4 (100%)	106 (± 0.29)
	8	1325	1643	5/8 (63%)	24 (± 2.66)
	11	432	527	3/6 (50%)	22 (± 3.39)
	20	3479	4210	4/6 (67%)	21 (± 2.36)

[a]The spleen and MLN were removed from various aged C57BL/6J male mice immunized intragastrically 14 days before with 500 μg of TNP-BGG in CFA. The tissues were processed and analysed for IgM, IgG, and IgM anti-TNP as previously described (36). The degree of response augmentation by free TNP was assessed by including 10^{-9}–10^{-5} M TNP-EACA in the IgG PFC reaction mixture. The enhancement of baseline PFC responses by hapten has been correlated with the suppression of PFC responses by surface-bound anti-idiotypic antibody (37,55,56).
[b]The results are presented as the geometric mean of IgG PFC/10^8 cells determined in the absence and presence of free TNP-EACA.
[c]The degree of response augmentation over the number of baseline PFC (no free hapten) is presented as the geometric mean (GM ± standard deviation of log-transformed data) from at least three independent experiments evaluating the immune response of individual animals.

animals, but also for its escape from suppressive auto-anti-idiotypic antibody regulation normally induced by other routes of stimulation.

IV. SUMMARY OF RESULTS

Collectively, the work discussed above (36,37,40; Tables 1-5) indicates that the mucosal lymphoid apparatus fully retains into old age the ability to produce a heterogeneous, elevated PFC response to a T-cell-dependent antigen. We have discussed work that suggests that unimpaired responses can also be observed in the secondary response to TNP-BGG (I.P.-I.P. or I.P.-I.G.), and in the primary response to T-independent type-2 antigens (I.P.) or TNP-BGG (I.G.). This characteristic did not appear to result from an elevation of lyt-1^+ T-cell numbers in the mucosa of old animals. The disparity in the effect of aging on systemic and mucosal B-cell responses is clearly demonstrated if the PFC levels in these two areas are compared after I.P. immunization of young and old mice with TNP-BGG (Table 1 and Ref. 38).

When the appearance of HA-PFC, as a measure of auto-anti-idiotypic antibody regulation, was monitored during the primary response, we found undetectable levels in the mucosal-associated lymph nodes at all ages, in contrast to a rapid age-associated rise in the spleen of the same animals. The hypothesized deviation, with age, in the systemic and mucosal anti-TNP idiotype repertoire was supported by our findings of selective suppression of splenic (and not mucosal) PFC responses by immune serum from old mice. Furthermore, a study examining the responses generated after direct antigenic stimulation of the gut suggested that under these conditions, a novel responding cell population was recruited in this area since HA-PFC were not produced in either the spleen or MLN of old mice immunized intragastrically in contrast to the high splenic levels generated following I.P. immunization.

In conclusion, our studies employing I.P. and I.G. immunization of aged mice reveal major differences in the effect of aging on systemic and mucosal lymphoid areas. Although the mucosal immune system does demonstrate a change in some immune parameters with age [e.g., a reduction of Thy 1.2^+, lyt-1^+, and lyt-2^+ cell numbers occurs in old nonimmune mice (see above), and HA-PFC are generated in the response to TNP-BGG in only young mice following I.G. immunization (Table 5)], the available evidence clearly suggests that this area remains relatively free of most age-associated defects. If true, it follows that the stem cell, B-cell, and T-cell compartments must retain the ability to function normally in the aged animal. Since this places into question the prevailing opinion that intrinsic lymphocyte defects account for approximately 90% of the immune deficits seen with age (20,67,68), we provide in Section V a brief literature review that discusses accumulating evidence for a major (micro)environmental role in this decline. In particular, we present evidence for a reduced responding cell frequency in the spleen but not the bone marrow or thymus of old animals (27,69–75), and we document work showing restoration of T-cell function in the aged mouse with either thymic hormones (8,28,76–79) or interleukin 2 (IL-2) (26,29,80–83). Consequently, we hypothesize that the reduction in immune potential of systemic areas in old mice is more a function of its aged environment, which (a) is defective in promoting the maturation but not differentiation of T helper cells and (b) plays a role in the expression or modification of regulatory mechanisms (idiotypic?) that serve to change the frequency of responding cells in an immune response. The suggestion that the expressed idiotype repertoire is nonoverlapping in mucosal and systemic immune responses of old mice would argue that the inductive signals responsible for the depressed immunity in systemic areas of aged mice either are not triggered or are not effective in the mucosal immune system.

V. INFLUENCE OF THE AGED ENVIRONMENT

In assessing the participation of environmental influences in the depression of systemic immunity in old mice, the status of the lymphoid precursors in the bone marrow and the thymus must first be shown to retain the potential of expressing the same clonotypic and idiotypic repertoire of stem cells in young mice. If this is demonstrated, productive efforts can be directed toward the evaluation of changes and extrinsic influences that occur after these cells leave their respective primary lymphoid microenvironments and enter the systemic or mucosal lymphoid apparatus. We have recently published a detailed discussion on the status of stem cells and B cells in the aged mouse (17); however we take this opportunity to update this information and provide recent evidence for the unimpaired T-cell differentiative ability of the thymus in aged individuals.

A. Development of B Cells

The functional status of stem cells in the BM of aged mice remains a controversial subject, possibly resulting from alleged experimental artifact in many reports, since the techniques employed in these studies necessarily involve disruptive procedures and removal of the cells from their resident microenvironment (84–87). In terms of the repopulating ability of BM stem cells, Harrison et al. have developed a novel technique that directly compares the proliferative abilities of BM from young and old mice; in this work they reconstituted irradiated recipients with competing stem cell populations from young and old mice and compared the relative numbers of each cell population after a suitable recovery period (88,89). These studies have revealed no difference in the hematopoietic (89) or erythropoietic (88) abilities of BM from young and old mice.

In terms of their ability to produce functional cells, Harrison and his colleagues (85,89–92) have found that the BM from old mice transplanted into young recipients will, after a stabilization period, generate PFC (89,93) and proliferate to phytohemagglutinin (PHA) and lipopolysaccharide (LPS) (85,89) to the same extent as transplanted BM from young mice. In other studies utilizing this technique, the number of endogenous or LPS-stimulated PFC to a number of antigens (94), and the frequency of SRBC-specific PFC (67) or dinitrophenyl (DNP)-specific B cells (70) in young recipients of old BM were not greatly altered from numbers determined for recipients of young BM. In one of these studies (94), minor differences between young and old BM were observed in the number of endogenous and LPS-stimulated PFC to some antigens. However, when in vitro limiting dilution analysis was performed with BM populations from a number of strains, the frequency of endogenous and LPS-stimulated B cells reacting to a large panel of antigens was judged to be equal in young and old mice (95). The available evidence, therefore, indicates that stem cells from old animals demonstrate little, if any, change in their clonotypic or functional B-cell repertoire during senescence if allowed to develop in a young environment.

This is evidently not the case, however, if stem cells from old mice mature, in an old environment (72,91,94,96,97), in vitro (24,84), or in young recipients with an insufficient period allowed for recovery (96). The acute sensitivity of these cells for the suppressive influences of their old environment is best shown in experiments that examined the responses of aged recipients injected with either young or old BM (91,94). In such studies, the recipients of BM from old animals always demonstrated a greater impairment in their immune response, as compared to the young → old chimeras. Since BM from young (but not old) mice can, under certain conditions, show normal responses in irradiated old recipients, it is clear that the stem cells of old mice (a) are not identical to those in young mice and (b) become functionally depressed during maturation in the aged environment when responsiveness is measured in the recipient spleen. Most important, the BM of old mice likely retains the potential to produce the available receptor repertoire of stem cells from young mice.

B. Development of T Cells

Unfortunately, there are a paucity of reports that examine the function of T cells derived from recipients of aged BM. Harrison et al. have shown that under these conditions, spleen cells from old → young chimeras give comparable responses to PHA as spleen cells from young → young chimeras (85,89). Gorczynski et al. (74), studying the generation of allogeneic cytotoxic T lymphocytes (CTL) from C57BL/6J mice under limiting dilution conditions, found that changes occurred with age in the frequency and proliferative capacity of splenic precursor CTL (pCTL) to a number of antigens. These changes could also be observed in either young or aged recipients injected with BM from old mice, indicating that the alterations were intrinsically programmed within the stem cell population. A further study from this laboratory (75) similarly indicated that the alloantigen-specific CTL repertoire developing from BM of either young or old animals was different, and furthermore, that the host environment had little effect on its expression. It was additionally observed in this study that higher numbers of suppressor cells for allo-CTL were generated from BM of old mice both in vivo and in vitro (75). In both these studies (74,75), the differentiation of BM from young animals in aged recipients allowed the development of CTL that were identical with those developing in young recipients.

These studies demonstrate some interesting findings: (a) apparently, BM from young mice can differentiate normally within the involuted thymus of old mice, and (b) there appear to be programmed alterations in the BM of old mice that are not reversed upon maturation within the thymic environment of young recipients.

In a further series of experiments, Chang and Gorczynski (71) examined the alloantigen-specific CTL repertoire in the thymus and spleen of young and old DBA/2J mice. In accord with previous findings (73), they reported that although the CTL repertoire in the spleen of old mice showed high individual variation, it was statistically different from the repertoire expressed in the spleen of young mice (71). In the thymus, however, a high degree of concordance was found in the diversity of CTL from young and old mice. From the data, the authors hypothesized that the pCTL repertoire in the thymus was similar in young and old mice, but that postthymic diversification in the periphery of young mice was greater than in old animals. This hypothesis was directly tested in a companion study (72) by injecting BM from either young or old mice into young and aged recipients. When the CTL repertoire of the thymus and spleen was examined after 60 days, it was found that the results closely paralleled those of Astle and Harrison (91) in their examination of BM B-cell generation. Specifically, it was found that young recipients of BM from either young or old animals expressed the heterogeneous CTL repertoire in their spleen and thymus normally associated with young animals. Transfer of BM cells (young or old) into aged recipients, however, resulted in a splenic CTL repertoire that was more characteristic of old mice. In these experiments, BM from old mice demonstrated a much greater susceptibility to the aged environment in the development of its cell repertoire in accord with the findings of Astle and Harrison (91).

It was concluded that precursor T cells in the BM of old mice, while not identical with those of young mice, retained the potential to express a "young" repertoire in the thymus of old recipients, and in the spleen and thymus of young recipients. Development of the altered CTL repertoire found in the spleen of old animals was attributed to defective postthymic repertoire diversification (72), which is thought to play a major role in the determination of the functional T-cell repertoire (98).

Unfortunately, reasons for the inconsistent results in the foregoing studies (71,72,74,75) have not been directly addressed; it is suspected however, that the analysis of individual animals in the latter papers (71,72), as opposed to grouped responses in the former (75,74), probably is more representative of aging events within the T-cell compartment of old animals.

Collectively, the work indicates that BM stem cells from old animals retain the potential to generate T- and B-cell repertoires that are indistinguishable from those of young mice. They distinguish themselves from stem cells of young animals, however, through a heightened sensitivity to suppressive influences within their peripheral systemic environment. A number of reports have documented findings of a altered responding cell frequency in the spleen of old mice in antigen-responsive B (67,70,94,99,100) or T (27,74,83,101) cells [although this may not be a general phenomenon (30,33,95,102)]. With reports of unchanged function per cell (69,70,100,101,103), it is apparent that age-associated reductions in immune reactivity may, in some cases, simply reflect the smaller responding cell set that develops in the spleen of old animals.

Perhaps the most interesting finding to come out of the studies above (71, 72) is that the involuted thymus of old mice (104,105) allows for relatively normal T-cell differentiation from stem cells in mice of any age. It is noteworthy in this regard that detailed histological studies of thymic tissue from old mice have identified no reason to prevent this (106,107). As pointed out by Baroni et al. (108), morphological involution of the thymus has a real significance only if conclusive correlations between the histology and functional properties of this tissue can be demonstrated. A number of studies have observed various deficiencies in the thymus of old individuals (105,109-112), but these have relied on measurements of in vitro grown (10,110), or transplanted (105,111,112) thymuses; consequently it is not immediately apparent whether these changes are paralleled or relevant in vivo. To our knowledge, there is no evidence to contradict the hypothesis that the involuted thymus of old animals allows for normal T-cell repertoire development in situ.

A second function of the thymus is the release of hormones that effect the differentiation and maturation of T cells (100,113). A number of studies have identified a slight reduction (104), or no change (76,114) in the circulating thymic hormones of aged individuals. It is interesting therefore that (a) increased numbers of circulating immature T cells are found in aged individuals (115) and (b) enhanced immune responses of aged individuals are observed with exogenous thymic hormones in vitro (8,76) or in vivo (28,77-79). The implied impairment of thymic T (helper?)-cell differentiation is supported by a large number of studies reporting the augmentation of CTL (27,29,81,116-118), T-suppressor (82), NK (119), and T-cell-dependent antibody (80,81) formation, or T-cell proliferation (26,29,81,120) after the addition of IL-2. Although a reduction in IL-1 synthesis (118,121) by macrophages with age may account for part of the defect in IL-2 production by cell of old mice, the impairment of Th cell maturation probably plays a greater role (118). The reduction of this immune function is likely a further reason for the reduced immune reactivity of old mice.

VI. CONCLUSIONS

The focus of past immunological aging research has been on the involuting thymus and its responsibilities in the generally depressed immunity of aged individuals (20,123). Recent reports demonstrate, however, that (a) this organ is fully capable of producing cells with an unchanged diversity when involuted (71, 72) and (b) peripheral T cells within the old animal probably retain full cell function (69). Consequently, it is unclear what responsibility the involuting thymus really has in promoting many of the immunological defects in aged individuals. Accumulating evidence suggests that the aged environment plays an underestimated role in promoting alterations in peripheral cell frequency (70-72,94), and possibly suppressive immune regulation (62). Findings of an unimpaired immune response in mucosal lymphocytes (Refs. 36 and 40; Tables 1-3) would also also support this conclusion. In addition, we have stressed that stem cells in old individuals are likely to retain the potential to produce fully functional cells that bear a receptor repertoire unchanged from that of stem cells in young mice. It appears that the environment in which these cells mature is the determining factor in their eventually expressed receptor repertoire and frequency.

The gastrointestinal system has been shown to undergo a number of age-associated changes in morphology (123-126) and function (125); however our studies on the immunological responsiveness of this area have identified no overt impairment in function with age (Refs. 36 and 40; Tables 1-3). It is apparent that the age-related change in the idiotype repertoire of cells within the systemic immune system (35,61) is not mirrored in cells within the mucosa (Ref. 37; Table 4). This immune system, by way of its unique cell populations and responses, compartmentalized nature, and milieu (17), may speculatively provide the necessary environment for the unimpaired maturation, differentiation, and maintenance of cell populations in old individuals. In this regard, it is interesting to observe that the small intestine, with its highly organized lymphoid system, is relatively exempt from the age-associated exponential rise in carcinogenic transformation occurring in the abutting stomach and colon (127). Our results regrettably, do not provide an explanation for the increased incidence of mucosal-associated infections in the elderly.

These studies highlight the importance of considering tissues other than those of the systemic immune system in studies of aging. It is hoped that further examination of the age-associated changes in mucosal immunity will provide a greater understanding of the alterations occurring in systemic immunity, and in particular, anti-idiotypic regulation in the aged animal.

ACKNOWLEDGMENTS

We gratefully acknowledge the expert technical assistance of Karen Norwood. This work was supported by a grant-in-aid of research from the Medical Research Council of Canada, MA7347. Dr. Szewczuk is a Career Scientist of the Ontario Ministry of Health. Dr. Wade was the recipient of a Ontario Graduate Scholarship.

REFERENCES

1. Gottesman, S.R.S., K. Y. Hall, and R. L. Walford. 1982. A thesis of genetic linkage of immune regulation and aging: The major histocompatibility complex as a supergene system. *In* Developmental Immunology: Clinical Problems and Aging. E. L. Cooper and M.A.B. Brazier, editors. Academic Press, Orlando, Fla. 247–261.
2. Verghese, A., and S. L. Berk. 1983. Bacterial pneumonia in the elderly. *Medicine (Baltimore)*. 62:271.
3. Blumenthal, H. T. 1983. The aging-disease connection in retrospect and prospect. *In* Handbook of Diseases of Aging, H. T. Blumenthal, editor. Van Nostrand, Reinhold, New York. 3–44.
4. Silverberg, E. 1985. Cancer statistics. *CA*. 35:19.
5. Yoshikawa, T. T. 1984. Aging and infectious diseases: State of the art. *Gerontology*. 30:275.
6. Kohn, R. R. 1982. Causes of death in very old people. *JAMA*. 247:2793.
7. Yoshikawa, T. T. 1983. Geriatric infectious diseases: An emerging problem. *J. Am. Geriatr. Soc.* 31:34.
8. Ershler, W. B., A. L. Moore, and M. A. Socinski. 1984. Influenza and aging: Age related changes and the effects of thymosin on the antibody response to influenza vaccine. *J. Clin. Immunol.* 4:445.
9. Nagami, P. H., and T. T. Yoshikawa. 1983. Tuberculosis in the geriatric patient. *J. Am. Geriatr. Soc.* 31:356.
10. Cantrell, M., and T. T. Yoshikawa. 1983. Aging and infective endocarditis. *J. Am. Geriatr. Soc.* 31:216.
11. Yoshikawa, T. T. 1984. Unique aspects of urinary tract infection in the geriatric population. *Gerontology*. 30:339.
12. Norman, D. C., and T. T. Yoshikawa. 1984. Intraabdominal infection: Diagnosis and treatment in the elderly patient. *Gerontology*. 30:327.
13. Hirokawa, K., M. Utsuyama, H. Goto, and K. Kuramoto. 1984. Differential rate of age-related decline in immune functions in genetically defined mice with different tumor incidence and life span. *Gerontology*. 30:223.
14. Smith, I. M. 1983. Infectious disease problems in the elderly. *In* Clinical Aspects of Aging. W. Reichel, editor. Williams & Wilkins, Baltimore. 218–234.
15. Makinodan, T., S. J. James, T. Inamizu, and M.-P. Chang. 1984. Immunological basis for susceptibility to infection in the aged. *Gerontology*. 30: 279.
16. Phair, J. P. 1979. Aging and infection: A review. *J. Chronic Dis.* 32:535.
17. Wade, A. W., and M. R. Szewczuk. 1984. Aging, idiotype repertoire shifts, and compartmentalization of the mucosal-associated lymphoid system. *Adv. Immunol.* 36:143.
18. Szewczuk, M. R., and A. W. Wade. 1983. Cellular aging, idiotype repertoire

changes and mucosal-associated lymphoid system. *Monogr. Dev. Biol.* 17: 122.
19. Weksler, M. E., and G. W. Siskind. 1983. The cellular basis of immune senescence. *Monogr. Dev. Biol.* 17:110.
20. Makinodan, T., and M.M.B. Kay. 1980. Age influence on the immune system. *Adv. Immunol.* 29:287.
21. Allardyce, R. A., and J. Bienenstock. 1984. The mucosal immune system in health and disease, with an emphasis on parasitic infection. *Bull. WHO.* 62:7.
22. Bienenstock, J. 1984. The mucosal immunological network. *Ann. Allergy.* 53:535.
23. Ogra, P. L. and R. Dhar. 1985. Local immune responses. *Br. Med. Bull.* 41: 28.
24. Duwe, K., J. C. Roder, and S. K. Singhal. 1979. Immunological senescence. II. Normal in vitro colony formation by B cells from old mice. *Immunology.* 37:293.
25. Callard, R. E., and A. Basten. 1977. Immune function in aged mice. I. T-cell responsiveness using phytohaemagglutinin as a functional probe. *Cell. Immunol.* 31:13.
26. Chang, M.-P., T. Makinodan, W. J. Peterson, and B. L. Strehler. 1982. Role of T cells and adherent cells in age-related decline in murine interleukin 2 production. *J. Immunol.* 129:2426.
27. Zharhary, D., Y. Segev, and H. E. Gershon. 1984. T-cell cytotoxicity and aging: Differing causes of reduced response in individual mice. *Mech. Ageing Dev.* 25:129.
28. Frasca, D., M. Garavini, and G. Doria. 1982. Recovery of T-cell functions in aged mice injected with synthetic thymosin-α_1. *Cell. Immunol.* 72: 384.
29. Thoman, M. L., and W. O. Weigle. 1982. Cell-mediated immunity in aged mice: An underlying lesion in IL-2 synthesis. *J. Immunol.* 128:2358.
30. Callard, R. E., A. Basten, and L. K. Waters. 1977. Immune function in aged mice. II. B-cell function. *Cell. Immunol.* 31:26.
31. DeKruyff, R. H., Y. T. Kim, G. W. Siskind, and M. E. Weksler. 1980. Age related changes in the in vitro immune response: Increased suppressor activity in immature and aged mice. *J. Immunol.* 125:142.
32. Callard, R. E., B. Fazekas De St. Groth, A. Basten, and I.F.C. McKenzie. 1980. Immune function in aged mice. V. Role of suppressor cells. *J. Immunol.* 124:52.
33. Callard, R. E., and A. Basten. 1978. Immune function in aged mice. IV. Loss of T cell and B cell function in thymus-dependent antibody responses. *Eur. J. Immunol.* 8:552.
34. Goidl, E. A., J. B. Innes, and M. E. Weksler. 1976. Immunological studies of aging. II. Loss of IgG and high avidity plaque-forming cells and increased suppressor cell activity in aging mice. *J. Exp. Med.* 144:1037.
35. Szewczuk, M. R., and R. J. Campbell. 1980. Loss of immune competence with age may be due to auto-anti-idiotypic antibody regulation. *Nature.* 286:164.
36. Szewczuk, M. R., R. J. Campbell, and L. K. Jung. 1981. Lack of age-

associated immune dysfunction in mucosal-associated lymph nodes. *J. Immunol.* 126:2200.
37. Szewczuk, M. R., and R. J. Campbell. 1981. Lack of age-associated auto-anti-idiotypic antibody regulation in mucosal-associated lymph nodes. *Eur. J. Immunol.* 11:650.
38. Szewczuk, M. R., and A. W. Wade. 1983. Aging and the mucosal-associated lymphoid system. *Ann. N.Y. Acad. Sci.* 409:333.
39. Kishimoto, S., T. Takahama, and H. Mizumachi. 1976. In vitro immune response to the 2,4,6-trinitrophenyl determinant in aged C57BL/6J mice: Changes in the humoral immune response to, avidity for the TNP determinant and responsiveness to LPS effect with aging. *J. Immunol.* 116:294.
40. Szewczuk, M. R., and R. J. Campbell. 1981. Differential effect of aging on the heterogeneity of the immune response to a T-dependent antigen in systemic and mucosal-associated lymphoid tissues. *J. Immunol.* 126:472.
41. DeKruyff, R., and G. W. Siskind. 1979. Studies on the control of antibody synthesis. XIV. Role of T cells in regulating antibody affinity. *Cell. Immunol.* 47:134.
42. Kraal, G., I. L. Weissman, and E. C. Butcher. 1983. Differences in in vivo distribution and homing of T cell subsets to mucosal vs. nonmucosal lymphoid organs. *J. Immunol.* 130:1097.
43. Tseng, J. 1984. Repopulation of the gut lamina propria with IgA-containing cells by lymphoid cells isolated from the gut lamina propria. *Eur. J. Immunol.* 14:420.
44. Husband, A. J., and M. L. Dunkley. 1985. Lack of site of origin effects on distribution of IgA antibody-containing cells. *Immunology.* 54:215.
45. Chin, Y.-H., R. Rasmussen, A. G. Cakiroglu, and J. J. Woodruff. 1984. Lymphocyte recognition of lymph node high endothelium. VI. Evidence of distinct structures mediating binding to high endothelial cells of lymph nodes and Peyer's patches. *J. Immunol.* 133:2961.
46. Gallatin, W. M., I. L. Weissman, and E. C. Butcher. 1983. A cell-surface molecule involved in organ-specific homing of lymphocytes. *Nature.* 304:30.
47. Tseng, J. 1981. Transfer of lymphocytes of Peyer's patches between immunoglobulin allotype congenic mice: Repopulation of the IgA plasma cells in the gut lamina propria. *J. Immunol.* 127:2039.
48. Pierce, N. F., and J. L. Gowans. 1975. Cellular kinetics of the intestinal immune response to cholera toxoid in rats. *J. Exp. Med.* 142:1550.
49. Gerbase-DeLima, M., J. Wilkinson, G. S. Smith, and R. L. Walford. 1974. Age-related decline in thymic-independent immune function in a long-lived mouse strain. *J. Gerontol.* 29:261.
50. Smith, A. M. 1976. The effects of age on the immune response to type III pneumococcal polysaccharide (SIII) and bacterial lipopolysaccharide (LPS) in BALB/c, SJL/J, and C3H mice. *J. Immunol.* 116:469.
51. Mond, J. J., P. K. A. Mongini, D. Sieckmann, and W. E. Paul. 1980. Role of T lymphocytes in the response to TNP-AECM-Ficoll. *J. Immunol.* 125:1066.

52. Mosier, D. E., and B. Subbarao. 1982. Thymus-independent antigens: Complexity of B-lymphocyte activation revealed. *Immunol. Today.* 3:217.
53. Pure, E., and E. S. Vitetta. 1980. The murine B cell response to TNP-polyacrylamide beads: The relationship between the epitope density of the antigen and the requirement for T cell help and surface IgD. *J. Immunol.* 125:420.
54. Delovitch, T. L., K. Kaufman, G. M. Gorczynski, and G. D. Sinclair. 1983. In vitro analysis of allogeneic lymphocyte interactions. VIII. Characterization of helper components of allogeneic effect factor (AEF) that activate lyb 5^+ and lyb 5^-B cells to respond to thymus-dependent and thymus-independent antigens. *J. Immunol.* 131:2246.
55. Goidl, E. A., T. Hayama, G. M. Shepherd, G. W. Siskind, and G. J. Thorbecke. 1983. Production of auto-anti-idiotypic antibody during the normal immune response. VI. Hapten augmentation of plaque formation and hapten-reversible inhibition of plaque formation as assays for anti-idiotypic antibody. *J. Immunol. Methods.* 58:1.
56. Goidl, E. A., A. F. Schrater, G. W. Siskind, and G. J. Thorbecke. 1979. Production of auto-anti-idiotypic antibody during the normal immune response to TNP-Ficoll. II. Hapten-reversible inhibition of anti-TNP plaque-forming cells by immune serum as an assay for auto-anti-idiotypic antibody. *J. Exp. Med.* 150:154.
57. Goidl, E. A., A. F. Schrater, G. J. Thorbecke, and G. W. Siskind. 1980. Production of auto-anti-idiotypic antibody during the normal immune response. IV. Studies of the primary and secondary responses to thymus-dependent and -independent antigens. *Eur. J. Immunol.* 10:810.
58. Szewczuk, M. R. 1984. Strain differences in the development of auto-anti-idiotypic antibody regulation with age: Genetic linkage to the Igh-C locus. *Cell. Immunol.* 84:393.
59. Goidl, E. A., C. Samarut, A. Schneider-Gadicke, N. L. Hochwald, G. J. Thorbecke, and G. W. Siskind. 1984. Production of auto-anti-idiotypic antibody during the normal immune response. IX. Characteristics of the auto-anti-idiotype antibody and its production. *Cell. Immunol.* 85:25.
60. Szewczuk, M. R. 1983. Selective suppression by auto-anti-idiotypic antibody of B-cell idiotype repertoires generated after stimulation with the same hapten on T-dependent and T-independent carriers. *Cell. Immunol.* 83:282.
61. Goidl, E. A., G. J. Thorbecke, M. E. Weksler, and G. W. Siskind. 1980. Production of auto-anti-idiotypic antibody during the normal immune response: Changes in the auto-anti-idiotypic antibody response and the idiotype repertoire associated with aging. *Proc. Natl. Acad. Sci. USA.* 77: 6788.
62. Goidl, E. A., J. W. Choy, J. J. Gibbons, M. E. Weksler, G. J. Thorbecke, and G. W. Siskind. 1983. Production of auto-antiidiotypic antibody during the normal immune response. VII. Analysis of the cellular basis for the increased auto-antiidiotypic antibody production by aged mice. *J. Exp. Med.* 157:1635.

63. Boyd, A. W., and J. W. Schrader. 1984. Mechanism of effector cell blockade. IV. Induction by monoclonal anti-μ or anti-idiotypic antibody, role of secreted IgM and mechanism of decreased secretion. *Mol. Immunol.* 21:119.
64. Thorbecke, G. J., B. S. Bhogal, and G. W. Siskind. 1984. Possible mechanism for down-regulation of auto-antibody production by auto-anti-idiotype. *Immunol. Today.* 5:92.
65. Szewczuk, M. R. 1982. Synergistic cooperation between T and B lymphocytes from old mice in the production of auto-anti-idiotypic antibody regulation in adult irradiated hosts. *Can. J. Aging.* 1:3.
66. Szewczuk, M. R., and A. W. Wade. 1985. Age-related strain differences in the development of auto-anti-idiotypic antibody regulation in the splenic and mucosal-associated lymphoid systems. *Gerontology.* 31:251.
67. Price, G. B., and T. Makinodan. 1972. Immunological deficiencies in senescence. I. Characterization of intrinsic deficiencies. *J. Immunol.* 108: 403.
68. Price, G. B., and T. Makinodan. 1972. Immunological deficiencies in senescence. II. Characterization of extrinsic deficiencies. *J. Immunol.* 108:413.
69. Miller, R. A. 1984. Age-associated decline in precursor frequency for different T-cell-mediated reactions, with preservation of helper or cytotoxic effect per precursor cell. *J. Immunol.* 132:63.
70. Zharhary, D., and N. R. Klinman. 1983. Antigen responsiveness of the mature and generative B cell population of aged mice. *J. Exp. Med.* 157: 1300.
71. Chang, M.-P., and R. M. Gorczynski. 1984. Peripheral (somatic) expansion of the murine cytotoxic T lymphocyte repertoire. I. Analysis of diversity in recognition repertoire of alloreactive T cells derived from the thymus and spleen of adult or aged DBA/2J mice. *J. Immunol.* 133:2375.
72. Gorczynski, R. M., and M.-P. Chang. 1984. Peripheral (somatic) expansion of the murine cytotoxic T lymphocyte repertoire. II. Comparison of diversity in recognition repertoire of alloreactive T cells in spleen and thymus of young or aged DBA/2J mice transplanted with bone marrow cells from young or aged donors. *J. Immunol.* 133:2381.
73. Gorczynski, R. M., M. Kennedy, and S. MacRae. 1982. Ontogeny of diversity in the receptor repertoire of murine cytotoxic lymphocytes. I. Comparison of recognition patterns of activated T cells of B10.D_2 and B10.BR mice of different ages and analysis of changes in F_1 hybrid and bone marrow radiation chimeras. *Cell. Immunol.* 73:44.
74. Gorczynski, R. M., M. Kennedy, and S. MacRae. 1983. Alteration in lymphocyte recognition repertoire during aging. II. Changes in the expressed T-cell receptor repertoire in aged mice and the persistence of that change after transplantation to a new differentiative environment. *Cell. Immunol.* 75:226.
75. Gorczynski, R. M., M. Kennedy, and S. MacRae. 1984. Altered lymphocyte recognition repertoire during aging. III. Changes in MHC restriction

patterns in parental T lymphocytes and diminution in T suppressor function. *Immunology*. 52:611.

76. Ershler, W. B., A. L. Moore, M. P. Hacker, J. Ninomiya, P. Naylor, and A. L. Goldstein. 1984. Specific antibody synthesis in vitro. II. Age-associated thymosin enhancement of antitetanus antibody synthesis. *Immunopharmacology*. 8:69.
77. Pandolfi, F., I. Quinti, F. Montella, M. C. Voci, A. Schipani, G. Urasia, and F. Aiuti. 1983. T-dependent immunity in aged humans. II. Clinical and immunological evaluation after three months of administering a thymic extract. *Thymus*. 5:235.
78. Verhaegen, H., W. De Cock, J. Cree, and G. Goldstein. 1981. Restoration of the impaired lymphocyte stimulation in old people by thymopoietin pentapeptide. *J. Clin. Lab. Immunol.* 6:103.
79. Weksler, M. E., J. B. Innes, and G. Goldstein. 1978. Immunological studies of aging. IV. The contribution of thymic involution to the immune deficiencies of aging mice and reversal with thymopoietin. *J. Exp. Med.* 148:996.
80. Thoman, M. L., and W. O. Weigle. 1981. Lymphokines and aging: Interleukin-2 production and activity in aged animals. *J. Immunol.* 127:2102.
81. Thoman, M. L., and W. O. Weigle. 1985. Reconstition of in vivo cell-mediated lympholysis responses in aged mice with interleukin 2. *J. Immunol.* 134:949.
82. Thoman, M. L., and W. O. Weigle. 1983. Deficiency in suppressor T cell activity in aged animals. Reconstitution of this activity by interleukin 2. *J. Exp. Med.* 157:2184.
83. Miller, R. A., and O. Stutman. 1982. Limiting dilution analysis of IL-2 production: Studies of age, genotype, and regulatory interactions. *Lymphokine Res.* 1:79.
84. Lipschitz, D. A., S. K. McGinnis, and K. B. Udupa. 1983. The use of long-term bone marrow culture as a model of the aging process. *Age*. 6:122.
85. Harrison, D. E., and C. M. Astle. 1982. Loss of stem cell repopulating ability upon transplantation. Effect of donor age, cell number, and transplantation procedure. *J. Exp. Med.* 156:1767.
86. Wolf, N. S., J. R. MacMillan, and G. V. Priestley. 1983. Decline of colony-forming units with serial bone marrow cell passage: Intrinsic or extrinsic causation? *Blood Cells*. 9:515.
87. Micklem, H. S. 1983. Factors affecting serially transplanted bone marrow. *Blood Cells*. 9:527.
88. Harrison, D. E., C. M. Astle, and C. Lerner. 1984. Ultimate erythropoietic repopulating abilities of fetal, young adult, and old adult cells compared using repeated irradiation. *J. Exp. Med.* 160:759.
89. Harrison, D. E., C. M. Astle, and J. W. Doubleday. 1977. Stem cell lines from old immunodeficient donors give normal responses in young recipients. *J. Immunol.* 118:1223.
90. Harrison, D. E. 1975. Normal function of transplanted marrow cell lines from aged mice. *J. Gerontol.* 30:279.

91. Astle, C. M., and D. E. Harrison. 1984. Effect of marrow donor and recipient age on immune responses. *J. Immunol.* 132:673.
92. Harrison, D. E., and J. W. Doubleday. 1975. Normal function of immunologic stem cells from aged mice. *J. Immunol.* 114:1314.
93. Gutowski, J. K., J. Innes, and M. E. Weksler. 1984. Induction of DNA synthesis in isolated nuclei by cytoplasmic factors. II. Normal generation of cytoplasmic stimulatory factors by lymphocytes from aged humans with depressed proliferative responses. *J. Immunol.* 132:559.
94. Gorczynski, R. M., M.-P. Chang, M. Kennedy, S. MacRae, K. Benzing, and G. B. Price. 1984. Alterations in lymphocyte recognition repertoire during aging. I. Analysis of changes in immune response potential of B lymphocytes from non-immunized aged mice, and the role of accessory cells in the expression of that potential. *Immunopharmacology.* 7:179.
95. Hooijkaas, H., A. A. Pressman, A. Van Oudenaren, R. Benner, and J. J. Haaijman. 1983. Frequency analysis of functional immunoglobulin C and V gene expression in murine B cells at various ages. *J. Immunol.* 131:1629.
96. Chen, M. G. 1971. Age-related changes in hematopoietic stem cell populations of a long-lived hybrid mouse. *J. Cell. Physiol.* 78:225.
97. Peterson, W. J., K. Onari, T. Akawaga, and T. Makinodan. 1983. Increase with age in the number of mitotically quiescent bone marrow stem cells. *Gerontologist.* 23(suppl.):248.
98. Miller, R. A., and O. Stutman. 1984. T cell repopulation from functionally restricted splenic progenitors: 10,000-fold expansion documented by using limiting dilution analyses. *J. Immunol.* 133:2925.
99. Andersson, J., A. Coutinho, and F. Melchers. 1977. Frequencies of mitogen-reactive B cells in the mouse. I. Distribution in different lymphoid organs from different inbred strains of mice at different ages. *J. Exp. Med.* 145:1511.
100. Abraham, C., Y. Tal, and H. Gershon. 1977. Reduced in vitro response to concanavalin A and lipopolysaccharide in senescent mice: A function of reduced number of responding cells. *Eur. J. Immunol.* 7:301.
101. Nordin, A. A., and G. D. Collins. 1983. Limiting dilution analysis of alloreactive cytotoxic precursor cells in aging mice. *J. Immunol.* 131:2215.
102. Zharhary, D., and N. R. Klinman. 1984. B cell repertoire diversity to PR8 influenza virus does not decrease with age. *J. Immunol.* 133:2285.
103. Staiano-Coicco, L., Z. Darzynkiewicz, M. R. Melamed, and M. E. Weksler. 1984. Immunological studies of aging. IX. Impaired proliferation of T lymphocytes detected in elderly humans by flow cytometry. *J. Immunol.* 132:1788.
104. Lewis, V. M., J. J. Twomey, P. Bealmear, G. Goldstein, and R. A. Good. 1978. Age, thymic involution, and circulating thymic hormone activity. *J. Clin. Endocrinol. Metab.* 47:145.
105. Hirokawa, K., and T. Makinodan. 1975. Thymic involution: Effect on T cell differentiation. *J. Immunol.* 114:1659.
106. Steinmann, G. S., and H.-K. Muller-Hermelink. 1984. Lymphocyte differ-

entiation and its microenvironment in the human thymus during aging. *Monogr. Dev. Biol.* 17:142.
107. Steinmann, G. G., and H.-K. Muller-Hermelink. 1984. Immunohistological demonstration of terminal transferase (TdT) in the age-involuted human thymus. *Immunobiology.* 166:45.
108. Baroni, C. D., M. Valtieri, A. Stoppacciaro, L. P. Ruco, S. Uccini, and C. Ricci. 1983. The human thymus in ageing: Histological involution paralleled by increased mitogen response and by enrichment of OKT3$^+$ lymphocytes. *Immunology.* 50:519.
109. Small, M., L. Barr-Nea, and M. Aronson. 1984. Culture of thymic epithelial cells from mice and age-related studies on the growing cells. *Eur. J. Immunol.* 14:936.
110. Sato, K., M.-P. Chang, and T. Makinodan. 1984. Influence of age on the ability of thymic adherent cells to produce factors in vitro which modulate immune responses of thymocytes. *Cell. Immunol.* 87:473.
111. Hirokawa, K., K. Sato, and T. Makinodan. 1982. Influence of age of thymic grafts on the differentiation of T cells in nude mice. *Clin. Immunol. Immunopathol.* 24:251.
112. Leiner, H., U. Greinert, W. Scheiwe, R. Bathmann, and H.-K. Muller-Hermelink. 1984. Repopulation of lymph nodes and spleen in thymus chimeras after lethal irradiation and bone marrow transplantation: Dependence on the age of the thymus. *Immunobiology.* 167:345.
113. Goldstein, A. L., T. L. K. Low, G. B. Thurman, M. M. Zatz, N. Hale, J. Chen, S.-K. Hu, P. B. Naylor, and J. E. McClure. 1981. Current status of thymosin and other hormones of the thymus gland. *Recent Prog. Horm. Res.* 37:369.
114. Fabris, N., E. Mocchegiani, L. Amadio, M. Zannotti, F. Licastro, and C. Franceschi. 1984. Thymic hormone deficiency in normal ageing and Down's syndrome: Is there a primary deficiency of the thymus? *Lancet.* 1:983.
115. Hallgren, H. M., D. R. Jackola, and J. J. O'Leary. 1983. Unusual pattern of surface marker expression on peripheral lymphocytes from aged humans suggestive of a population of less differentiated cells. *J. Immunol.* 131:191.
116. Effros, R. B., and R. L. Walford. 1983. The immune response of aged mice to influenza: Diminished T-cell proliferation, interleukin 2 production and cytotoxicity. *Cell. Immunol.* 81:298.
117. Miller, R. A., and O. Stutman. 1981. Decline, in aging mice, of the anti-2,4,6-trinitrophenyl (TNP) cytotoxic cytotoxic T cell response attributable to loss of lyt-2$^-$, interleukin 2-producing helper cell function. *Eur. J. Immunol.* 11:751.
118. Bruley-Rosset, M., and I. Vergnon. 1984. Interleukin-1 synthesis and activity in aged mice. *Mech. Ageing Dev.* 24:247.
119. Saxena, R. K., Q. B. Saxena, and W. H. Adler. 1984. Interleukin-2 induced activation of natural killer activity in spleen cells from old and young mice. *Immunology.* 51:719.

120. Kennes, B., D. Brohee, and P. Neve. 1983. Lymphocyte activation in human aging. V. Acquisition of response to T cell growth factor and production of growth factors by mitogen-stimulated lymphocytes. *Mech. Ageing Dev.* 23:103.
121. Inamizu, T., M.-P. Chang, and T. Makinodan. 1983. Decline in interleukin-1 production with age. *Gerontologist.* 23(suppl.):249.
122. Kay, M.M.B. 1979. The thymus: Clock for immunological aging? *J. Invest. Dermatol.* 73:29.
123. Andrew, W., and N. V. Andrew. 1957. An age involution in the small intestine of the mouse. With a description of the fundamental process of lymphoepithelial metamorphosis in intestinal mucosa. *J. Gerontol.* 12:136.
124. Cornes, J. S. 1965. Number, size, and distribution of Peyer's patches in the human small intestine. Part 2. The effect of age on Peyer's patches. *Gut.* 6:230.
125. McDougal, J. N., M. S. Miller, and T. F. Burks. 1984. Age-related changes in colonic function in rats. *Am. J. Physiol.* 247:G542.
126. Schmucker, D. L., R. Gilbert, A. L. Jones, G. T. Hradek, and H. Bazin. 1985. Effect of age on the hepatobiliary transport of dimeric immunoglobulin A in the male Fischer rat. *Gastroenterology.* 88:436.
127. Potten, C. S. 1984. Clonogenic, stem and carcinogen-target cells in small intestine. *Scand. J. Immunol.* 19(suppl. 104):3.

7

The Effect of Aging on Acquired Immunological Tolerance in Mice

Gail S. Habicht

State University of New York
Stony Brook, New York

I. INTRODUCTION

One of the chief characteristics of aging is a decline in the ability to deal with environmental stress. This is revealed by an increased incidence of certain diseases including cancer, cardiovascular disease, and some bacterial and viral infections. The immune system provides the primary mechanism with which the organism can deal with environmental stress. As the body ages, this system also undergoes an immunological senescence that is characterized by decreasing ability to produce antibodies or to mount a cell-mediated immune response. Paradoxically, however, there is an increased incidence of autoantibody formation both in human beings and experimental animals. We are interested in the cellular mechanisms of immune senescence whereby responses to foreign antigens decline while those to self antigens are enhanced. Specifically, we are interested in the mechanisms by which self-tolerance fails during aging.

II. ANTIBODY FORMATION DECLINES DURING SENESCENCE

A. Cellular Basis

Several studies have addressed the cellular basis of the age-related decline in antibody formation. That the decrease was due to changes in lymphoid cells rather than to the extralymphoid environment was shown by adoptive transfer studies in which splenocytes largely maintained their aged or young immune phenotypes when transferred into lethally irradiated syngeneic aged or young hosts (1,21). However, peripheral lymphoid cells such as splenocytes may have already suffered the effects of the aged internal environment, therefore not representing a true test of the lymphoid cells-lymphoid environment question. Adoptively transferred bone marrow cells, on the other hand, assumed the immune potential of the host (3,4).

The functions of both T and B lymphocytes have been shown to decline with advancing age (5-8), although the T helper cells were most sensitive to the ravages of aging (5,9). In contrast, in most experiments using human or animal cells both nonspecific and antigen-specific T suppressor cell activities actually increased during senescence (10-18), although in other systems, decreased T suppressor cell function occurred (19). Some investigators have demonstrated the existence of suppressor cells in aged animals that are not of the T-cell lineage (20,21). Sensitivity of antibody synthesis to antigen-specific suppression has been found to be either increased (15) or decreased (18) in aged mice. A causal relationship between increased suppressor cell function and decreased longevity has been suggested by preliminary experiments in which long-term treatment of mice with anti-I-J antibodies, which should reduce suppressor cell numbers and functions, elevated T helper function and increased life span (22).

B. Role of Lymphokines

The role of lymphokines in immune senescence is the subject of current investigation. Both human and rodent T lymphocytes produced less interleukin 2 (IL-2) in response to challenge with mitogens or allogeneic cells (23-28). Not only was IL-2 production impaired in aging, but responsiveness to IL-2 also declined (28). However, in one study IL-2 production in response to interleukin 1 was not impaired in aged rats (29). That declining IL-2 production may be responsible for reduced immune function was shown by experiments in which in vivo IL-2 administration caused restoration of cytotoxic T-lymphocyte formation by aged animals to the level attained in young adults (30).

IL-1 is produced by macrophages in response to a variety of challenges including whole bacteria, endotoxin, tumor promoters, and phagocytosis (31). Most reports have shown that macrophage function is unchanged during aging (5) and, consonant with these observations, the ability to produce IL-1 is maintained during aging (29,32; Leichtling and Habicht, unpublished observations). In addition, IL-1 responsiveness as measured by thymocyte proliferation or pyrogenicity was actually elevated in senescent mice (Leichtling and Habicht, unpublished observations).

III. AUTOANTIBODY FORMATION RISES DURING AGING

In marked contrast to the declining ability to mount an immune response to foreign antigens during the aging process is the rising incidence of autoimmune phenomena in humans (33-39). These observations have been extended by studies in experimental animals that showed that exposure to polyclonal B-cell activators either in vivo or in vitro preferentially induced autoantibody formation by cells from aged mice (4,40,41). Injection of hapten-modified murine erythrocytes induced autoantibody formation in aged mice while failing to do so in young animals (42). However, other antigens such as cross-reacting xenogeneic thyroglobulin or erythrocytes failed to induce any more autoantibody formation in old mice than in young mice (41). Whether autoantibody formation during senescence represents a physiological mechanism for disposing of effete cells (43) or is causally related to the aging process (44) remains to be determined. The observation by Goidl et al. (45) that auto-anti-idiotypic antibody formation increased with advancing age may, in part, explain the apparent paradox of declining antibody responses to foreign antigens in the presence of increased ability to mount an autoantibody response. In this model the fundamental age-related change, namely, an increased ability to mount an *auto*immune response, could also account for suppression of antibody responses to foreign antigens through the anti-idiotypic network.

Why are more autoantibodies formed in the aged individual? We are interested in the immune mechanisms involved in this decreased ability to maintain self-tolerance. Several theoretical possibilities are immediately apparent. Since the immunological repertoire is being regenerated throughout life, it follows that the induction of self-tolerance is an ongoing process. Thus, any age-related failure in the tolerance-induction mechanism will result in the loss of self-tolerance and the potential for the development of autoimmunity. Alternatively, molecular wear and tear associated with the aging process, perhaps due to disease or to accumulated physicochemical modification of macromolecules, could result in the formation of neoantigens that are immunologically cross-reactive with their normal counterparts. A third possibility is that lymphoid cells lose the capacity to maintain the tolerant state so that otherwise innocuous insults—bacterial infection, for example—might induce autoantibody formation through the release of polyclonal B-cell activators.

IV. FAILURE OF IMMUNOLOGICAL TOLERANCE IN AGED MICE

We, and others, have investigated the various mechanisms for tolerance failure in aged animals by studying the induction and maintenance of acquired immunological tolerance. Most of the studies have involved the use of heterologous, deaggregated immunoglobulins as the tolerogen. This system has been well characterized in young adult mice. Both B and T lymphocytes become unresponsive without the intervention of a suppressor cell (46,47). Tolerance in one cell population is sufficient to maintain the tolerant phenotype in the intact animal (46). While the heterologous immunoglobulin model system affords advantages for studies of the ease of tolerance induction through quantitation of tolerogen required and for studies of the loss of tolerance, it has been criticized with regard to its physiological relevance because, among the most studied systems, it is unique in the ease with which tolerance is induced in adult animals in the absence of suppressor cells. However, in many respects tolerance to immunoglobulins mimics self-tolerance. In support of this model as physiologically relevant are the observations that defects in experimental tolerance to heterologous immunoglobulin are associated with defects in self-tolerance in both aging and in autoimmune-prone strains of mice (48).

A. Induction of Tolerance

In view of the age-related decline in immunoresponsiveness to foreign antigens and the increase in suppressor cell activities, it might be predicted that induction and maintenance of immunological tolerance would become easier with advancing age. However, the results of several studies have shown that aged mice become more resistant to tolerance induction (49–62). The age of onset of tolerance resistance varied with the strain, the antigen, and whether T- or B-cell tolerance was the subject of investigation. In general, autoimmune-prone strains such as SJL or MRL lpr/lpr became tolerance resistant at an earlier age (51,59) and long-lived strains were more tolerance sensitive at an early age (62).

We have studied the induction of tolerance in C_{57}Bl/6 mice, a relatively long-lived, tolerance-susceptible strain and Balb/c mice, a normal strain that is relatively tolerance resistant and has a shorter life span. Deaggregated human IgG (DHGG) was used as the tolerogen. Mice of 2, 12 and 22–24 months of age were injected with doses of DHGG ranging from 1 μg to 10 mg and were challenged with 400 μg of AHGG on days 21 and 36 after tolerance induction. The splenic plaque-forming cell (PFC) response was measured 5 days after the second challenge injection and compared to that in age-matched animals not receiving the tolerogen. The results showed that Balb/c mice became tolerance resistant by 12 months of age and C_{57}Bl/6 mice evidenced a dramatic loss of tolerance sensitivity such that 24-month-old mice required 10-fold more tolerogen for a given degree of unresponsiveness than did 12-month-old animals. In turn, 12-month-old mice required 10-fold more tolerogen than did 2-month animals (Table 1) (56,62).

The exact temporal pattern for the loss of tolerance sensitivity varied according to strain and to the tolerogen used. In a series of studies, Cinader and his

Table 1 Dose of Tolerogen (DHGG) Required for 50% Unresponsiveness in $C_{57}Bl/6$ Mice of Different Ages

Age (months)	Dose of DHGG (μg)
2	3
12	32
24	372

colleagues (50,52,53,58,59) examined age-related changes in the induction of unresponsiveness to rabbit IgG in several mouse strains. All strains became tolerance resistant, but at different ages. The temporal pattern of sensitivity to tolerance induction varied independent of the age-related variation in antibody-forming capacity (58), and autoimmune-prone strains, such as SJL and MRL/Mp-lpr/lpr, became tolerance resistant early, i.e., by 8–10 weeks of age (51,59). Our studies and those of Cinader's group have shown that neither tolerance induction nor the age-related change in tolerance susceptibility was regulated by genes in the major histocompatibility complex (18,63).

Cinader's group has also shown that not only did deaggregated heterologous immunoglobulins fail to induce tolerance in aged mice, but they actually primed the immune system for a secondary response upon further challenge with the antigen (56,60). In early studies of the DHGG system, it was found that months after tolerogen exposure, when B cells from young adult A/J mice lost the tolerant state, they became hyperresponsive to the aggregated form of the antigen (65). Thus, immunity following tolerogen exposure is not restricted to aged animals.

B. Cellular Basis for the Difference in Tolerance Sensitivity Between Young and Aged Mice

Weksler and his colleagues have looked specifically at the induction of T-cell tolerance in aged mice (54) and have found that the pattern of declining sensitivity directly reflected the declining sensitivity of the intact aged mouse. They demonstrated that 6 months was the inflection point in a curve relating tolerance sensitivity and age. Studies from the same laboratory on the induction of B-cell tolerance to a hapten (dinitrophenyl [DNP] derivative of the copolymer of D-glutamic acid and D-lysine) showed that B-cell tolerance resistance also began at about 6 months in Balb/c mice (55,57). However, a large part of the decline could be accounted for by the declining response to immunogen in aged mice, so that, although there was no difference in response to dinitrophenylated bovine γ-globulin (DNP-BGG) between tolerogen-treated young and aged mice, the percentage of unresponsiveness was reduced because of the reduced response to the immunogen in aged mice. McIntosh and Segre (49) used DNP coupled to mouse immunoglobulin to induce B-cell tolerance in BC_3F_1 mice and also found that a smaller dose was required to produce reduced B-cell responsiveness to DNP-HGG in young mice than was needed in old (2 years) animals. A thymus-independent antigen, type III pneumococcal polysaccharide, was more effective in producing immunological paralysis in young animals than in old (64).

C. Role of Suppressor Cells in Acquired Tolerance During Senescence

The role of suppressor cells in the induction and maintenance of tolerance in aged mice has been investigated in several systems. Acquired unresponsiveness, induced with deaggregated heterologous immunoglobulins, does not require suppressor cell activity, although suppressor T lymphocytes have been observed during the induction phase and at the time of tolerance loss (47,66,67). To determine whether differences in suppressor cell function could account for the age-related loss of tolerance sensitivity, we examined the activity of suppressor cells during the induction phase by using adoptive transfer of splenocytes from tolerogen-treated and normal donors into lethally irradiated syngeneic hosts (4). Suppressor cells were found in both $C_{57}Bl/6$ and Balb/c splenocytes pooled from aged tolerogen-treated donors (Table 2). There is a great deal of variability between aged mice in their response to tolerogen and it was possible that individual aged mice contained highly active suppressor cells that were dominant in the pooled splenocytes from tolerogen-treated donors. The suppressor activity was either not present ($C_{57}Bl/6$) or significantly less (Balb/c) in cells from young

Table 2 Development of Suppressor Cells in Spleens of Tolerogen-Treated Donors of Different Ages

Strain	Age (months)	% Suppression[a]
Balb/c	2	61.3
	12	71.4
	24	95.8
$C_{57}Bl/6$	2	-45.8
	12	18.7
	24	41.0

[a]Calculated by comparing the splenic PFC response to AHGG of lethally irradiated mice which received 70×10^6 splenocytes from normal donors (NS) with that in mice that received both NS and 70×10^6 splenocytes from tolerogen-treated, age-matched donors (TS) according to the following formula:

$$\% \text{ suppression} = 1 - \frac{\text{NT} + \text{TS}}{\text{NS}}$$

donors. To test the hypothesis that spleens from individual aged mice might contain highly active suppressor cells that were dominant in the pooled splenocytes from tolerogen-treated donors, the adoptive transfer experiment was repeated using individual tolerogen-treated or normal old donors. Splenocytes from these animals were injected into the adoptive hosts along with splenocytes from a pool of normal young donors. The results showed that both Balb/c and $C_{57}Bl/6$ tolerogen-treated aged mice produced suppression (average of 44 and 88% respectively), but in Balb/c mice the expression was variable, with only 43% of the aged donors possessing suppressor cell activity.

Since aged mice, especially $C_{57}Bl/6$ mice, were more resistant to tolerance induction in spite of the presence of antigen-specific suppressor cells in tolerogen-treated animals, it was necessary to consider the possibility that cells from aged mice were less sensitive to the effects of suppressor cells. To test this, a pool of suppressor cells from young Balb/c mice was adoptively transferred into lethally irradiated syngeneic hosts along with either pooled splenocytes from normal young donors or cells from individual aged (24 months) donors. The results showed that contrary to the original hypothesis, splenocytes from aged animals were more susceptible to suppression (Table 3).

Suppression could not be aborted in aged mice by low doses of cyclophosphamide (25 mg/kg) and, in fact, both 25 and 200 mg/kg enhanced the induction of tolerance and suppressed antibody formation in normal aged mice. Mice of all ages withstood two injections of 200 mg/kg cyclophosphamide without weight loss or other indications of ill effects (Table 4).

Amagai et al. (60) have studied the induction of suppressor cells in the thymus in 1- and 8-month-old $C_{57}Bl/6$ mice treated with deaggregated rabbit γ-globulin (DRGG). They found that thymocytes from young treated donors

Table 3 Capacity of Splenocytes from Young and Old Balb/c Donors to be Suppressed

Cells transferred	$PFC/10^6$ splenocytes in adoptive host	% Suppression
70×10^6 normal, 2 month	50 ±25	–
70×10^6 normal, 24 month	222 ±167	–
70×10^6 normal, 2 month + 70×10^6 tolerant, 2 month[a]	101 ±36	0
70×10^6 normal, 24 month + 70×10^6 tolerant, 2 month	21 ±12	91

[a]That the tolerogen-treated young mice were, in fact, unresponsive was shown by challenging part of the donor group with AHGG. There was 91% unresponsiveness (24 $PFC/10^6$ splenocytes in tolerogen-treated mice vs. 263 $PFC/10^6$ splenocytes in normal AHGG-challenged animals).

Table 4 Effect of Cyclophosphamide on Tolerance Induction in 12-Month-Old $C_{57}Bl/6$ Mice

Dose of tolerogen (μg)	% Unresponsiveness	
	With cyclophosphamide[a]	Without cyclophosphamide
1	48	0
10	62	0
100	75	100
1000	96	100

[a]Cyclophosphamide-treated mice received 25 mg/kg 5 days prior to tolerogen injection.

were suppressive as measured by both PFC responses and in vivo degradation of ^{125}I[RGG]. Small numbers of thymocytes from tolerogen-treated donors actually enhanced responsiveness to aggregated RGG and only relatively large numbers (2.5 times the number of splenocytes that were the target for the suppression) sufficed to produce suppression. Slightly elevated suppression was found in the spleens of tolerogen-treated old mice.

Doria et al. (15) induced suppression by injecting azobenzene arsonate (ABA)-coupled syngeneic splenocytes into $(C_{57}Bl/10 \times DBA/2)F_1$ mice of 3-4 and 20-21 months of age. Results of these experiments indicated that antigen-specific suppressor T cells were slightly more active in spleens of aged mice and that lymph node cells from old animals were considerably less sensitive to suppression. The latter result differs from ours, but the difference may be attributable either to the nature of the tolerogen or to the use of lymph node cells rather than splenocytes as the suppressor effector cells. It is of great interest that none of the studies on tolerogen-induced suppression has revealed an excess of functional nonspecific or naturally occurring suppressor cells in aged mice.

D. Duration of Tolerance in Aged Mice

The duration of the tolerant state following treatment with heterologous IgGs has been found to be reduced, at least in B lymphocytes, in aged mice (18). Failing B-cell tolerance was revealed in 2-year-old mice 90 days post-tolerogen by challenging with a combination of AHGG plus lipopolysaccharide (LPS, endotoxin) (Table 5). From the combined evidence of reduced sensitivity of B cells to tolerance induction and maintenance, as well as increased suppressor cell function and increased sensitivity to suppression, we and others have concluded that the primary lymphocyte defect in the tolerance mechanism in aged mice lies in the B cell (18,60).

Table 5 Duration of T- and B-Lymphocyte Tolerance in $C_{57}Bl/6$ Mice

Age (months)	% Unresponsiveness			
	T cells		B cells	
	Day 50	Day 90	Day 50	Day 90
2	83	100	95	99
12	100	98	100	75
24	92	88	99	19

E. Role of Extralymphoid Factors in Tolerance Induction During Senescence

It is also possible that a tolerance defect in aging lies outside the lymphoid system, i.e., that the environment of the lymphocyte in the aged animal affects its response to tolerogen. This problem has been addressed by examining the induction of tolerance in lymphocytes adoptively transferred to syngeneic hosts. [It has been shown that less tolerogen is required for the induction of unresponsiveness in adoptively transferred splenocytes and bone marrow cells (4,68). This was true whether the donor cells came from young or aged animals.] Splenocytes from 2- and 24-month-old $C_{57}Bl/6$ mice were injected into lethally irradiated syngeneic young hosts. Cells from 2-month-old donors were pooled, while those from old mice were not. Two days later various doses of DHGG ranging from 1 μg to 1 mg were injected intraperitoneally. The mice were challenged 3 weeks later and the splenic PFC response determined. No significant difference in tolerance sensitivity between young and old splenocytes was found (Table 6). Since splenocytes from an individual old donor could be transferred to more than one recipient, it was possible to test both tolerogen and immunogen

Table 6 Dose of Tolerogen (DHGG) Required for Induction of 50% Unresponsiveness in Adoptively Transferred Cells

Donor age (months)	Cells transferred	Dose of DHGG (μg)
2	50×10^6 splenocytes	3.0
24	50×10^6 splenocytes	1.3
2	20×10^6 bone marrow cells	0.01
12	20×10^6 bone marrow cells	0.02
24	20×10^6 bone marrow cells	0.02

sensitivity in the cells from a single donor. When the results were examined, no correlation was found between immunogen and tolerogen sensitivity in aged mice. When the experiment was repeated using bone marrow cells, the dose of tolerogen required for the induction of unresponsiveness was reduced to 10–20 ng for cells from 2-, 12-, and 24-month-old donors. The bone-marrow-reconstituted mice were fully immunologically competent, since the responses to the challenge injection of aggregated HGG in mice not treated with tolerogen were equivalent to those in intact mice. However, the age-related decline in responsiveness to AHGG was also found in the recipients of bone marrow cells from aged donors. Preliminary results of the reciprocal experiment in which splenocytes from young donors were transferred into young or old irradiated recipients showed that cells in the young hosts were more sensitive to tolerogen as measured by the dose of tolerogen required for induction of unresponsiveness.

F. Role of Gram-Negative Bacterial Endotoxin in Promoting Loss of Tolerance During Aging

The nature of the extralymphoid environmental component to reduced tolerance sensitivity in the aged mouse is yet to be determined. One such factor that is known to influence tolerance induction (69,71) and maintenance (72) is gram-negative bacterial endotoxin (LPS). LPS produces a variety of immunoregulatory effects. It acts as a B-cell mitogen, as an adjuvant, and as a polyclonal B-cell activator. In addition, endotoxin may have indirect effects on immunoresponsiveness by inducing interleukin 1 (IL-1) formation (31), or by modulating the immune response by affecting body temperature, by causing a production of immunoregulatory acute phase reactants, or by producing tissue damage resulting in increased exposure of autoantigens to the immune system.

The effects of LPS in acquired immunological tolerance and in autoantibody formation by cells from aged mice have been investigated by several laboratories. We have shown that LPS administered 3 h after tolerogen (DHGG) blocked tolerance induction with equal efficiency in young and aged mice as revealed by immunogenic challenge (AHGG) 3 weeks after exposure to DHGG plus LPS (Table 7). Endotoxin also acts as an adjuvant to convert DHGG from a tolerogen to an immunogen (70). When this effect was studied in 2- and 20-month-old C_{57}B1/6 mice, it was found that as little as 5 μg of LPS rendered DHGG immunogenic in aged mice, while 50 μg was required in young mice. Thus, in our studies, although LPS present at challenge was no more efficient at terminating tolerance in old mice, it was more effective at converting the tolerogen into a potent immunogen in these animals. It should be noted that LPS regulatory effects on tolerance induction are restricted to thymus-dependent antigens (73). Studies of the effects of LPS on the termination of acquired

Table 7 Abrogation of Tolerance Induction by Lipopolysaccharides (LPS) in 2- and 20-Month-Old $C_{57}Bl/6$ Mice

Age	Treatment[a]	% of control PFC response
2 months	None	100
	1 mg DHGG	0
	1 mg DHGG + 5 μg LPS	32
	1 mg DHGG + 20 μg LPS	109
	1 mg DHGG + 50 μg LPS	284
20 months	None	100
	1 mg DHGG	3
	1 mg DHGG + 5 μg LPS	46
	1 mg DHGG + 20 μg LPS	135
	1 mg DHGG + 50 μg LPS	214

[a]All mice were challenged twice with 0.4 mg of AHGG beginning at 21 days after tolerogen exposure and splenic PFC were determined 5 days after the second challenge.

tolerance in aged mice have shown that because B-cell tolerance breaks down more rapidly, an LPS-plus-antigen challenge can terminate the tolerant state earlier in old animals (18,60).

There are several possible mechanisms whereby LPS could be more efficacious in terminating unresponsiveness in aged mice. Is it more efficient as a polyclonal B-cell activator in these animals? Several investigators have addressed this question. Meredith et al. (40) studied in vitro polyclonal B-cell activation by LPS of splenocytes from Balb/c and $C_{57}Bl/6$ mice of different ages. They found a larger increase in PFC specific for a variety of antigens in aged $C_{57}Bl/6$ mice but no increase in old Balb/c mice, in which LPS was a very poor B-cell activator. Goidl et al. (41) also found that LPS was a more potent activator of B cells from aged mice. We have obtained similar results following in vivo activation of B cells with LPS (4). Both in vitro and in vivo polyclonal B-cell activation may be secondary to the induction of IL-1 formation by LPS. It is known that IL-1 acts directly on murine B cells to enhance their proliferation (74). Although IL-1 formation is no more efficient in aged animals (29; Leichtling and Habicht, unpublished observations), sensitivity to IL-1 is increased as measured by thymocyte proliferation and pyrogenicity (Leichtling and Habicht, unpublished observations).

Several studies have addressed the specificity of PFC following polyclonal B-cell activation either in vivo or in vitro. Most have revealed a disproportionate number of PFC specific for autoantigens including IgG (rheumatoid factor), DNA, and bromelain-treated erythrocytes (4,41,75,77). A study by Kawaguchi

(78) showed that the kinetics of responsiveness to bromelain-treated erythrocytes differed from those of PFC to foreign antigens. Responsiveness to self preceded responses to foreign antigens. When the response to LPS was studied in aged mice, not only was the polyclonal B-cell activation greater as measured by the reverse PFC assay (79), but responses to autoantigens were selectively increased (4,40,41,74).

Although other stimuli are effective in terminating the tolerant state, e.g., introduction of a cross-reacting immunogen (80,81), LPS is of particular interest because of its potential physiological role in the induction of autoimmunity. Lambert et al. (82) have noted that bacterial infection triggers anti-DNA antibody formation in systemic lupus erythematosus patients. Autoantibody formation in apparently normal aging may be the result of increased exposure to LPS from the gastrointestinal tract, elevated incidence of gram-negative bacteremia, or urinary tract infections that occur in the aged (83-85). Thus, either increased exposure or sensitivity to LPS during aging may be a prime factor in the termination of self-tolerance.

V. CONCLUSION

Immunological tolerance is both more difficult to induce and more fragile in aged animals. Both these factors result in a reduced ability to maintain self-tolerance during immunological senescence. Lymphoid stem cells from the bone marrows of young and aged mice are equipotent in their potential for developing acquired immunological tolerance. This suggests that factors outside the lymphoid system act to reduce the tolerance potential. One such factor, perhaps the major one, is enhanced sensitivity to gram-negative bacterial endotoxin. Horan and Fox (85) have suggested that aging is accompanied by an abnormal endotoxin load resulting from increased or altered bacterial colonization of the gastrointestinal or urinary tracts, superimposed on a reduced capacity of liver Kupffer cells to clear LPS from the portal blood. Endotoxin that reaches the systemic circulation will act on a variety of target tissues, including the cells of the immune system, to produce adjuvanicity and polyclonal B-cell activation. Endotoxin in sufficient concentration is cytotoxic and may cause the release of otherwise sequestered antigens so that they may stimulate an autoimmune response. The latter may be facilitated by the adjuvant properties of LPS (86) (Figure 1). Although autoantibody formation increases because of the breakdown of self-tolerance, responsiveness to foreign antigens may be reduced by prolonged or prior exposure to LPS (75,87,88). Thus, altered LPS exposure might account for both the enhanced autoimmunity and the reduced antibody-forming potentials of aging.

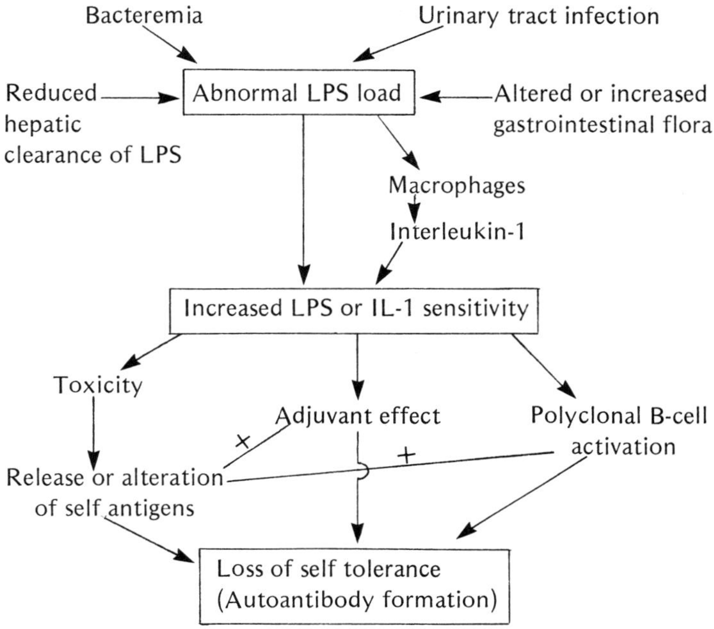

Figure 1 Factors leading to the loss of tolerance during immunological senescence. Several age-related changes have the potential for increasing the amount of endotoxin in the circulation. Endotoxin in turn accelerates the breakdown of self-tolerance either directly or through the agency of interleukin 1. Adjuvanicity and polyclonal B-cell activation effected by either LPS or IL-1 in combination with exposure to cryptic or altered self antigens may account for much of the autoantibody formation associated with aging of the immune system.

ACKNOWLEDGMENT

This work was supported in part by grant AG-00801 from the National Institute on Aging.

REFERENCES

1. Heidrick, M. L., and T. Makinodan. 1972. Nature of cellular deficiencies in age-related decline of the immune system. *Gerontologia.* 18:305.

2. Price, G. B., and T. Makinodan. 1972. Immunologic deficiencies in senescence. II. Characterization of extrinsic deficiencies. *J. Immunol.* 108:413.
3. Astle, C. M., and D. E. Harrison. 1984. Effects of marrow donor and recipient age on immune responses. *J. Immunol.* 132:673.
4. Habicht, G. S. 1985. Acquired immunological tolerance in aged mice. III. The contribution of lymphoid cells and their environments to the age related resistance to tolerance induction. *Mech. Ageing Dev.* 30:37.
5. Makinodan, T., and M.M.B. Kay. 1980. Age influence on the immune system. *Adv. Immunol.* 29:287.
6. Gerbase-DeLima, M., J. Wilkinson, G. S. Smitti, and R. L. Walford. 1974. Age-related decline in thymic independent immune function in a long-lived mouse strain. *J. Gerontol.* 29:261.
7. Callard, R. E., and A. Basten. 1977. Immune function in aged mice. I. T-cell responsiveness using phytohemagglutinin as a functional probe. *Cell. Immunol.* 31:13.
8. Callard, R. E., and A. Basten. 1978. Immune function in aged mice. IV. Loss of T cell and B cell function in thymus-dependent antibody responses. *Eur. J. Immunol.* 8:552.
9. Liu, J., M. Segre, and D. Segre. 1982. Changes in suppressor, helper and B cell functions in aging mice. *Cell. Immunol.* 66:372.
10. Goidl, E. A., J. B. Innes, and M. E. Weksler. 1976. Immunological studies of aging. II. Loss of IgG and high avidity plaque forming cells and increased suppressor cell activity in aging mice. *J. Exp. Med.* 144:1037.
11. Segre, D., and M. Segre. 1976. Humoral immunity in aged mice. I. Increased suppressor T cell activity in immunologically deficient old mice. *J. Immunol.* 116:735.
12. Makinodan, T., J. W. Albright, P. I. Good, C. P. Peter, and M. L. Heidrick. 1976. Reduced humoral immune activity in long-lived old mice: An approach to elucidating its mechanisms. *Immunology.* 31:903.
13. DeKruyff, R. H., Y. I. Kim, G. W. Siskind, and M. E. Weksler. 1976. Age related changes in the in vitro immune response: Increased suppressor activity in immature and aged mice. *J. Immunol.* 125:142.
14. Callard, R. E., B. Fazekas de St. Groth, A. Basten, and I.F.C. McKenzie. 1980. Immune function in aged mice. V. Role of suppressor cells. *J. Immunol.* 124:52.
15. Doria, G., C. Mancini, and L. Adorini. 1982. Immunoregulation in senescence: Increased inducibility of antigen-specific suppressor T cells and loss of cell sensitivity to immunosuppression in aging mice. *Proc. Natl. Acad. Sci. USA.* 79:3803.
16. Delfraissy, J. F., P. Gabraud, C. Wallon, J. F. Balavoine, and J. Dormont. 1982. Abolished in vitro antibody response in elderly: Exclusive involvement of prostaglandin induced T suppressor cells. *Clin. Immunol. Immunopathol.* 24:377.
17. Globerson, A., L. Abel, M. Barzilay, and I. Zan-Bar. 1982. Immunoregulatory cells in aging mice. I. Concanavalin A-induced and naturally occurring suppressor cells. *Mech. Ageing Dev.* 19:293.

18. Habicht, G. S. 1985. Acquired immunological tolerance in aged mice. II. The cellular basis of the loss of tolerance sensitivity. *Mech. Ageing Dev.* 30:23.
19. Thoman, M. L., and W. O. Weigle. 1983. Deficiency in suppressor T cell activity in aged animals. *J. Exp. Med.* 157:2184.
20. Segre, D., E. H. Greeley, and M. Segre. 1982. Cyclophosphamide induction of non-T suppressor cells and their possible role in self-tolerance. *In* Immunological Aspects of Aging. D. Segre and L. Smith, editors. Marcel Dekker, New York. 151.
21. Roder, J. C., A. K. Duwe, D. A. Bell, and S. K. Singhal. 1978. Immunological senescence. I. The role of suppressor cells. *Immunology.* 35:837.
22. Liu, J. J., D. Segre, H. B. Gelberg, A. H. Fudenberg, K. Y. Tsang, N. Khansari, C. R. Waltenbaugh, and M. Segre. 1984. Effects of long-term treatment with anti-I-J monoclonal antibody and dialyzable leukocyte extraction immune function and life span. *Mech. Ageing Dev.* 27:359.
23. Gillis, S., R. Kozak, M. Durante, and M. E. Weksler. 1981. Immunological studies of aging. Decreased production and response to T cell growth factor by lymphocytes from aged humans. *J. Clin. Invest.* 67:937.
24. Miller, R. A., and O. Stutman. 1981. Decline, in aging mice, of the anti 2,4,6-trinitrophenyl (TNP) cytotoxic T cell response attributable to loss of Lyt 2^-, interleukin 2-producing helper cell function. *Eur. J. Immunol.* 11:751.
25. Thoman, M., and W. Weigle. 1982. Cell mediated immunity in aged mice: An underlying lesion in IL-2 synthesis. 1982. *J. Immunol.* 128:2358.
26. Joncourt, F., Y. Wang, F. Kristensen, and A. L. deWeck. 1982. Aging and immunity: Decrease in interleukin-2 production and interleukin-2 dependent RNA-synthesis in lectin-stimulated murine spleen cells. *Immunobiology.* 163:521.
27. Gilman, S. C., J. S. Rosenberg, and J. D. Feldman. 1982. T-lymphocytes of young and aged rats. II. Functional defects and the role of interleukin-2. *J. Immunol.* 128:644.
28. Thoman, M. L., and W. O. Weigle. 1981. Lymphokines and aging: Interleukin-2 production and activity in aged animals. *J. Immunol.* 127:2102.
29. Rosenberg, J. S., S. C. Gilman, and J. D. Feldman. 1983. Effects of aging on cell cooperation and lymphocyte responsiveness to cytokines. *J. Immunol.* 130:1754.
30. Thoman, M. L., and W. O. Weigle. 1985. Reconstitution of in vivo cell-mediated lympholysis response in aged mice with interleukin 2. *J. Immunol.* 134:949.
31. Dinarello, C. A. 1984. Interleukin-I. *Rev. Infect. Dis.* 6:51.
32. Bruley-Rosset, M., and I. Vergnon. 1984. Interleukin 1 synthesis and activity in aged mice. *Mech. Ageing Dev.* 24:247.
33. Helmer, R., F. M. Levin, and E. Rudd. 1963. Globulins resembling rheumatoid factor in serum of the aged. *Am. J. Med.* 5:175.
34. Cammarata, R. J., G. P. Rodman, and R. H. Fennell. 1967. Serum anti-γ-globulin and antinuclear factors in the aged. *J. Am. Med. Assoc.* 199:455.

35. Rowley, M. J., H. Buchanan, and I. R. Mackay. 1968. Reciprocal change with age in antibody to extrinsic and intrinsic antigens. *Lancet.* 2:24.
36. Hooper, B., S. Whittingham, J. D. Matthews, I. R. Mackay, and D. H. Curnow. 1972. Autoimmunity in a rural community. *Clin. Exp. Immunol.* 12:79.
37. Matthews, J. D., S. Wittingham, B. M. Hooper, and I. R. Mackay. 1973. Association of autoantibodies with smoking, cardiovascular morbidity and death in the Brusselton population. *Lancet.* 2:754.
38. Hallgren, H. M., C. E. Buckley III, V. A. Gilbertsen, and E. J. Yunis. 1973. Lymphocyte phytohemagglutinin responsiveness, immunoglobulins and autoantibodies in aging humans. *J. Immunol.* 111:1101.
39. Hijmans, W., J. Radl, G. F. Bottazzo, and D. Doniach. 1984. Autoantibodies in highly aged humans. *Mech. Ageing Dev.* 26:83.
40. Meredith, P. J., J. A. Kristie, and R. L. Walford. 1979. Aging increases expression of LPS-induced autoantibody secreting B cells. *J. Immunol.* 123:87.
41. Goidl, E. A., M. A. Michelis, G. W. Siskind, and M. E. Weksler. 1981. Effect of age on the induction of autoantibodies. *Clin. Exp. Immunol.* 44:24.
42. Naor, D., B. Bonavida, and R. L. Walford. 1976. Autoimmunity and aging: The age related response of mice of a long-lived strain to trinitrophenylated syngeneic mouse red blood cells. *J. Immunol.* 117:2204.
43. Grabar, P. 1975. Hypothesis: Auto-antibodies and immunological theories: An analytical review. *Clin. Immunol. Immunopathol.* 4:453.
44. Walford, R. L. 1969. The Immunologic Theory of Aging. Williams & Wilkins, Baltimore.
45. Goidl, E. A., J. W. Choy, J. J. Gibbons, M. E. Weksler, G. J. Thorbecke, and G. W. Siskind. 1983. Production of autoanti-idiotypic antibody during the normal immune response. VII. Analysis of the cellular basis for the increased autoanti-idiotypic antibody production by aged mice. *J. Exp. Med.* 157:1635.
46. Chiller, J. M., G. S. Habicht, and W. O. Weigle. 1971. Kinetic differences in unresponsiveness of thymus and bone marrow cells. *Science.* 171:813.
47. Parks, D. E., M. V. Doyle, and W. O. Weigle. 1978. Induction and mode of action of suppressor cells generated against human gamma globulin. I. An immunologic unresponsive state devoid of demonstrable suppressor cells. *J. Exp. Med.* 148:625.
48. Laskin, C. A., J. D. Taurog, P. A. Smathers, and A. D. Steinberg. 1981. Defective tolerance in murine lupus. *J. Immunol.* 127:1743.
49. McIntosh, K. R., and D. Segre. 1976. B- and T-cell tolerance induction in young adult and old mice. *Cell. Immunol.* 27:230.
50. Hosono, M., B. Cinader, and J. R. Ellerson. 1977. Tolerance induction as an index of age-related changes. *Immunol. Commun.* 6:239.
51. Hosono, M., and B. Cinader. 1977. Resistance to tolerance induction and age dependent cellular changes in SJL mice. *Int. Arch. Allergy Appl. Immunol.* 54:289.
52. Nakano, K., B. Cinader, and B. H. Sabiston. 1979. Age-dependent changes

in tolerizability with rabbit gamma-globulin in the Biozzi high and low responder lines of mice. *Eur. J. Immunol.* 9:1014.
53. Nakano, K., and B. Cinader. 1980. A strain survey of age-dependent changes in antigen elimination, antibody formation and tolerance. *J. Immunogenet.* 7:183.
54. DeKruyff, R., E. A. Rinnooy Kan, M. E. Weksler, and G. W. Siskind. 1980. Effect of aging on T cell tolerance induction. *Cell. Immunol.* 56:58.
55. Dobken, J. H., M. E. Weksler, and G. W. Siskind. 1980. Effect of age on B-cell tolerance induction. *Cell. Immunol.* 55:66.
56. Habicht, G. S., and D. A. Jerrard. 1981. Tolerance to HGG in mice of different age groups. *In* Immunological Aspects of Aging. D. Segre and L. Smith, editors. Marcel Dekker, New York. 127.
57. Weksler, M. E., R. DeKruyff, J. Dobken, and G. W. Siskind. 1981. Ease of tolerance induction in mice of different ages. *In* Immunological Aspects of Aging. D. Segre and L. Smith, editors. Marcel Dekker, New York. 119.
58. Amagai, T., K. Nakano, and B. Cinader. 1981. Diversity of age-dependent changes of antibody formation and of tolerance decrease. *Immunol. Lett.* 3:329.
59. Amagai, T., and B. Cinader. 1981. Resistance of MRL/Mp-lpr mice to tolerance induction. *Eur. J. Immunol.* 11:923.
60. Amagai, T., Nakano, K., and B. Cinader. 1982. Mechanisms involved in age-dependent decline of immune responsiveness and apparent resistance against tolerance induction in C_{57}Bl/6 mice. *Scand. J. Immunol.* 16: 217.
61. Cinader, B., T. Amagai, T. Matsuzawa, and K. Nakano. 1981. Genetic programmes for change in immune responsiveness in adult life. *In* Cellular and Molecular Mechanisms of Immunologic Tolerance. T. Hraba and M. Hasek, editors. Marcel Dekker, New York. 187.
62. Habicht, G. S. 1982. Acquired immunological tolerance in aged mice. I. The dose–response relationship. *Mech. Ageing Dev.* 19:53.
63. Fujiwara, M., and A. Karyione. 1977. Lack of correlation between tolerance inducibility and major histocompatibility gene complex. *Jap. J. Exp. Med.* 47:525.
64. Smith, A. M. 1976. The effect of age on the immune response to type III pneumococcal polysaccharide (SIII) and bacterial lipopolysaccharide in Balb/c, SJL/L and C3H mice. *J. Immunol.* 116:469.
65. Parks, D. E., and W. O. Weigle. 1980. Maintenance of immunologic unresponsiveness to human γ-globulin: Evidence for irreversible inactivation in B lymphocytes. *J. Immunol.* 124:1230.
66. Doyle, M. V., D. E. Parks, and W. O. Weigle. 1976. Specific suppression of the immune response by HGG tolerant cells. I. Parameters affecting the level of suppression. *J. Immunol.* 116:1640.
67. Benjamin, D. C. 1977. Suppressor cells in tolerance to HGG: Kinetics and cross-suppression in high dose tolerance—absence in low dose tolerance. *J. Immunol.* 118:2125.
68. Schleimer, R. P., R. J. Scibierski, H. F. Vollger, and E. Benjamini. 1982.

Induction of tolerance to a soluble antigen following irradiation and bone marrow reconstitution. *Int. Arch. Allergy Appl. Immunol.* 69:199.
69. Golub, E. S., and W. O. Weigle. 1967. Studies on the induction of immunologic unresponsiveness. *J. Immunol.* 98:1241.
70. Louis, J. A., J. M. Chiller, and W. O. Weigle. 1973. The ability of bacterial lipopolysaccharide to modulate the induction of unresponsiveness to a state of immunity. *J. Exp. Med.* 138:1481.
71. Parks, D. E., S. M. Walker, and W. O. Weigle. 1981. Bacterial lipopolysaccharide (endotoxin) interferes with the induction of tolerance and primes thymus-derived lymphocytes. *J. Immunol.* 126:938.
72. Chiller, J. M., and W. O. Weigle. 1973. Termination of tolerance to human gamma globulin in mice by antigen and bacterial lipopolysaccharide (endotoxin). *J. Exp. Med.* 137:740.
73. Scott, D. W., and E. Diener. 1976. Effect of lipopolysaccharide on the induction of tolerance to polymerized flagellin. *J. Immunol.* 116:1220.
74. Howard, M., S. B. Mizel, L. Lachman, J. Ansel, B. Johnson, and W. E. Paul. 1983. Role of interleukin 1 in anti-immunoglobulin induced B cell proliferation. *J. Exp. Med.* 157:1529.
75. Fujiwara, M., and A. Kariyone. 1981. Lipopolysaccharide-induced autoantibody response. II. Age-related change in plaque-forming cell response to bromelain-treated syngeneic erythrocytes. *Int. Arch. Allergy Appl. Immunol.* 66:161.
76. Dziarski, R. 1982. Preferential induction of autoantibody secretion in polyclonal activation by peptidoglycan and lipopolysaccharide. I. In vitro studies. *J. Immunol.* 128:1018.
77. Dziarski, R. 1982. Preferential induction of autoantibody secretion in polyclonal activation by peptidoglycan and lipopolysaccharide. II. In vivo studies. *J. Immunol.* 128:1026.
78. Kawaguchi, S. 1981. Ontogenical studies on kinetics of lipopolysaccharide induced response to bromelain treated mouse erythrocytes in mouse spleen cells. I. Differences from the response of total IgM secreting cells. *Cell. Immunol.* 65:293.
79. Gronowicz, E., A. Coutinho, and F. Melchers. 1976. A plaque assay for all cells secreting Ig of a given type or class. *Eur. J. Immunol.* 6:588.
80. Weigle, W. O. 1963. Termination of acquired immunological tolerance to protein antigens following immunization with altered protein antigens. *J. Exp. Med.* 116:913.
81. Habicht, G. S., J. M. Chiller, and W. O. Weigle. 1975. Termination of acquired and natural immunological tolerance with specific complexes. *J. Exp. Med.* 142:312.
82. Lambert, P. H., J. A. Louis, S. Izui, and T. Kobayakawa. 1979. Relevance of polyclonal antibody formation to the development of autoimmunity in particular relation to murine lupus. *In* 6th International Convocation of Immunology (1978). F. Milgrom and B. Albini, editors. Karger, Basel. 191.
83. Craven, D. E., B. E. Kreger, and W. R. McCabe. 1979. Adult bacteremia caused by gram-negative bacilli. *Clin. Obstet. Gynecol.* 22:361.

84. Kaye, D. 1980. Urinary tract infections in the elderly. *Bull. N.Y. Acad. Med.* 56:209.
85. Horan, M. A., and R. A. Fox. 1984. Aging and the immune response–A unifying hypothesis? *Mech. Ageing Dev.* 26:165.
86. Louis, J. A., and P. H. Lambert. 1979. Lipopolysaccharides–From immunostimulation to autoimmunity. *Springer Semin. Immunopathol.* 2:215.
87. Nakano, M., M. J. Tanabe, T. Saito, and T. Shimizu. 1976. Immunosuppressive effect of bacterial lipopolysaccharides on antibody response. *Jap. J. Microbiol.* 20:53.
88. Venkataraman, M., and D. W. Scott. 1979. B-cell subsets responsive to fluorescein-conjugated antigens. III. Differential effect of *E. coli* lipopolysaccharide on T-dependent and T-independent response in vivo. *Immunology.* 38:519.

8

Immunoregulation of Antibody Responses in Aging Mice

Gino Doria, Luciano Adorini, and Daniela Frasca

Laboratory of Pathology
ENEA, C.R.E. Casaccia
Rome, Italy

I. INTRODUCTION

The expression of effector immune functions against exogenous and self antigens is modulated by cellular and molecular interactions in a complex immunoregulatory network. The expression of the remarkably wide repertoire of antibody specificities encoded in the B-cell genome is induced by macrophage-processed antigen and modulated by signals passed among cells of different types (isotype, allotype, and idiotype) that regulate antibody quality, as well as intensity and duration of the antibody response. Cellular members of the immune network bear membrane receptors specific for exogenous antigens and for self structures encoded by the major histocompatibility complex (MHC) and immunoglobulin heavy chain (Igh) genes, as well as membrane markers associated with genetically programmed functions. The main cell types involved in activation and regulation of B-cell antibody responses are antigen-presenting accessory cells or macrophages, helper T cells, suppressor T cells, and contrasuppressor T cells. B cells, macrophages, and T cells are all derived from a common stem cell through distinct maturation pathways, some of which are conditioned by the lymphoid microenvironment, where the maturation process occurs independently from the presence of exogenous antigens (1,2).

During senescence the immune system undergoes profound alterations associated with progressive decline of immune responsiveness to exogenous antigens and increasing incidence of autoimmune phenomena.

The age-related immunologic alterations seem to play a major role in the biological processes of aging (3). The maximum life span has been shown to be significantly influenced by the MHC (4), which controls immunoregulatory cell functions and interactions (5). Furthermore, genes within the MHC together with other MHC-related genes regulating superoxide dismutase, mixed function oxidases, and the level of cyclic nucleotides have been postulated to constitute a multigene family exerting a multifactorial influence on the aging process (6). Beside affecting immune functions, this multigene family appears to regulate enzymes protecting from free-radical-induced damage, which accumulates in aging (7), as well as cyclic nucleotides involved in cell proliferation and differentiation, which show marked age-related alterations (8). Although etiological theories of aging have proposed stochastic and programmed events to explain the biological processes of aging, convincing evidence favors genetic programming, encoded in a small portion of the genome, as the major mechanism of aging (6). Regardless of the etiology of the age-dependent events and mechanisms affecting MHC or MHC-related genes, most of the major diseases observed in senescence have an immunological pathogenesis associated with the decline of immune responsiveness and increased propensity to autoimmune reactivity (3).

Age-related immune dysfunctions result mainly from alterations in cell populations of the immune system rather than from changes in the animal milieu during senescence (9). The decrease in immune reactivity with increasing age may reflect multiple events, affecting cell proliferation and differentiation, leading to reduction in cell number and function within one or more cell populations (10). Precursor frequency analysis of immunocompetent cells, by limiting dilution microculture techniques, indicates that the fraction of responding precursors declines with aging, but the progeny of each cell precursor maintains full proliferative capacity and immunocompetence (11).

II. STEM CELLS

Stem cells, the progenitors of lymphocytes and accessory cells, have been thoroughly investigated to detect changes in their proliferative and differentiative capacities but were found in most studies to be unimpaired by aging. Apart from some subtle defects that have been unmasked in old mice, the bulk of information indicates that stem cells as well as other rapidly dividing cells, such as intestinal crypt cells and germinal cells, maintain their cell population size in aging by selection of fully functional self-replicating units (12,13). This conclusion disagrees with the prediction from in vitro studies with fibroblasts (14) that somatic cells should age as a result of intrinsic limits on their proliferative capacity. In a conclusive study (15) on stem cells from fetal, young, and old mice it has been found that aging is not intrinsic to stem cells but may affect their proliferation and differentiation in a genetically controlled way.

III. MACROPHAGES

Macrophages bind, ingest, and degrade antigen but also process and present it in immunogenic form to antigen-specific lymphocytes. As reviewed by Unanue (16), antigen presentation to helper T cells requires that macrophages process antigen, express on their membrane class II molecules (Ia) controlled by genes in the I-A and I-E subregions of the MHC, present antigenic determinants in association with class II MHC products, and synthesize and release interleukin 1 (IL-1).

Protein antigens enter the macrophage and then an acid vesicle, where they are degraded in immunogenic fragments that are subsequently transported and anchored to the cell membrane. The immunogenic fragment may interact, with some degree of specificity, with the polymorphic domains of the Ia molecule or may complex, through its hydrophobic portion, with the nonpolymorphic domains of Ia.

The percentage of Ia-positive macrophages varies extensively from tissue to tissue: 10–20% of resident macrophages in the peritoneal cavity, 50% in the spleen and liver, and 75% in the thymus. The expression of Ia on macrophages is induced by T-cell-dependent (γ-interferon) and T-cell-independent (undefined factors accounting for a normal percentage of Ia-positive macrophages in nude athymic mice) stimuli, which are continuously required to prevent the Ia-positive macrophage from reverting to the Ia-negative state. The expression of Ia on macrophages is inhibited by prostaglandin E (PGE2), α-fetoprotein, and glucocorticoids, the first two probably accounting for the low number of Ia-positive macrophages during neonatal development.

The relationship between IL-1 production and antigen-presenting activity of the macrophage is not yet well established, since some experiments indicate that IL-1 secretion is necessary for antigen presentation and T-cell activation, whereas other experiments deny such a role of IL-1. It appears that virgin T-cell activation requires IL-1, whereas primed T cells and T-cell clones are effectively restimulated by antigen and accessory cells in the absence of IL-1.

While recognition of antigen in the context of both I-A and I-E products is required for helper T-cell activation, various suppressor T-cell subsets appear to recognize antigen and suppressor factors presented in association with I-J molecules expressed on macrophages that also bear I-A molecules. It is unclear whether the concomitant presence of I-A molecules is instrumental for suppressor T-cell activation. On the other hand, antigen-presenting cells that induce T cells mediating delayed-type hypersensitivity (DTH), helper T cells, and cytotoxic T lymphocytes (CTL) exhibit I-A but lack I-J molecules. The coexistence of I-A and I-J molecules on the same antigen-presenting cell may reflect a peculiar state of cell activation or the existence of a transitional cell type (17,18).

Studies on the fate of antigen injected in aging animals have revealed an increased rate of antigen elimination (19,20) as well as a decreased antigen localization in lymphatic follicles (21) and in liver (19). These observations are consistent with the finding that the activity of macrophage lysosomal enzymes gradually increases with age (22). However, despite many attempts to detect alterations in phagocytosis and antigen presentation, no changes have been thus far observed in senescence (23-25).

Age-related changes in antigen presentation by resident peritoneal macrophages from (C57BL/10×DBA/2)F1 male (BDF1) mice was investigated by an antigen-specific T-cell proliferation assay (26). Briefly, 4×10^5 popliteal lymph node cells (LNC) from four mice 8 days after priming by footpad injection of 0.1-ml emulsion containing 100 μg of trinitrophenyl-azobenzene arsonate-keyhold limpet hemocyanin (TNP-ABA-KLH) or chicken ovalbumin (OVA) in saline and an equal volume of complete Freund's adjuvant were cultured for 5 days with graded numbers ($0.2-30 \times 10^4$) of antigen-pulsed macrophages (Mϕ) from unprimed syngeneic mice. Both LNC and Mϕ were obtained from mice at 3 (young) or 24 (old) months of age. The Mϕ were selected from among resident peritoneal cells by plastic adherence and were treated with mitomycin after antigen pulsing. Proliferative response of LNC was assessed by tritiated thymidine incorporation during the last 18 h of culture. After cells had been harvested and transferred onto filter disks and radioactivity had been counted, this response was expressed as mean counts per minute (cpm) from quadruplicate cultures, plus or minus standard error (± SE). Results from a typical experiment in which LNC from young mice primed with TNP-ABA-KLH were cultured with Mϕ from young or old mice after 2 h pulsing with TNP-ABA-KLH (100 μg/ml) are illustrated in Figure 1. Macrophages from old mice are more efficient than Mϕ from young mice in presenting antigen in form suitable to trigger T-cell proliferation. The difference in antigen presentation is small but consistent at all antigen-pulsed Mϕ concentrations. This finding was confirmed in similar experiments showing enhanced antigen presentation by Mϕ from old mice, regardless of whether LNC donors were young or old mice (Table 1). This difference between Mϕ from young and old mice is unaffected by increasing the antigen concentration (from 100 to 1000 μg/ml) during the 2 h pulsing, regardless of the antigen used (TNP-ABA-KLH or OVA) and the age of the LNC donors (data not shown). Thus, the observed difference seems to reflect changes in surface properties of the Mϕ rather than in rate of intracellular catabolism.

The possibility that the difference in antigen presentation between Mϕ from young and old mice may result from a difference in IL-1 production and release was also investigated. Peritoneal Mϕ (1×10^6) from young or old mice were cultured for 24 h without or with lipopolysaccharide (LPS) (20 ng/ml) to induce IL-1 production. Culture supernatants were dialyzed twice against phosphate-buffered saline (PBS) and once against medium, two-fold serially

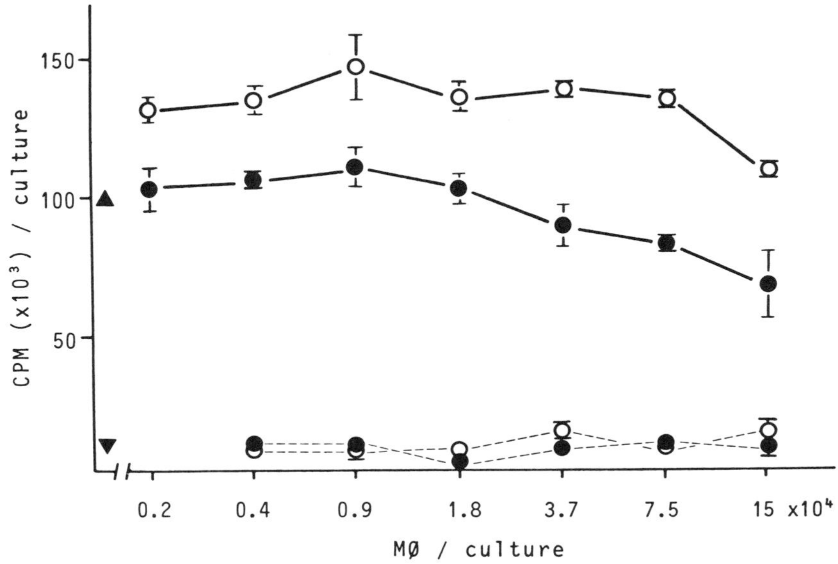

Figure 1 Enhanced antigen presentation by macrophages (Mϕ) from old mice. Proliferative responses of LNC, from young mice primed with TNP-ABA-KLH, cultured with: no antigen (▼); soluble antigen, 100 μg/ml (▲); antigen-pulsed Mϕ from young (●——●) or old (○——○) mice; antigen-unpulsed Mϕ from young (●- - - ●) or old (○- - - ○) mice. Vertical bars represent one SE of the mean cpm from quadruplicate cultures.

Table 1 Enhanced Antigen Presentation by Macrophages from Old Mice

Experiment number	Primed LNC	Pulsed macrophages (mean cpm $(\times 10^{-3})$ from quadruplicate cultures ±SE)[a] Young	Old
1	Young	8.7 ±1.1	36.8 ±1.9
2	Young	24.9 ±3.1	38.4 ±3.7
3	Young	12.8 ±3.0	23.7 ±3.8
	Old	4.1 ±1.2	9.9 ±1.2
4	Young	39.6 ±2.0	56.2 ±1.9
	Old	29.8 ±5.9	43.3 ±6.5

[a]Peak proliferative responses of LNC from TNP-ABA-KLH-primed mice cultured with antigen-pulsed macrophages.

diluted, and tested for mitogenic activity on thymocytes (1×10^6) cultured for 72 h with phytohemoagglutinin (PHA) (3 μg/ml). Cell proliferation was assessed by tritiated thymidine incorporation during the last 18 h of culture and expressed as described above (mean cpm from triplicate cultures ±SE). The thymocytes used in the assay were obtained from 30-day-old BDF1 or C3H/HeJ mice, the latter strain being unresponsive to LPS. The titration data reported in Figure 2, showing similar mitogenic activity in the culture supernatants of LPS-stimulated or -unstimulated Mϕ from young and old mice, rule out age-related changes in IL-1 production by Mϕ.

Since antigen presentation by Mϕ requires expression of class II MHC molecules on the cell surface, a cytotoxic assay was performed on plastic-adherent resident peritoneal Mϕ from young and old mice to assess whether the number of Ia-positive Mϕ, as determined by monoclonal antibodies and rabbit complement (C) killing, is increased in old mice. Titration data obtained with

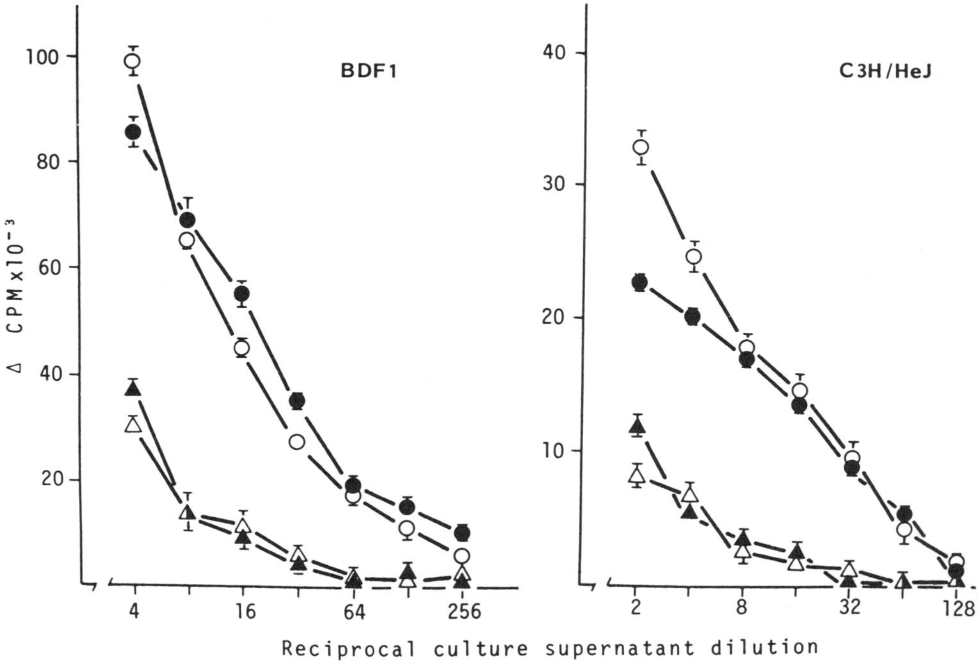

Figure 2 IL-1 titration on BDF1 or C3H/HeJ thymocytes: proliferative response induced by IL-1 released by LPS-stimulated Mϕ from young (●) or old (○) mice; unstimulated Mϕ from young (▲) or old (△) mice. Vertical bars represent one SE of the mean cpm from triplicate cultures after subtraction of mean cpm from thymocyte cultures that received medium instead of Mϕ supernatant.

Table 2 Specificity of Macrophage (Mϕ) Killing by anti-I-A Monoclonal Antibody and Complement

Macrophage treatment	% cytotoxicity			Cytotoxic index[a]		
	BDF1, 20 months	BDF1, 2 months	C3HeB/FeJ, 2 months	BDF1, 20 months	BDF1, 2 months	C3HeB/FeJ, 2 months
αI-A^b + C[b]	27.5	18.2	2.5	21.6	14.2	0.4
MOPC 21 + C[b]	5.1	4.4	1.8	0	0	0
C alone[c]	7.5	4.6	2.2	–	–	–

[a] $\frac{\text{Killed M}\phi - \text{total M}\phi\ (\%\ \text{C} - \text{killed M}\phi)}{\text{Total M}\phi - \text{total M}\phi\ (\%\ \text{C} - \text{killed M}\phi)} \times 100.$

[b] Final dilution of αI-A^b and MOPC 21 ascitic fluids, 1:400. The latter fluid was obtained from the peritoneal cavity of BALB/c mice transplanted with a mineral-oil-induced plasmacytoma.

[c] Final dilution of rabbit complement, 1:10.

anti-I-A^b monoclonal IgG_{2a} antibody (ascitic fluid 25-9-17S, gift from D. H. Sachs) are expressed in term of cytotoxic index as defined in Table 2. The results, pooled from four independent experiments and reported in Figure 3, indicate higher expression of I-A molecules in Mϕ populations from mice 20–24 months old than in Mϕ populations from mice 2–3 months old. The maximum values of cytotoxic index, as observed at 1:400 antibody dilution, were 25.7 ±4.4 for Mϕ from old mice and 17.5 ±0.5 for Mϕ from young mice, the difference being statistically significant ($p < .05$). Analysis of the specificity of BDF1 Mϕ killing by the anti-I-A^b monoclonal antibody and C is reported in Table 2. Since in each experiment approximately the same number of Mϕ could be recovered from the peritoneal cavity of young or old mice, the 50% higher cytotoxic index observed for Mϕ from old mice represents an increase in percentage and absolute number of I-A-positive Mϕ in aged mice. This finding provides a satisfactory explanation for the observed increase in antigen presentation by Mϕ from aging mice.

A similar assay was performed to determine the cytotoxic index for I-J-positive Mϕ from mice 2–3 and 20–24 months old by use of anti-I-J^b monoclonal IgM antibody (ascitic fluid D7, gift from M. Taniguchi) and C. Titration data pooled from four independent experiments demonstrate higher cytotoxic index for Mϕ from old than for Mϕ from young mice (Figure 4). Maximum values of cytotoxic index, as observed at 1:1000 antibody dilution, were 12.4

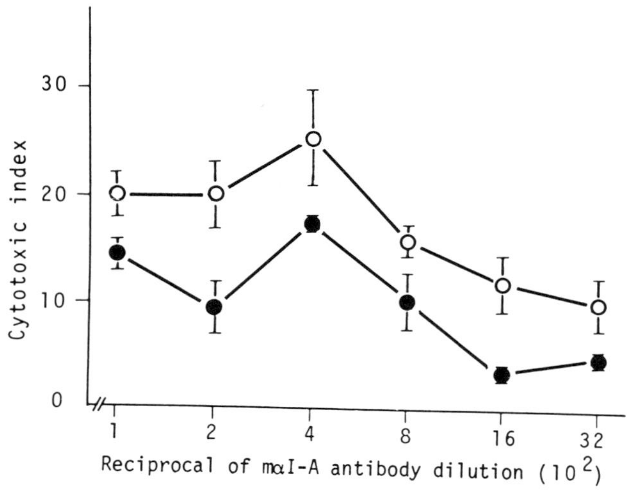

Figure 3 BDF1 killing of young (●) and old (○) Mϕ by anti-I-A monoclonal (mαI-A) antibody and complement. Vertical bars represent one SE of the mean cytotoxic index from four experiments. Cytotoxic index is defined in Table 2.

Table 3 Specificity of Macrophage (Mϕ) Killing by anti-I-A Monoclonal Antibody and Complement

Macrophage treatment	% cytotoxicity			Cytotoxic index[a]		
	BDF1, 23 months	BDF1, 2 months	C3HeB/FeJ, 2 months	BDF1, 23 months	BDF1, 2 months	C3HeB/FeJ, 2 months
αI-J^b + C[b]	12.8	10.1	4.5	9.3	5.4	0
MOPC 21 + C[b]	3.9	4.3	6.2	0	0	0
C alone[c]	3.8	5.0	6.4	–	–	–

[a] $\frac{\text{Killed M}\phi - \text{total M}\phi\ (\%\ \text{C} - \text{killed M}\phi)}{\text{Total M}\phi - \text{total M}\phi\ (\%\ \text{C} - \text{killed M}\phi)} \times 100.$

[b] Final dilution of αI-J^b and MOPC 21 ascitic fluids, 1:500.

[c] Final dilution of rabbit complement, 1:10.

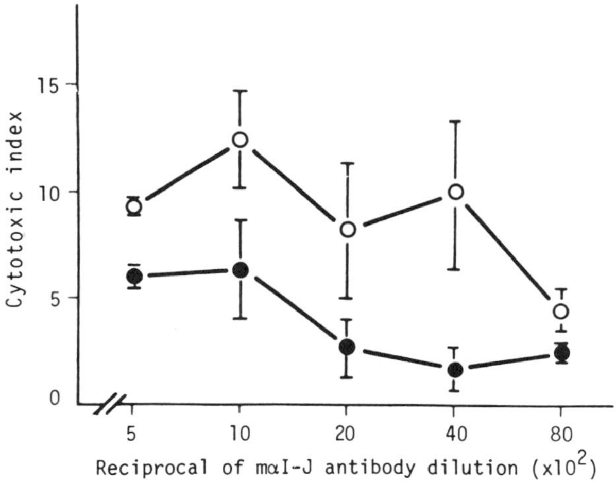

Figure 4 BDF1 killing of young (●) and old (○) Mϕ by anti-I-J monoclonal (mαI-J) antibody and complement. Vertical bars represent one SE of the mean cytotoxic index from four experiments. Cytotoxic index is defined in Table 2.

±2.3 for old and 6.4 ±2.4 for young mice, the difference being statistically significant ($p < .05$). Results from a control experiment reported in Table 3 show that BDF1 Mϕ killing by the anti-I-J^b monoclonal antibody and C was highly specific. Since in these experiments the same number of Mϕ was obtained from the peritoneal cavity of young and old mice, it appears that in aged mice I-J-positive Mϕ double in percentage and in absolute number. Whether the anti-I-A or anti-I-J antibody and C kill Mϕ expressing either one or both Ia molecules was not established in these experiments. However, the age-related increase in number of I-J-positive Mϕ, regardless of whether the same cells also express I-A molecules, suggests enhanced antigen presentation to suppressor T cells and therefore increased propensity to activation of immunosuppressive cell circuits in aging mice. This possibility has been supported by our studies (27) on immunosuppression in senescence (see below).

IV. B CELLS

B lymphocytes have been typed by surface markers in several subsets characterized by different modes of activation and representing different stages of differentiation or commitment to express a particular idiotype, allotype, or isotype. B cells are responsive to soluble growth factors after activation by antigen, lectin, or anti-Ig antibodies. Among these factors, the T-cell-produced B-cell growth factor (BCGF), more recently designated as B-cell stimulatory factor (BSF) (28), and the macrophage-produced IL-1 support the early phase of splenic B-cell polyclonal proliferation but do not lead to the development of Ig-secreting cells in the absence of additional factors (29). In contrast, B-cell differentiation factors (BCDF), including also the T-cell-replacing factor (TRF), act on the late process of B-cell differentiation by inducing active Ig secretion (30). Furthermore, macrophage-derived IL-1 and T-cell-derived IL-3 act on pre-B cells, the former by inducing the synthesis of light chains and the expression of surface Ig (31), the latter by supporting in vitro cell growth (32). Moreover, proliferation and differentiation of antigen-stimulated B cells is enhanced by helper T-cell-derived IL-2 (33).

Age-related changes in B-cell responses to a variety of mitogens and immunogens are likely to reflect defects in T-cell regulatory signals. However, experiments carried out under conditions that exclude aging effects on T-cell regulation of B-cell responses to T-dependent antigens, such as TNP- or dinitrophenyl (DNP)-carrier conjugates (34,35), or to T-independent antigens, such as pneumococcal polysaccharide type III (SIII) or LPS (36,37), have demonstrated B-cell defects in aged mice. Since neither the total number of B cells nor the number of specific antigen-binding B cells is affected by aging, the reduced antigen-specific B-cell responses observed in old mice cannot be attributed to cell depletion. The role of environmental factors is also excluded by the persistent impairment of the antibody response of B cells from old mice upon adoptive transfer into young irradiated recipients (37). More recent studies have shown that mature, DNP-specific splenic B cells from old mice give rise to clones of antibody-forming cells that are fully normal in terms of amount and affinity of the anti-DNP antibody produced. Yet, the proportion of DNP-responsive, Ig-bearing cells in the spleen of old mice is significantly reduced as compared to the spleen of young mice (38). Conversely, the frequency of B cells responsive to viral antigens seems to be unaffected by aging (39). Also the frequency of LPS-reactive B cells from spleen and bone marrow of young and old mice is only slightly decreased by aging, while B cells maintain full capacity to switch from IgM to IgG_1 synthesis (40). Yet, the existence of intrinsic B-cell defects in aged mice is definitely supported by the finding of increased resistance to B-cell tolerance induction (41), whereas neonatal B cells are more susceptible than B cells from adult mice to tolerance induction by most, but not all antigens (42).

Antigen-binding B cells with a full range of affinity heterogeneity have been found to have the same frequency early in development as in the adult mouse (43). The capacity to respond to different antigens, however, is acquired in a programmed stepwise manner (44). Thus, from birth to adulthood B cells display a pattern of functional changes that is similar, but not identical, in different strains and for different T-dependent and T-independent antigens. This pattern spans from an antibody response of relatively restricted affinity heterogeneity to a higher antibody response with greater average affinity and wider affinity heterogeneity (45). In aged mice, antibody affinity was found decreased in average value and heterogeneity upon immunization with T-dependent antigens (34,46,47). The decline in antibody affinity observed in all these studies may reflect aging effects on both B and T cells. However, the protocol used in our experiments (47) allows a more direct association between antibody affinity and B-cell changes. Spleen cells from mice 10–720 days old were transferred and stimulated with trinitrophenylated horse red blood cells (TNP-HRBC) in lethally irradiated, syngeneic 90-day-old recipients, carrier-primed by injection of HRBC before irradiation. The anti-TNP antibody response of the donor cells was estimated from the number of direct plaque-forming cells (PFC) per recipient spleen, while affinity was evaluated by PFC inhibition assay. It is noteworthy that the anti-TNP antibody response in carrier-primed recipients was negligible, implying that B cells from young or old donors could express their immune potential only after interaction with radioresistant primed T cells of the young recipients. It was found that antibody response and affinity rise and fall with age. Affinity heterogeneity was maximal at 180 days, when average affinity and PFC response also reached maximum values, and equally restricted at 10 and 720 days of age. The parabolic change in affinity heterogeneity with age does not support the theory of antibody diversity as result of somatic mutation (48), since this predicts a continuous increase in B-cell heterogeneity through the life span of the animal. Restriction in heterogeneity of the B-cell population in old mice could reflect accumulation of non-sense B-cell mutants, loss of high-affinity B cells, or impairment in the expression of the B-cell repertoire. The same degree of restriction observed in affinity heterogeneity of B cells from very young and old mice is likely to reflect different mechanisms. Upon LPS stimulation, neonatal B cells can convert their immune response of restricted heterogeneity into a more heterogeneous response of adult type (49), whereas injection of LPS in old mice does not increase but rather decreases the heterogeneity of antibody affinity (46). Age-related changes in the B-cell repertoire at the idiotype level have been shown by use of hapten-reversible inhibition of plaque formation as an assay for anti-idiotype antibody and idiotype-bearing antibody-secreting cells. Sera from old mice immunized with TNP-Ficoll significantly inhibit plaque formation, in a hapten-reversible manner, by spleen cells from TNP-Ficoll-immunized old mice. However, these sera inhibit much less efficiently plaque formation by cells from similarly immunized young mice. Likewise, sera from TNP-Ficoll-immunized young mice consistently inhibit formation of plaques by cells from immunized young donors but only rarely inhibit plaque formation by cells from old mice (50).

Intrinsic changes in B cells have been well documented in most, although not in all, studies on aging mice. Extensive work on rats has demonstrated decreased densities of surface antigens B, Ia, and FcR (51) as well as μ, γ, and α

chains (52) in old animals. Capping of the former three membrane structures is slower in old rats owing to defects in the microtubule network and to decrease in membrane fluidity (51). Studies in humans (53) have shown in B lymphocytes freshly withdrawn from old individuals and in diploid fibroblasts after several in vitro doublings the appearance of extrachromosomal circular copies of an inter-Alu DNA-unstable sequence. This finding could be taken as evidence for age-related loss of genome stability if circular copies were derived from chromosomal DNA. The B-cell biosynthetic machinery for antibody production has been shown to undergo alterations in aging mice leading to reduction of more than 40% in Ig-specific messenger RNA (54). These intrinsic defects of B cells may result from error accumulation, codon restriction, exhaustion of redundant messages, or transcription error (55). However, the possibility that B-cell functions, such as antibody affinity and heterogeneity, decline in old mice as a consequence of an increased immunosuppression is not ruled out by many studies, including our own (47), but is made unlikely by the results of our experiments (27) on immunosuppression in senescence (see below).

V. HELPER T CELLS

The antibody response of B cells to T-dependent immunogens has been shown in the mouse to require the participation of antigen-specific Lyt-1^+, 2^- T cells exerting helper activity. Antigen-specific helper T cells (Th) have been classified in two types, based on different properties such as surface phenotype, presence of anti-isotype, -allotype, and -idiotype receptors, MHC restriction, nylon-wool adherence, radiosensitivity, and mode of action. One cell type (Th1), nonadherent to nylon, recognizes epitopes of the antigen molecule in association with MHC-controlled class II antigens (Ia) and interacts with B cells through an antigen bridge of physically linked carrier and hapten determinants (cognate B-cell activation). The other cell type (Th2), adherent to nylon, recognizes isotypic, allotypic, and idiotypic markers on B cells, is not MHC restricted, and does not require physical linkage of carrier and hapten determinants for effective cooperation between T and B cells (polyclonal B-cell activation). Both mechanisms may operate synergistically (56). These interactions imply transduction of activating signals from T cells to B cells via helper factors produced and released by T cells. Lymphokines are a major series of soluble factors acting sequentially and amplifying B-cell activation and differentiation (57). At the onset of the antibody response, antigen-stimulated macrophages release IL-1, which in turn induces the release of IL-2 from activated helper T cells. Furthermore, binding of antigen to specific receptors on T cells induces the expression of IL-2 receptors. IL-2 promotes the proliferation of activated T and B cells that express IL-2 receptors which, in turn, are modulated by IL-2. IL-2 also enhances the production of immune interferon (IFN-γ) by activated T cells, which favors antigen presentation by macrophages and stimulates helper T cells to increase IL-2 production and release. Once B cells have been activated first by antigen and then by helper factors released by antigen-activated T cells, their proliferation is amplified by IL-1, IL-2, and BSF, while their differentiation to antibody-producing cells is sustained by BCDF and IL-2 (57).

Profound defects have been detected in the Th cell population of old mice (35,58). Furthermore, an age-related decline in the degree of T-T cell cooperation has been described and attributed to reduction either in the pool size of Th1 and Th2 cells or in their ability to interact synergistically in the generation of helper activity (59,60). The decrease in helper T-cell activity has been attributed to thymus involution (61) and subsequent reduced concentration of thymic factors involved in T-cell maturation (62). The precursor frequency of helper T cells is, indeed, decreased in old mice, although the progeny of each precursor cell maintain full capacity to produce IL-2 and to proliferate (11).

In a series of experiments recently carried out in our laboratory (63,64) helper T-cell activity in aging BDF1 mice was evaluated as follows. Mice were carrier primed by intravenous injection of 2×10^5 HRBC in 0.2 ml of PBS to induce helper T cells. Helper activity of spleen cells from these mice was titrated in vitro 4 days later. In each experiment triplicate culture wells received 0.1 ml of medium containing 2×10^5 TNP-HRBC and 1×10^6 nucleated spleen cells from a pool of 8-10 uninjected 3-month-old mice. Culture wells of one group received no further cells and were used as background control, while wells of other groups received graded numbers ($5\text{-}20 \times 10^4$) of nucleated spleen cells pooled from four to six carrier-primed mice of a given age. The anti-TNP antibody response of cells pooled from triplicate wells was evaluated at days 4 and 5 of culture and the peak response expressed as direct PFC per culture. The PFC response of 1×10^6 nucleated spleen cells from the unprimed 3-month-old mice was subtracted from the PFC responses exhibited by the same spleen cells cocultured with $5\text{-}20 \times 10^4$ spleen cells from carrier-primed mice. Helper activity was evaluated from the anti-TNP PFC versus primed cells per culture regression coefficient plus or minus standard error of a straight line forced through the origin by the least-squares method (Figure 5).

Control experiments demonstrated that helper activity of the carrier-primed spleen cells is mediated by T cells, not by B cells or macrophages, nor is it influenced by T cells of the unprimed spleen cell population. Since helper activity was titrated by adding limiting numbers of T cells from aging mice to an excess of macrophages and B cells from young mice, different regression coefficients should reflect age-related changes in helper T-cell activity. In each experiment carried out to assess helper activity of spleen cells from mice of a given age, helper activity of spleen cells from 3-month-old mice was also evaluated and used as standard age control. The decline of helper T-cell activity with increasing age is described in Figure 6, showing the ratios between regression

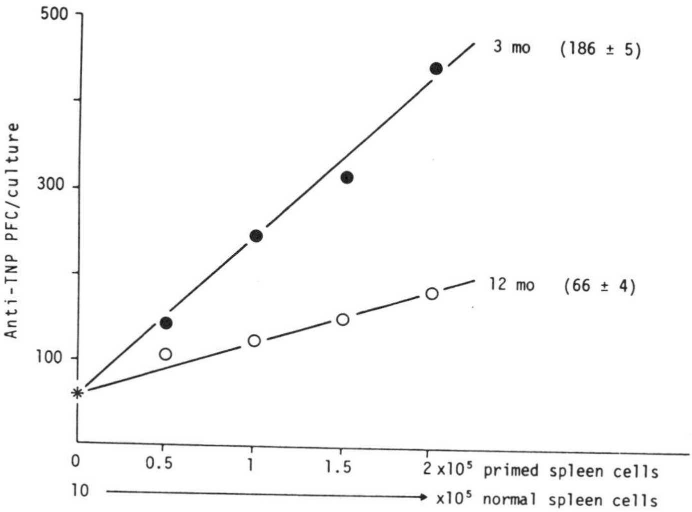

Figure 5 Titration of helper activity of spleen cells from HRBC-primed young (3 months) and old (12 months) mice. Limiting numbers of these cells were cultured with TNP-HRBC and a constant number of spleen cells from unprimed (normal) young mice. The background control response of normal spleen cells alone was subtracted from the responses in mixed cultures and linear regressions forced through the origin were calculated. After regression calculations, the control response was added back to each experimental value to show the original data. The regression coefficients ±SE are given in parentheses.

coefficients: old (6–24 months)/young (3 months). It is noteworthy that helper T-cell activity is already reduced to 64% at 6 months but is not completely lost (30% residual activity) at 24 months of age.

Lyt-1^+,2^- helper T cells produce IL-2 in response to antigens, mitogens, and other lymphokines (57). IL-2 production is decreased in old mice (65), rats (66), and humans (67), this decline accounting to a large extent for the impairment of helper T-cell activity.

Production of IL-2 by spleen cells from aging BDF1 mice has been evaluated in our laboratory (68) as follows. Spleen cells (1×10^7/ml) were stimulated in culture with 2 μg of concanavalin A (Con A) per milliliter and 10 ng of phorbol myristic acetate (PMA) per milliliter. After 48 h culture supernatants were collected and titrated for IL-2 activity. The assay was based on a method previously described (69) but involved statistical validation of titration data according to the principles of the biological assay by parallel lines as applied to probit analysis of quantitative responses. Briefly, supernatants were two fold serially diluted in medium from 1:2 to 1:256, and 100-μl samples from each

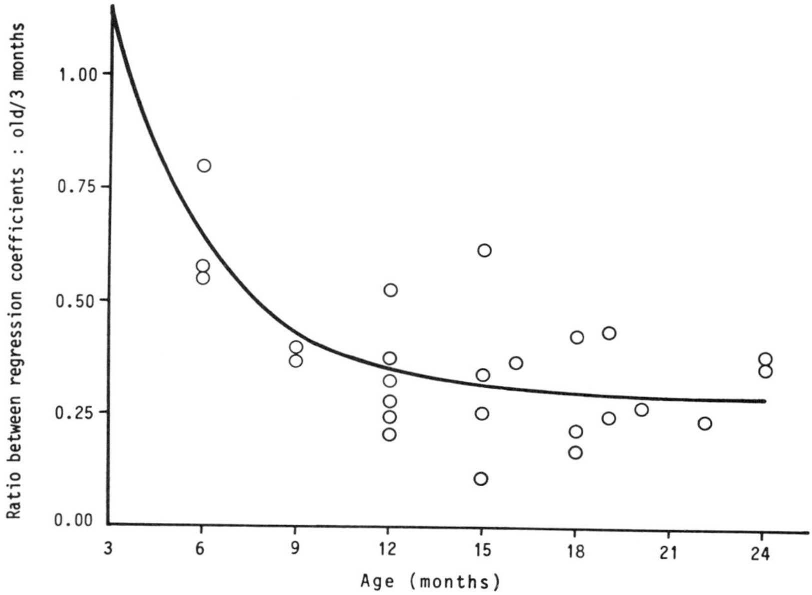

Figure 6 Decline of helper T-cell activity in aging mice. Each point refers to a separate experiment and represents the ratio between anti-TNP PFC versus primed cells per culture regression coefficients: old (6–24 months)/young (3 months). The logistic function $y = 2.09 \exp(-0.30x) + 0.295$ was fitted through individual points by the least-squares method.

dilution were added to triplicate microwells containing 100 μl of IL-2-dependent cytotoxic T lymphocyte line (CTLL) cell suspension (1×10^4/well). Triplicate cell control wells received 100 μl of medium, containing no IL-2, instead of dilution samples. After incubation for 20 h, all cultures received tritiated thymidine and, after 4 h, cell proliferation was assessed and expressed as counts per minute (see Section III, "Macrophages"). The mean cpm from CTLL cells cultured in the absence of IL-2 was subtracted from cpm in each well. Net cpm were then referred, as percent, to the maximum cpm observed in the assay. Sigmoid curves fitting percent of the maximum response as a function of the reciprocal of supernatant $\log_2$ final dilutions were transformed in straight lines by substituting percentage with probit value for each well. In each titration assay, probit transformation was applied to dilution of a standard supernatant (from a culture of MLA 144 line), arbitrarily defined to contain 10 units of gibbon IL-2 per milliliter and to experimental dilutions of spleen cell culture supernatants. Parallelism between the standard regression and each experimental regression as well as linearity of the two combined regressions were verified by analysis of variance. The potency of the experimental supernatant relative to that of the standard supernatant was calculated as the antilog$_2$ of the horizontal distance between the experimental and standard lines. Then, the relative potency was multiplied by 10 to estimate the IL-2 titer of the experimental supernatant in terms of units per milliliter. A factor by which the titer should be multiplied or divided to obtain the variation due to one standard error was also calculated. Results reported in Table 4 show that aging negatively affects IL-2 production by mouse spleen cells. It should be noted that the decline of IL-2 production in mice from 3 to 22 months of age is 170-fold, whereas the decline in helper T-cell activity is only 4-fold (Figure 6). Thus, the dependence of helper activity from IL-2 is not absolute, since other factors, probably less affected by aging, compensate the decreased IL-2 production and contribute to the maintenance of a reduced helper T-cell activity in old mice.

IL-2 responsive cells appear in the fetal thymus as soon as it has been colonized by prethymocytes. After birth, the response of thymocytes to IL-2 is fivefold greater than that of thymocytes from adult mice. These observations (70,71) suggest that T cells expressing IL-2 receptors appear before birth and their number rapidly increases thereafter. Cell expression of IL-2 receptors seems to decrease with advancing age, since mitogen-activated spleen and lymph node cells from old mice are less effective than cells from young mice in absorbing out IL-2 activity from culture supernatants (72). This decline in IL-2 absorption may reflect a decreased number or affinity of IL-2 receptors or a decreased number of IL-2 receptor-bearing cells.

The decline of IL-2 receptors on mitogen-activated spleen cells from aging BDF1 mice has been investigated in our laboratory by a radioimmunoassay (RIA). Microwells of flexible microtiter plates were pretreated with a solution of poly-L-lysine hydrobromide and then received 50 μl of a cell suspension

Table 4 IL-2 Production by Spleen Cells from Mice of Different Ages[a]

Age (months)	IL-2 (U/ml $\overset{\times}{\div}$ SE)
3	15.48 $\overset{\times}{\div}$ 1.10
6	8.63 $\overset{\times}{\div}$ 1.07
12	0.33 $\overset{\times}{\div}$ 1.42
22	0.09 $\overset{\times}{\div}$ 1.59

[a]Data refer to mitogen-activated spleen cells pooled from four mice of ages given.

(4×10^6/ml) in balanced salt solution (BSS). The cells used in each assay were mouse spleen cells activated by mitogens as described above for IL-2 production, P3X63 Ag8.653 non-Ig-producing mouse myeloma cells (negative control), and CTLL cells (positive control). Each cell suspension was distributed in a series of wells and then treated with glutaraldehyde for cell fixation. Cell-coated triplicate wells were washed with 2% fetal calf serum in PBS (RIA buffer, RIAB) and then were given 100-μl samples of rat IgM monoclonal antibody 7D4 (from E. M. Shevach), specific for the mouse IL-2 receptor, twofold serially diluted in RIAB from 1:200 to 1:12,800. For each cell population, additional triplicate wells received 100 μl of RIAB containing no monoclonal antibody. After incubation for 1 h, unbound antibody was flicked off and cell-coated wells were washed three times with RIAB before receiving 100 μl of rabbit antibodies anti-rat Ig (RARIg) diluted 1:1000 in RIAB. After incubation for 1 h, unbound RARIg was removed by repeated washings of the plates with RIAB. Finally, all wells received 100 μl of RIAB containing ^{125}I-Protein A (1×10^5 cpm) from *Staphylococcus aureus*, and after 45 min unbound radioactivity was removed by washing the plates four times with RIAB. Wells were cut and radioactivity was measured as counts per minute in a gamma counter. Results are expressed as net cpm: mean cpm from triplicate wells with 7D4 minus mean cpm from triplicate wells without 7D4. Results in Table 5 indicate that mitogen-activated spleen cells from mice 6–18 months old have lost the capacity to express IL-2 receptors detectable by 7D4 monoclonal antibody. Preliminary observations (data not shown) by fluorescence-activated, cell-sorting analysis support an age-related loss of IL-2 receptor-bearing cells.

Table 5 Expression of IL-2 Receptors on Mitogen-activated Spleen Cells[a]

Age (months)	^{125}I-Protein A bound (net cpm ±SE)[b,c]
3	1435 ±24
6	318 ±105
12	208 ±62
18	367 ±192

[a]Mitogen-activated spleen cells pooled from four mice of the ages given were incubated stepwise with rat monoclonal antibody 7D4 (dilution 1:200), rabbit antibodies anti-rat Ig, and ^{125}I-protein A.

[b]"Net cpm" represents the difference between mean cpm from triplicate wells containing 7D4 and mean cpm from triplicate wells in which 7D4 has been replaced by RIAB.

[c]Net cpm ±SE in controls: P3X63 Ag8.653 cells, 355 ±88; CTLL cells, 5883 ±322.

VI. SUPPRESSOR AND CONTRASUPPRESSOR T CELLS

Antigen-specific suppressor T cells that modulate a variety of immune responses involving both humoral and cellular immunity have been intensively studied since their discovery in 1970 (73). The analysis of immunosuppression has clearly revealed the existence of multiple interactions among T-cell subsets. Several experimental systems have been used to examine such interactions and, as a result, several related but nonidentical regulatory pathways have been described. Integration of many results from different systems into a single overall scheme has been attempted (74). Yet, the identification of T cells with different phenotypes and soluble factors with different immunochemical and biological properties is still controversial, and it remains difficult to reconcile different views from various laboratories working on different experimental systems. Moreover, the model systems suitable to unmask suppressive pathways require subtle experimental conditions that may be difficult to reproduce consistently, even in the same laboratory. Beside these considerations, information from the major experimental systems (SRBC, KLH, ABA, and NP or 4-hydroxy-3-nitrophenyl acetyl) has indicated some features that may be common to most of these systems. All these systems are characterized by sequential interaction of several T-cell subsets. As to the NP system (17,75), antigen presentation by I-J$^+$, I-A$^+$ Mϕ activates an inducer T cell, Ts1 (Lyt-1$^+$, 2$^-$; I-J$^+$; Id$^+$), which produces an antigen-specific factor TsF1 (I-J$^+$; Id$^+$; nonrestricted by MHC and Igh genes; antigen binding). In the absence of antigen TsF1 presented by I-J$^+$, Mϕ activates amplifier or transducer T cells, Ts2 (Lyt-1$^+$, 2$^+$; I-J$^+$; Id$^-$), which recognize TsF1 by anti-Id receptors and are restricted by I-J and Igh genes. Activated Ts2 cells produce a factor, TsF2 (I-J$^+$; anti-Id; restricted by I-J and Igh genes), which, if presented by I-J$^+$ Mϕ, activates effector cells, Ts3 (Lyt-1$^-$, 2$^+$; I-J$^+$; Id$^+$), that bind antigen specifically. Ts3 cells produce a factor, TsF3 (I-J$^+$; Id$^+$; restricted by I-J and Igh genes; antigen binding), which, if presented by I-J$^+$ Mϕ and antigen, activates effector Ts4 cells (Lyt-1$^-$, 2$^+$; I-J$^+$). Activated Ts4 cells release an antigen-nonspecific factor, TsF4, which suppresses Th cells nonspecifically and in a genetically unrestricted way.

Within the SRBC system, a novel immunoregulatory activity interfering with suppression has been described and designated "contrasuppression" (76). The relevant circuit is composed of an inducer T cell (Lyt-1$^-$, 2$^+$; I-J$^+$; Qal$^+$) that produces an I-J$^+$ factor able to bind antigen nonspecifically and to act on a transducer T cell (Lyt-1$^+$, 2$^+$; I-J$^+$; Qal$^+$). The transducer T cell is required for the expression of effector contrasuppressor T cells (Lyt-1$^+$, 2$^-$; I-J$^+$), which interferes with immunosuppression of Th cells (Lyt-1$^+$, 2$^-$; I-J$^-$) by blocking the suppressive activity of soluble mediators released by effector suppressor T cells.

Some experimental observations together with imaginative interpretations have led us to postulate the necessity for the existence of a second level of suppression, constituted by inducer (Lyt-2^+; I-J^+), transducer (Lyt-1^+, 2^+; I-J^+), and effector (Lyt-2^+; I-J^+) T cells. Accordingly, level-1 suppression, as triggered by subimmunogenic doses of antigen, leads to nonresponsiveness (low-zone tolerance); contrasuppression, as stimulated by immunogenic doses of antigen, counteracts level-1 suppression and leads to responsiveness; level-2 suppression, as activated by very high doses of antigen, inactivates contrasuppression and leads to nonresponsiveness (high-zone tolerance) (77). Perseverance along these lines of thought and research may soon provide experimental evidence to prove or reject these fascinating views of immunoregulation.

The incidence of autoantibodies shows a dramatic increase with aging (50, 78). The high percentage of T cells binding autologous erythrocytes (79) and the increased response to chemically altered syngeneic erythrocytes (80) in old mice indicate an enhanced propensity to lose self tolerance during senescence. Beside the intrinsic B-cell resistance to tolerance induction in old mice (41), age-related deficiency in immunosuppression may account for expression of autoreactive clones. This mechanism is supported by the decline in suppressor T-cell activity found in aging NZB mice that are prone to autoimmunity and accelerated senescence (81). However, increased immunosuppression with aging has been repeatedly described in other strains of mice (46,82,83). This controversial issue has been examined in our laboratory to establish whether changes in immunosuppression occur in aging mice (27). It has been found that antigen-specific suppressor T cells are more easily induced in old than in young mice. The enhanced inducibility of antigen-specific suppressor T cells is consistent with the finding of a higher percentage of I-J^+ macrophages in old mice (Figure 4) and may reconcile the coexistence of an increased number of suppressor T cells with thymus involution (61,62). However, the enhanced inducibility of suppressor T cells appears in contrast with the higher incidence of autoimmune reactivity in senescence. This discrepancy has been settled by the results of our experiments (27), which demonstrate a loss of cell sensitivity to suppression in lymphoid cell populations from carrier-primed old mice. The in vitro immune response of these primed cells is resistant to suppression when cultured not only with suppressor cells from young mice but also with suppressor cells from old mice, which are very effective in exerting in vitro suppressive activity on the immune response of primed cells from young mice. This age-related loss of sensitivity to immunosuppression not only may explain the development of autoreactive clones (50, 78), but it also rules out a contribution of suppressor T cells to the decline of immune responsiveness to exogenous antigens in old mice. Resistance to immunosuppression may be explained by several mechanisms that have been discussed in detail elsewhere (27). Among them, resistance to immunosuppression may reflect an increased contrasuppressive activity that renders Lyt-1^+,

2^- helper T cells resistant to level-1 immunosuppression. This possibility is supported by the following observation (84). When spleen cells from old mice are cultured for 5 days, they generate cells capable of interfering with suppression produced by precultured adult cells. This contrasuppressive activity arising from cells of old mice is sensitive to treatment with anti-I-J antibodies and C. In addition, a monoclonal anti-I-J antibody, which blocks contrasuppression but not suppression, inhibits this contrasuppressive activity when added to culture. It is possible that cells of level-2 suppression, which regulates contrasuppression, are lost in old mice. Hence, contrasuppression may dominate and lead to suppression resistance and, perhaps, to autoimmunity.

VII. RECONSTITUTION OF T-CELL FUNCTIONS BY IMMUNOREGULATORY MOLECULES

During the past few years several studies have been carried out in our laboratory to investigate the effects of injecting old mice with immunoregulatory molecules synthesized by solid phase or recombinant DNA technology. Cellular changes induced in vivo by these molecules have been analyzed in vitro to assess whether age-related alterations of T-cell functions can be corrected to a significant extent. The immunoregulatory molecules used in these studies are thymosin α_1, IL-2, and IFN-γ.

A. Thymosin α_1

The calf thymus extract fraction 5 (85) contains several immunoregulatory peptides including thymosin α_1, which has been purified to homogeneity, sequenced (86), and synthesized (87). This peptide, consisting of 28 amino acid residues (mol wt 3108), has an important role in promoting T-cell maturation in several experimental animal models and clinical trials (88,89).

In our initial studies, injection of immunodeficient old mice with thymosin α_1 has been shown to restore defects in helper activity of spleen cells (90) and of Th1 and Th2 cell subpopulations (60,63). Moreover, injection of thymosin α_1 appears to stimulate a population of nylon wool-adherent, Lyt-2^+, suppressor T cells that negatively affect the helper activity of Th1 and Th2 cells (64). Therefore, thymosin α_1 injection in old mice enhances helper and suppressor T-cell activities, although enhancement of helper activity is the prevailing effect.

These studies on the immunoregulatory role of thymosin α_1 in aging BDF1 mice have been continued and extended in our laboratory. Helper activity of spleen cells was induced by injecting aging mice with HRBC, titrated in vitro 4 days later, and expressed by the anti-TNP PFC versus primed cells per culture regression coefficient as described above (Figure 5). Three days before HRBC priming, these mice were left uninjected or were injected intraperitoneally with 0.2 ml of saline solution containing 10 μg of thymosin α_1, or 5 μg of N_{14} (*N*-terminal amino acid residues 1-14) or 5 μg of C_{14} (*C*-terminal amino acid residues 15-28) synthetic fragments of the α_1 molecule (all provided by A. L. Goldstein). Mice of different ages (3, 6, 12, 18, and 24 months) were assayed in separate experiments. In each experiment the regression coefficient for pooled HRBC-primed spleen cells of each group was referred, as a percentage, to the coefficient for HRBC-primed spleen cells of uninjected 3-month-old mice, which served as age controls. Results from five experiments are reported in Table 6 and illustrate that helper T-cell activity is impaired by aging but is restored to a large extent by a single injection of 10 μg of thymosin α_1. Injection of an equimolar amount of the N_{14} fragment is at least as effective as the entire α_1 molecule in restoring helper T-cell activity in mice 6-24 months old, whereas the injection of the C_{14} fragment has no effect. Control experiments showed that anti-Thy-1.2 monoclonal antibody and C treatment of spleen cells from uninjected or thymosin α_1-injected, carrier-primed 12-month-old mice completely abrogates helper activity, demonstrating that the activity induced in old mice by thymosin α_1 is T-cell dependent (data not shown). It is noteworthy that both thymosin α_1 and its N_{14} fragment are devoid of activity when injected in 3-month-old mice, suggesting that these molecules are effective only in T-cell-deficient mice.

The remarkable effect of thymosin α_1 injection on helper activity in old mice need not conflict with the marginal effects induced by other thymic factors (91,92) on the immune response of old mice, since the different potency of the tested molecules may reflect only the differing efficiencies of the experimental designs. In our experiments, indeed, B cells from unprimed young mice were

Table 6 Effects of Thymosin α_1, N_{14}, or C_{14} Peptide Injection on Helper T-Cell Activity[a]

Material injected	Effects[b] at given ages (months)				
	3	6	12	18	24
None	100 ±27	57 ±2	52 ±5	43 ±4	38 ±6
α_1 (10 μg)	107 ±28	74 ±5	79 ±6	74 ±8	79 ±5
N_{14} (5 μg)	106 ±23	105 ±3	114 ±9	86 ±8	86 ±4
C_{14} (5 μg)	111 ±28	59 ±4	43 ±3	46 ±4	50 ±4

[a]Helper activity of spleen cells pooled from four mice of ages given, uninjected or injected with a thymosin peptide 3 days before carrier priming: titrated 4 days after priming and defined as the anti-TNP PFC versus primed cells per culture regression coefficient. Mice of different ages were assayed in separate experiments.

[b]In each experiment regression coefficients were referred, as percentages, to the coefficient for primed cells from uninjected 3-month-old mice. The standard error of each percentage was calculated from the SE of the two regression coefficients.

used to titrate helper activity of T cells from HRBC-primed old mice as a fully responding cell population suitable to unmask the stimulatory effect of thymosin α_1 on T cells. Conversely, if spleen cells from HRBC-primed old mice are stimulated with TNP-HRBC, the in vitro anti-TNP PFC response is not significantly improved by thymosin α_1 injection (90). This is as expected, since B cells from old mice are unable to display higher antibody response as a result of increased T-cell help.

As reported in Table 4, IL-2 production by mitogen-activated spleen cells decreases with aging. The effects on both helper T-cell activity and IL-2 production of injecting 12-month-old mice with thymosin α_1 and its N_{14} and C_{14} fragments were investigated as follows. Eight BDF1 mice per group were left uninjected or were injected with 10 μg of thymosin α_1, 5 μg of N_{14}, or 5 μg of C_{14} fragment 3 days before HRBC-priming. Four days later, spleen cells from individual mice were assayed for helper activity and IL-2 production, as described above (Figure 5 and Table 4). Eight uninjected, HRBC-primed, 3-month-old mice served as an age-control group. Results reported in Table 7 demonstrate that when injected in old mice, thymosin α_1 and its N_{14} fragment, but not the C_{14} fragment, not only enhance spleen cell helper activity but also increase IL-2 production. Similar results were obtained when 6-month-old but not 3-month-old mice were used in the same type of experiment. These findings, showing that thymosin α_1 is effective in immunodeficient aging mice but not in young mice, are concordant with the inability of thymosin α_1 in vitro to increase IL-2 production by human (93) and murine (94) T cells from young individuals. Beside age-related differences in cell populations, thymosin α_1 may be more effective in vivo than in vitro in stimulating maturation of precursor T cells.

Our results suggest the possibility that thymosin α_1 and the N_{14} fragment enhance helper T-cell activity via an increased production of IL-2. Enhancement of IL-2 production could, in turn, favor the expression of IL-2 receptors. The effects of injecting aging mice with thymosin α_1 or its fragments on the expression of IL-2 receptors were investigated as follows. Four BDF1 mice per group at the age of 3, 6, 12, or 18 months were left uninjected or were injected with 10 μg of thymosin α_1, 5 μg of N_{14}, or 5 μg of C_{14} fragment 3 days before sacrifice. Spleen cells pooled from each group were activated in culture and assayed for expression of IL-2 receptors as described above (Table 5). Results in Table 8 show that injection of thymosin α_1 or its N_{14}, but not C_{14}, fragment greatly enhances the expression of IL-2 receptors on mitogen-activated spleen cells from mice 6, 12, and 18 months old, but not from 3-month-old mice. This effect on IL-2 receptors could, in turn, increase cell sensitivity to the IL-2 signal.

It is apparent from our studies that the observed biological activities of thymosin α_1 are restricted to the first 14 amino acid residues from the *N*-terminal end of the α_1 molecule, whereas the other half of the thymosin molecule is devoid of any demonstrable activity. Beside the interesting finding of the

Table 7 Effects of Thymosin α_1, N_{14}, or C_{14} Peptide Injection on Helper T-Cell Activity and IL-2 Production

Age (months)	Material injected	Anti-TNP PFC vs. primed cells/culture regression coefficient ± SE[a]	p	IL-2 production (U/ml ± SE)[a]	p
3	None	429.6 ±12.4		6.59[b]	
12	None	143.2 ±29.8		0.93 ±0.07	
12	α_1 (10 μg)	375.7 ±61.1	$<.01$	5.57 ±0.44	$<.001$
12	N_{14} (5 μg)	315.7 ±13.7	$<.001$	6.94 ±0.49	$<.001$
12	C_{14} (5 μg)	151.9 ±31.6	$>.90$	0.90 ±0.11	$>.80$

[a] Figures refer either to single values from a pool of four mice (3 months old) or to mean values from eight individual mice per group (12 months old).

[b] To obtain the variation due to one standard error, the IL-2 units should be multiplied or divided by 1.16.

Table 8 Effects of Thymosin α_1, N_{14}, or C_{14} Peptide Injection on the Expression of IL-2 Receptors on Mitogen-activated Spleen Cells[a]

Material injected	Effects[b] at given ages (months)			
	3	6	12	18
None	100 ±2	22 ±7	14 ±4	26 ±13
α_1 (10 μg)	106 ±5	78 ±6	100 ±3	122 ±16
N_{14} (5 μg)	70 ±16	106 ±2	141 ±9	115 ±10
C_{14} (5 μg)	101 ±2	9 ±6	21 ±6	18 ±4

[a]Experimental conditions and control values are the same as reported in Table 5.
[b]Figures are percentages ± SE of net cpm from ^{125}I-Protein A bound as referred to the control value 1435 ±24 cpm for uninjected 3-month-old mice.

molecular localization of important biological activities of thymosin α_1, the inactivity of the C_{14} fragment indicates that this fragment may be used as negative control for the activity of the N_{14} fragment in well-balanced experimental designs.

The results of our studies altogether indicate that thymosin α_1-induced enhancement of helper T-cell activity in old mice may be mediated by increased IL-2 production and expression of IL-2 receptors. Thus, the effect of thymosin α_1 in old mice may result from precursor cell maturation leading, upon T cell activation, to increased number of IL-2 receptor-bearing cells and to enhanced production of IL-2 that up-regulates the expression of IL-2 receptors. Since IL-2 is a necessary signal not only for the expansion of helper T cells but also for the production of other lymphokines required for the generation of effector cells (57), modulation of IL-2 production by thymosin α_1 provides a rational basis for therapeutic intervention in age-related immunodeficiencies.

B. Interleukin 2

Our results from the preceding section have indicated the possibility that thymosin α_1 injection in old mice enhances helper T-cell activity through increased IL-2 production. Synthesis of this lymphokine is, indeed, markedly reduced in aging mice, as shown in Table 4. The effect on helper T-cell activity of injecting BDF1 mice with recombinant human interleukin 2 (rHuIL-2 from Hoffmann-La Roche, Basel) was investigated as follows. Four mice per group at the age of 3 or 16 months were left uninjected or were injected subcutaneously with 1, 10, or 100 units of rHuIL-2 in 0.2 ml of saline solution immediately before HRBC priming. Four days later, helper activity of pooled spleen cells was assessed as previously described (Figure 5). Results in Table 9 show that injection of IL-2 enhances helper T-cell activity in young and old mice. This finding is in line with the observation that although IL-2 production is decreased in old mice, the

Table 9 Enhanced Helper Activity of Spleen Cells[a] from Mice Injected with IL-2

Material injected	Activity[b] at given ages (months)	
	3	16
None	100 ±10	37 ±5
rHuIL-2 (1 U)	169 ±16	79 ±7
rHuIL-2 (10 U)	199 ±38	129 ±10
rHuIL-2 (100 U)	359 ±32	173 ±29

[a]Helper activity of spleen cells from HRBC-primed mice was titrated as described in Figure 5.
[b]Figures are percentages ±SE calculated as in Table 6.

ability to respond to IL-2 is unimpaired, as evidenced by the reconstitution of their immune responses by injected exogenous IL-2 (63,95). It appears from these studies that thymosin α_1 is active only in T-cell-deficient old mice by inducing maturation of precursor T cells which, upon activation, become able to produce IL-2 and to respond to it. Conversely, exogenous IL-2 amplifies helper T-cell activity in both T-cell-deficient old mice and fully competent young mice.

C. Gamma Interferon

It has been shown (96) that administration of IFN-γ to mice enhances in vivo antibody responses to several antigens. This enhancing effect may be attributed not only to increased expression of cell surface I-A molecules and IL-1 production by macrophages (96,97) but also to activation of T cells to become IL-2 responsive via increased expression of IL-2 receptors (98).

In recent studies (63,99) carried out in our laboratory, young and old mice were injected with IFN-γ to assess whether this lymphokine is able to enhance helper T-cell activity. Four BDF1 mice per group were left uninjected or were injected intravenously with 0.2 ml of saline solution containing either IFN-γ produced by L12R4 T lymphoma (provided by S. Landolfo) or recombinant murine IFN-γ (rMuIFN-γ from Genentech, San Francisco) immediately before HRBC priming. Four days later, helper activity of spleen cells was evaluated as already described (Figure 5). Results of a typical experiment reported in Table 10 show that the two IFN-γ preparations are almost equally effective in restoring helper T-cell activity in 20-month-old mice. Other experiments (99) have also shown that IFN-γ enhances helper activity of separated Th1 and Th2 cells, regardless of whether it has been administered in vivo or in vitro. Furthermore, IFN-γ in vitro treatment was found to increase IL-2 production by mitogen-activated spleen cells. All these immunoregulatory effects of IFN-γ have been observed in both young and old mice, stressing the important

Table 10 Effect of IFN-γ on Helper Activity of Spleen Cells[a] from Old Mice

Age (months)	Material injected	Helper activity[a,b]
3	None	100 ±12
20	None	27 ±5
20	IFN-γ (10^3 U)	91 ±8
20	rMuIFN-γ (10^3 U)	102 ±12

[a]Helper activity of spleen cells from HRBC-primed mice was titrated as described in Figure 5.
[b]Figures are percentages ±SE calculated as in Table 6.

role of this lymphokine in helper T-cell amplification under normal and immunodeficient conditions.

VIII. CONCLUDING REMARKS

Age-related immune dysfunctions seem to reflect biochemical alterations in individual cells and changes in the relative proportion of immunoregulatory cells with distinct functions.

DNA repair capacity and maximum life span have been found to be positively correlated (100), and both have been shown to be under MHC control (101). Expression of this correlation at the single-cell level may be examplified by the finding that the number of doublings sustained by human peripheral T cells cultured in the presence of IL-2 declines with the increasing age of the lymphocyte donor (6). Moreover, T lymphocytes from aged mice (65; Table 4), as well as from aged rats (66) and humans (67), have been found defective in the ability to produce IL-2. Also the expression of IL-2 receptors appears to be decreased by aging (72; Table 6). At variance with other observations (11), these findings indicate that T cells display the Hayflick phenomenon (14), probably reflecting age-related DNA alterations. DNA instability, as described in human B cells from old individuals (53), may result in reduced transcription of Ig-specific mRNA (54) and in decreased expression of surface molecules (51,52), as well as in transcription of altered genetic information leading to the appearance of new antigenic determinants on the cell surface (102). Changes in cell surface properties in old animals is also likely to induce autoimmune responses to naturally hidden antigenic determinants (103). However, in contrast with the Hayflick phenomenon (14), no convincing evidence has been found for intrinsic limits imposed by aging on the proliferative capacity of stem cells (15).

Changes in relative pool size and reactivity of immunoregulatory cells with antithetic functions, such as helper T cells, suppressor T cells, contrasuppressor

T cells, as well as I-A$^+$, I-J$^-$, and I-A$^+$, I-J$^+$ macrophages, may also reflect alterations in their biochemical machinery required for cell replication, synthesis of immunoregulatory molecules, and maintenance of cell sensitivity to external regulatory signals. However, besides intrinsic alterations of these cells, age-related defects in other cells, such as thymus epithelial cells, reduce the effective concentration of the peptides required for T-cell maturation. The decline of these maturation factors contributes to a large extent to the upsetting of the physiological balance among several immunoregulatory cell subpopulations, thus ultimately affecting antigen recognition, cell activation, and cell interactions.

Results from experiments on reconstitution of T-cell functions by injecting old mice with thymosin α_1, IL-2, or IFN-γ demonstrate the possibility of repairing important immune functions up to the level of adult mice. These findings are very promising because they suggest possible ways of preventing or treating immune disorders in the elderly. However, suitable protocols should be devised to effectively increase immune responsiveness to exogenous antigens and to prevent expression of autoimmune reactivity. Maintenance of a normal balance of immune functions may prolong the duration of life and improve its biological quality.

ACKNOWLEDGMENTS

This work was supported by ENEA-Euratom contract; publication No. 2287 of the Euratom Biology Division.

REFERENCES

1. Fougereau, M., and J. Dausset, editors. 1980. Progress in Immunology, Vol. IV. Academic Press, Orlando, Fla.
2. Yamamura, Y., and T. Tada, editors. 1983. Progress in Immunology, Vol. V. Academic Press, Tokyo.
3. Walford, R. L. 1974. Immunologic theory of aging: Current status. *Fed. Proc.* 33:2020.
4. Smith, G. S., and R. L. Walford. 1977. Influence of the main histocompatibility complex on aging in mice. *Nature.* 270:727.
5. Dorf, M. E. 1981. The role of the major histocompatibility complex in immunobiology. *In* The Role of the Major Histocompatibility Complex in Immunobiology. M. E. Dorf, editor. Garland, New York.
6. Walford, R. L., R. H. Weindruch, S.R.S. Gottesman, and C. F. Tam. 1981. The immunopathology of aging. *Annu. Rev. Gerontol. Geriat.* 2:3.
7. Harman, D. 1981. The aging process. *Proc. Natl. Acad. Sci. USA.* 78:7124.
8. Tam, C. F., and R. L. Walford. 1978. Cyclic nucleotide levels in resting and mitogen-stimulated cell suspensions from young and old mice. *Mech. Ageing Dev.* 7:309.

9. Makinodan, T., and W. H. Adler. 1975. Effects of aging on the differentiation and proliferation potentials of cells of the immune system. *Fed. Proc.* 34:153.
10. Makinodan, T., J. W. Albright, P. I. Good, C. P. Peter, and M. L. Heidrick. 1976. Reduced humoral immune activity in long-lived old mice: An approach to elucidating its mechanisms. *Immunology.* 31:903.
11. Miller, R. A. 1984. Age-associated decline in precursor frequency for different T cell-mediated reactions, with preservation of helper or cytotoxic effect per precursor cell. *J. Immunol.* 132:63.
12. Callard, R. E. 1981. Aging of the immune system. *In* Handbook of Immunology in Aging. M.M.B. Kay and T. Makinodan, editors. CRC Press, Boca Raton, Fla. 103.
13. Kay, M.M.B., and T. Makinodan. 1982. The ageing immune system. *In* Lectures on Gerontology, Vol. 1. A. Viidik, editor. Academic Press, Orlando, Fla. 143.
14. Hayflick, L. 1968. Human cells and aging. *Sci. Am.* 218:32.
15. Harrison, D. E. 1983. Long-term erythropoietic repopulating ability of old, young and fetal stem cells. *J. Exp. Med.* 157:1496.
16. Unanue, E. R. 1984. Antigen-presenting function of the macrophage. *Annu. Rev. Immunol.* 2:395.
17. Dorf, M. E., and B. Benacerraf. 1984. Suppressor cells and immunoregulation. *Annu. Rev. Immunol.* 2:127.
18. Dorf, M. E., and B. Benacerraf. 1985. I-J as a restriction element in the suppressor T cell system. *Immunol. Rev.* 83:23.
19. Garvey, J. S., J. W. Shafer, and T. C. Caperna. 1980. Antigen handling in relation to ageing. *Mech. Ageing Dev.* 12:287.
20. Nakano, K., and B. Cinader. 1980. A strain survey of age-dependent changes in antigen elimination, antibody formation and tolerance. *J. Immunogenet.* 7:183.
21. Metcalf, D., R. Moulds, and B. Pike. 1967. Influence of the spleen and thymus on immune responses in ageing mice. *Clin. Exp. Immunol.* 2:109.
22. Heidrick, M. L. 1972. Age-related changes in hydrolase activity of peritoneal macrophages. *Gerontologist.* 12:28.
23. Perkins, E. H. 1971. Phagocytic activity of aged mice. *J. Reticuloendothel. Soc.* 9:642.
24. Heidrick, M. L., and T. Makinodan. 1973. Presence of impairment of humoral immunity in nonadherent spleen cells of old mice. *J. Immunol.* 111:1502.
25. Callard, R. E. 1978. Immune functions in aged mice. III. Role of macrophages and effect of 2-mercaptoethanol in the response of spleen cells from old mice to phytohemagglutinin, lipopolysaccharide and allogeneic cells. *Eur. J. Immunol.* 8:697.
26. Corradin, G., H. M. Etlinger, and J. M. Chiller. 1977. Lymphocyte specificity to protein antigens. I. Characterization of the antigen-induced in vitro T cell-dependent proliferative response with lymph node cells from primed mice. *J. Immunol.* 119:1048.

27. Doria, G., C. Mancini, and L. Adorini. 1982. Immunoregulation in senescence: Increased inducibility of antigen specific suppressor T cells and loss of cell sensitivity to immunosuppression in aging mice. *Proc. Natl. Acad. Sci. USA.* 79:3803.
28. Paul, W. E. 1984. Letter to the editor. *J. Immunol.* 132:1056.
29. Howard, M., L. Matis, T. R. Malek, E. Shevach, W. Kell, D. Cohen, K. Nakanishi, and W. E. Paul. 1983. Interleukin-2 induces antigen-reactive T cell lines to secrete BCGF-1. *J. Exp. Med.* 158:2024.
30. Hirano, T., T. Teranishi, H. Toba, N. Sakagushi, T. Fukukawa, and I. Tsuyuguchi. 1981. Human helper T cell factors (ThF). I. Partial purification and characterization. *J. Immunol.* 126:517.
31. Giri, J. G., P. W. Kincade, and S. B. Mizel. 1984. Interleukin 1-mediated induction of κ-light chain synthesis and surface immunoglobulin expression on pre-B cells. *J. Immunol.* 132:223.
32. Palacios, R., G. Henson, M. Steinmetz, and J. P. McKearn. 1984. Interleukin 3 supports growth of mouse pre-B-cell clones in vitro. *Nature.* 309: 126.
33. Muraguchi, A., J. H. Kehrl, D. L. Longo, D. J. Wolkman, K. A. Smith, and A. S. Fauci. 1985. Interleukin-2 receptors on human B cells. Implications for the role of interleukin-2 in human B cell function. *J. Exp. Med.* 161: 181.
34. Kishimoto, S., T. Takahama, and H. Mizumachi. 1976. In vitro immune response to 2,4,6-trinitrophenyl determinant in aged C57BL/6J mice: Changes in the humoral immune response to, avidity for the TNP determinant and responsiveness to LPS effect with aging. *J. Immunol.* 116: 294.
35. Callard, R. E., and A. Basten. 1978. Immune functions in aged mice. IV. Loss of T cell and B cell functions in thymus-dependent antibody responses. *Eur. J. Immunol.* 8:552.
36. Mason Smith, A. 1976. The effects of age on the immune response to type III pneumococcal polysaccharide (SIII) and bacterial lipopolysaccharide (LPS) in Balb/c, SJL/J, and C3H mice. *J. Immunol.* 116:469.
37. Callard, R. E., A. Basten, and L. K. Waters. 1977. Immune function in aged mice. II. B cell function. *Cell. Immunol.* 31:26.
38. Zharhary, D., and N. R. Klinman. 1983. Antigen responsiveness of the mature and generative B cell populations of aged mice. *J. Exp. Med.* 157: 1300.
39. Zharhary, D., and N. R. Klinman. 1984. B cell repertoire diversity to PR8 influenza virus does not decrease with age. *J. Immunol.* 133:2285.
40. Hooijkaas, H., A. A. Preesman, A. Van Oudenaren, R. Benner, and J. J. Haaijman. 1983. Frequency analysis of functional immunoglobulin C and V gene expression in murine B cells at various ages. *J. Immunol.* 131:1629.
41. Dobken, J., M. E. Weksler, and G. W. Siskind. 1980. Effect of age on ease of B cell tolerance induction. *Cell. Immunol.* 55:66.
42. Szewczuk, M. R., and G. W. Siskind. 1977. Ontogeny of B lymphocyte function. III. In vivo and in vitro studies on the ease of tolerance induction

in B lymphocytes from fetal, neonatal and adult mice. *J. Exp. Med.* 145:1590.

43. D'Eustachio, P., and G. M. Edelman. 1975. Frequency and avidity of specific antigen-binding cells in developing mice. *J. Exp. Med.* 142:1078.
44. Silverstein, A. M., J. W. Uhr, K. L. Kraner, and R. J. Lukes. 1963. Fetal response to antigenic stimulus. II. Antibody production by the fetal lamb. *J. Exp. Med.* 117:799.
45. Sherr, D. H., M. R. Szewczuk, A. Cusano, W. Rappaport, and G. W. Siskind. 1979. Ontogeny of B lymphocyte function. IX. Difference in the time of maturation of the capacity of B lymphocytes from fetal and neonatal mice to produce a heterogeneous antibody response to thymic-dependent and thymic-independent antigens. *Immunology.* 36:891.
46. Goidl, E. A., J. B. Innes, and M. E. Weksler. 1976. Immunological studies of aging. II. Loss of IgG and high avidity plaque-forming cells and increased suppressor cell activity in aging mice. *J. Exp. Med.* 144:1037.
47. Doria, G., G. D'Agostaro, and A. Poretti. 1978. Age-dependent variations of antibody avidity. *Immunology.* 35:601.
48. Gearhart, P. J. 1982. Generation of immunoglobulin variable gene diversity. *Immunol. Today.* 3:107.
49. Goidl, E. A., J. Klass, and G. W. Siskind. 1976. Ontogeny of B lymphocyte function. II. Ability of endotoxin to increase the heterogeneity of affinity of the immune response of B lymphocytes from fetal mice. *J. Exp. Med.* 143:1503.
50. Goidl, E. A., G. J. Thorbecke, M. E. Weksler, and G. W. Siskind. 1980. Production of auto-anti-idiotypic antibody during the normal immune response: Changes in the auto-anti-idiotypic antibody response and the isotype repertoire associated with aging. *Proc. Natl. Acad. Sci. USA.* 77:6788.
51. Woda, B. A., J. Yguerabide, and J. D. Feldman. 1979. Mobility and density of AgB, "Ia," and Fc receptors on the surface of lymphocyte from young and old rats. *J. Immunol.* 123:2161.
52. Woda, B. A., and J. D. Feldman. 1979. Density of surface immunoglobulin and capping on rat lymphocytes. *J. Exp. Med.* 149:416.
53. Shmookler Reis, R. J., C. K. Lumpkin, Jr., J. R. McGill, K. T. Raibowol, and S. Goldstein. 1983. Extrachromosomal circular copies of an "Inter-Alu" unstable sequence in human DNA are amplified during in vitro and in vivo ageing. *Nature.* 301:394.
54. Dupere, S. L. R., and B. J. Kolodziej. 1983. Cellular and molecular aspects of thymus dependent antibody production in aged C3H/HeBr mice. *Age.* 6:11.
55. Strehler, B. L. 1982. Ageing: Concepts and theories. *In* Lectures on Gerontology, Vol. 1. A. Viidik, editor. Academic Press, Orlando, Fla. 1.
56. Doria, G. 1982. Immunoregulatory cell interactions in the antibody response. *In* Immunogenetics and Immune Regulation. B. Benacerraf, editor. Masson, Milano. 109.
57. Farrar, J. J., W. R. Benjamin, M. L. Hilfiker, M. Howard, W. L. Farrar, and J. Fuller-Farrar. 1982. The biochemistry, biology, and role of inter-

leukin 2 in the induction of cytotoxic T cell and antibody-forming B cell responses. *Immunol. Rev.* 63:129.
58. Krogsrud, R. L., and E. H. Perkins. 1977. Age-related changes in T cell function. *J. Immunol.* 118:1607.
59. Doria, G., G. D'Agostaro, and M. Garavini. 1980. Age-dependent changes of B-cell reactivity and T cell–T cell interaction in the in vitro antibody response. *Cell. Immunol.* 53:195.
60. Doria, G., D. Frasca, and L. Adorini. 1983. Immunoregulation of antibody response in aging. *In* Progress in Immunology, Vol. 5. Y. Yamamura and T. Tada, editors. Academic Press, Tokyo. 1549.
61. Hirokawa, K., and T. Makinodan. 1975. Thymic involution: Effect on T-cell differentiation. *J. Immunol.* 114:1659.
62. Goldstein, A. L., T.L.K. Low, G. B. Thurman, M. M. Zatz, N. Hall, J. Chen, S. K. Hu, P. B. Naylor, and J. E. McClure. 1981. Current status of thymosin and other hormones of the thymus gland. *In* Recent Progress in Hormone Research, Vol. 37. R. O. Greef, editor. Academic Press, Orlando, Fla. 369.
63. Doria, G., L. Adorini, and D. Frasca. 1984. Recovery of T cell functions in aged mice by injection of immunoregulatory molecules. *In* Lymphoid Cell Functions in Aging. A. L. De Weck, editor. EURAGE, Rijswijk. 59.
64. Frasca, D., L. Adorini, and G. Doria. 1985. Enhancement of helper and suppressor T cell activities by thymosin α_1 injection in old mice. *Immunopharmacology.* 10:41.
65. Thoman, M. L., and W. O. Weigle. 1981. Lymphokines and aging: Interleukin-2 production and activity in aged animals. *J. Immunol.* 127:2102.
66. Gilman, S. C., J. S. Rosenberg, and J. D. Feldman. 1982. T lymphocytes in young and aged rats. II. Functional defects and the role of interleukin-2. *J. Immunol.* 128:644.
67. Gillis, S., R. Kozek, M. Durante, and M. E. Weksler. 1981. Immunological studies of aging. Decreased production of and response to T cell growth factor by lymphocytes from aged humans. *J. Clin. Invest.* 67:937.
68. Frasca, D., L. Adorini, and G. Doria. 1984. Production of and response to interleukin-2 in aging mice. Modulation by thymosin α_1. *In* Lymphoid Cell Functions in Aging. A. L. De Weck, editor. EURAGE, Rijswijk. 155.
69. Gillis, S., M. M. Ferm, W. Ou, and K. A. Smith. 1978. T cell growth factor: Parameters of production and a quantitative microassay for activity. *J. Immunol.* 120:2027.
70. Bocchieri, M. H., O. A. Batuman, S. P. Hauptman, I. M. Zitron, and J. B. Smith. 1983. Ontogeny of interleukin 2 responsive cells in the fetal thymus. *J. Immunol.* 131:533.
71. Raulet, D. H. 1985. Expression and function of interleukin-2 receptors on immature thymocytes. *Nature.* 314:101.
72. Chang, M. P., T. Makinodan, W. J. Peterson, and B. L. Strehler. 1982. Role of T cells and adherent cells in age-related decline in murine interleukin 2 production. *J. Immunol.* 129:2426.
73. Gershon, R. K., and K. Kondo. 1970. Cell interactions in the induction of tolerance. *Immunology.* 18:723.

74. Germain, R. N., and B. Benacerraf. 1981. A single major pathway of T-lymphocyte interactions in antigen-specific immune suppression. *Scand. J. Immunol.* 13:1.
75. Furusawa, S., M. Minami, D. H. Sherr, and M. E. Dorf. 1984. Analysis of the suppressor T cell cascade with products derived from T cell hybridomas. *In* Cell Fusion: Gene Transfer and Transformation. R. F. Beers and E. G. Bassett, editors. Raven Press, New York. 299.
76. Gershon, R. K., D. D. Eardley, S. Durum, D. R. Green, F. W. Shen, K. Yamauchi, H. Cantor, and D. B. Murphy. 1981. Contrasuppression. A novel immunoregulatory activity. *J. Exp. Med.* 153:1533.
77. Green, D. R., P. M. Flood, and R. K. Gershon. 1983. Immunoregulatory T-cell pathways. *Annu. Rev. Immunol.* 1:439.
78. Meredith, P. J., and R. L. Walford. 1979. Autoimmunity, histocompatibility and aging. *Mech. Ageing Dev.* 9:61.
79. Charreire, J., and J. F. Bach. 1975. Binding of autologous erythrocytes to immature T cells. *Proc. Natl. Acad. Sci. USA.* 72:3201.
80. Naor, D., B. Bonavida, and R. L. Walford. 1976. Autoimmunity and aging: The age-related response of mice of a long-lived strain to trinitrophenylated syngeneic mouse red blood cells. *J. Immunol.* 117:2204.
81. Barthoid, D. R., S. Kysela, and A. D. Steinberg. 1974. Decline in suppressor T cell function with age in female NZB mice. *J. Immunol.* 122:9.
82. Gerbase-De Lima, M., P. Meredith, and R. L. Walford. 1975. Age-related changes including synergy and suppression in the mixed lymphocyte reaction in long-lived mice. *Fed. Proc.* 34:159.
83. Segre, D., and M. Segre. 1976. Humoral immunity in aged mice. II. Increased suppressor T cell activity in immunologically deficient old mice. *J. Immunol.* 116:735.
84. Green, M. I., and R. K. Gershon. 1984. Contrasuppression: The second law of thymodynamics, revisited. *Adv. Cancer Res.* 42:277.
85. Hooper, J. A., M. C. McDaniel, G. B. Thurman, G. H. Cohen, R. S. Schulof, and A. L. Goldstein. 1975. The purification and properties of bovine thymosin. *Ann. N.Y. Acad. Sci.* 249:125.
86. Low, T.L.K., and A. L. Goldstein. 1979. The chemistry and biology of thymosin. II. Amino acid sequence analysis of thymosin α_1 and polypeptide β_1. *J. Biol. Chem.* 254:987.
87. Wang, S. S., I. Douvan Kulesha, and D. P. Winter. 1979. Synthesis of thymosin α_1. *J. Am. Chem. Soc.* 101:253.
88. Zatz, M. M., T.L.K. Low, and A. L. Goldstein. 1982. Role of thymosin and other thymic hormones in T-cell differentiation. *In* Biological Responses in Cancer, Vol. 1. E. Mihich, editor. Plenum Press, New York. 219.
89. Schulof, R. S., and A. L. Goldstein. 1983. Clinical applications of thymosin and other thymic hormones. *In* Recent Advances in Clinical Immunology. R. A. Thompson and N. R. Rose, editors. Churchill Livingstone, New York. 243.
90. Frasca, D., M. Garavini, and G. Doria. 1982. Recovery of T-cell functions in aged mice injected with synthetic thymosin α_1. *Cell. Immunol.* 72:384.

91. Bliznakov, E. G., Y.-P. Wan, D. Chang, and K. Folkers. 1978. Partial reactivation of impaired immune competence in aged mice by synthetic thymus factors. *Biochem. Biophys. Res. Commun.* 80:631.
92. Weksler, M. E., J. B. Innes, and G. Goldstein. 1978. Immunological studies of aging. IV. The contribution of thymic involution to the immune deficiencies of aging mice and reversal with thymopoietin 32–36. *J. Exp. Med.* 148:996.
93. Zatz, M. M., J. Oliver, C. Samuels, A. B. Skotnicki, M. B. Sztein, and A. L. Goldstein. 1984. Thymosin increases production of T cell growth factor by normal human peripheral blood lymphocytes. *Proc. Natl. Acad. Sci. USA.* 81:2882.
94. Zatz, M. M., and A. L. Goldstein. 1985. Mechanism of action of thymosin. I. Thymosin fraction 5 increases lymphokine production by mature murine T cells responding in a mixed lymphocyte reaction. *J. Immunol.* 134:1032.
95. Thoman, M. L., and W. O. Weigle. 1985. Reconstitution of in vivo cell-mediated lympholysis. Responses in aged mice with interleukin 2. *J. Immunol.* 134:949.
96. Nakamura, M., T. Manser, G.D.N. Pearson, M. J. Daley, and M. L. Gefter. 1984. Effect of IFN-γ on the immune response in vivo and on gene expression in vitro. *Nature* 307:381.
97. Wong, G.H.W., I. Clark-Lewis, A. W. Harris, and J. W. Schrader. 1984. Effect of cloned interferon-γ on expression of H-2 and Ia antigens on cell lines of hemopoietic, lymphoid, epithelial, fibroblastic and neuronal origin. *Eur. J. Immunol.* 14:52.
98. Johnson, H. M., and W. L. Farrar. 1983. The role of a gamma-interferon-like lymphokine in the activation of T cells for expression of IL-2 receptors. *Cell. Immunol.* 75:154.
99. Frasca, D., L. Adorini, S. Landolfo, and G. Doria. 1985. Enhancing effect of IFN-γ on helper T cell activity and IL-2 production. *J. Immunol.* 134:3907.
100. Hart, R. W., and R. B. Setlow. 1974. Correlation between deoxyribonucleic acid excision repair and lifespan in a number of mammalian species. *Proc. Natl. Acad. Sci. USA.* 71:2169.
101. Walford, R. L., and K. Bergmann. 1979. Influence of genes associated with the main histocompatibility complex on deoxyribonucleic acid excision repair capacity and bleomycin sensitivity in mouse lymphocytes. *Tissue Antigens.* 14:336.
102. Callard, R. E., A. Basten, and R. B. Blanden. 1979. Loss of immune competence with age may be due to a qualitative abnormality in lymphocyte membranes. *Nature.* 281:218.
103. Rivnay, B., A. Globerson, and M. Shinitzky. 1979. Viscosity of lymphocyte plasma membrane in aging mice and its possible relation to serum cholesterol. *Mech. Ageing Dev.* 10:71.

9

Effect of Thymic Hormones on Immunity and Life Span

Raymond N. Hiramoto, Vithal K. Ghanta, and Sen-jaw Soong

Veterans Administration Medical Center
and Comprehensive Cancer Center
University of Alabama
Birmingham, Alabama

I. INTRODUCTION

The last decade has witnessed an impressive growth in research directed at an understanding of aging processes. It is therefore not surprising that interventions are now being proposed to alter the rate of human aging and aging of the immune system. Several experimental models can be used to study aging of the immune system. Those that are in the realm of applicability are dietary manipulation and chemical therapy. Dietary restriction is primarily started early in life and its aim is preventive, while chemical therapy (i.e., the supplementation of thymic hormones or the use of double-stranded polynucleotides) would be used in an attempt to restore the activity of an already aging immune system. At this time, the only intervention that has been repeatedly demonstrated to alter the rate of aging of the immune system and aging in general in mammals is dietary restriction.

One of the concerns of the National Institute on Aging is to explore approaches to extend the vigorous and productive years of life. It is therefore important that we undertake to develop the appropriate technology for assessing interventions that affect aging. One of the proven markers of aging is the generalized decline in immune response and increased autoimmunity and cancer. The decline in immune response is preceded by the involution of thymus. The lymphoid cells that undergo maturation in the thymus are responsible for a variety of cell-mediated immune reactions, namely, response to T-cell mitogens, delayed-type hypersensitivity (DTH), surveillance against cancer cells, graft rejections, controlling viral infections, and regulating autoimmunity. Therefore, it is reasonable to believe that preservation of the immune system as the individual ages would provide a greater chance of living a long, healthy, useful life, free from disease.

Because it has been established that the thymus, in addition to providing T cells, has an endocrine function, we have set out to determine the effect of long-term treatment of mice (CFW, an outbred strain, and A/HeN and C57BL/6, inbred strains) with extracts of thymic tissue and synthetic analogues of the small fragments of thymic hormones on the changes in immune function and changes in survival with age. This study was initiated in 1979 and completed in 1984 and was supported by the National Institute on Aging. The thymic hormones and analogues were obtained from various scientists from this country and abroad who have extensive experience with thymic hormones and have characterized their material for its biological functions and biochemical properties.

The hormones used are the thymic humoral factor FTS (facteur thymique serique), TP5 (thymopoietin), TM4 (an enzyme-resistant variant of FTS), and TH (thymosin). The mice are treated with these preparations weekly starting from 2 months of age for their entire lifetime. These are extensive studies in which various immunological parameters were monitored repeatedly on individual animals. Such animals were maintained in a closely regulated environment (in temperature- and light-controlled rooms, housed in sterile cages), given regular food and sterile water to minimize infections, and handled with care. Under such ideal care, some mice lived longer than 3 years. From this study we found that one strain treated with the hormone TM4 had a median survival (time when half the animals in the group had died) of 31.1 months, which was significantly greater than in mice not treated with the hormone (24.9 months). This is an increase of 6.2 months or 25% increase in median survival. To put this into human perspective, if we assume that one day in the life of a mouse is equivalent to one month in man, a 6.2-month increase in median survival time is equivalent to adding 15.5 years to a man's life. These observations indicate that at least one of the analogues of thymic hormones can increase the median life span of one strain of mice and this mechanism, which increased life span, differs from that mediated through dietary restriction. These studies are still very preliminary, but overall the findings are encouraging.

The results indicate that in the laboratory the immune functions and survival of both short-lived and long-lived rodents can be manipulated by these experimental procedures. Thus, it appears that successful methods of immunological intervention are feasible. Progress in the next 10 years should resolve to what extent immunological aging and restoration of normal immune functions of aged individuals may have an effect on their disease pattern and life span.

II. AGING OF THE IMMUNE SYSTEM

Aging predisposes the individual to a decline in cell-mediated and antibody responses to foreign antigens, and the response to autoantigens is increased (1-3). With the age-related involution of the thymus, several T-cell responses are altered. There is a depression of the DTH reaction (3,4), a decline in responses to lectins (5-8) and allogeneic cells (9), a reduction in cytotoxic lymphocytes (10) and helper T-cell activity, and an increase in suppressor T-cell function (11-13). While the absolute number of circulating peripheral blood lymphocytes may remain stable (14,15), others have reported a decline (16). The percentage of circulating T cells has been reported to be unchanged (8,14,16). Decreased thymic hormone levels, lymphokine production (17,18), and interleukin 2 (IL-2) production (19) have been observed. However, the fact that no age-related differences in the expression of IL-2 receptors could be found (20) indicates that IL-2 supplementation might restore some of the reactivity of T-cell function in old animals. The B cells, on the other hand, show no loss in proliferative ability, and their number may be slightly increased or unaltered (21-23). The functional state of B cells however, appears to be altered. There is an increase in the incidence of autoantibody synthesis (24), which implies a selective increase in number and in type of subpopulations of B cells. With these alterations, a change in balance between idiotype and auto-anti-idiotype antibody production occurs (25).

The decline with age in immune responses is of great theoretical and practical importance. The theory of aging postulated by Walford (26) and Burnet (27) considers immunosenescence as the underlying basis for aging. The exact mechanisms of the decline of immunocompetence associated with aging are not clearly understood, although it is generally accepted that they are somehow related to depressed thymic hormone production (28-30). Thymic hormones, and thymosin in particular, have been widely used for treatment of primary immunodeficiency diseases (31-33). Thymosin treatment of aged individuals or patients with advanced stages of cancer has also produced improvement in T-cell functions (34,35).

The thymus gland plays a central role in the immune defense mechanism by producing effector and regulator T-lymphocytes and also polypeptide hormones. Thymic hormones have a differentiator role in lymphopoiesis (36,37). Since bone marrow stem cells from old mice are not defective in their regenerative capacity, it is possible that pre-T-stem level is intact, but the factors that provide the capacity to differentiate or proliferate these pre-T cells into mature T cells are deficient in aging mice. The number of pre-T stem cells is influenced by the thymus, the external environment, and the age of the host. An increase in pre-T stem is seen in nude mice and thymectomized mice. Pre-T stem can be detected by treating bone marrow or spleen cells in vitro with thymic extracts or chemicals that induce cell surface markers characteristic of T cells, including TL, Thy-1, and Lyt. Some of the thymic factors that can induce T-cell surface markers are thymosin, ubiquitin, and thymopoietin. Chemicals producing the same effects are cyclic adenosine monophosphate (AMP), dibutyryl cyclic AMP, polyadenosine/uracil, and endotoxin (38).

If the differentiation signals provided by the thymic hormones can be shown to be intact, it may well be that deficiency lies in the proliferative growth signals (IL-1, IL-2, or both). A recent study indicates that functional maturation of B cells is also directly controlled to some extent by thymic hormones (39) or IL-2. IL-2 has been shown to allow the in vivo induction of antierythrocyte autoantibody production in nude mice injected with rat erythrocytes (40).

These results indicate that the altered reactivity experienced during aging depends on selective loss or depletion of specific subsets of effector cells (T and B) and regulatory cells both in absolute numbers of cells and in the functional activity per cell and in their interactions.

III. LYMPHOKINES AND THEIR ROLE IN AGING

The importance of lymphokines in maintaining functional T cells, B cells, and macrophages must be emphasized. Lymphokines serve as the messengers that permit cellular interdependency to be fully realized in vivo. Defective macrophage, T-cell, and B-cell function in aging may conceivably be the indirect result of a thymic hormone deficiency. A study by Knop (41) provides evidence that the IL-producing ability of murine monocytes is associated with well-differentiated macrophages. The functional maturation of macrophages also requires a lymphokine, which can only be provided by mature T cells. The macrophage-Ia-recruiting factor (42–44) has been implicated in macrophage maturation. The close interrelationship of T cells with macrophages is apparent. T cells not only play a role in macrophage maturation (Ia induction), but it is believed that pre-T cell interacts with such Ia^+ cells to induce the former to produce IL-1, which in turn, in combination with Ia^+ cells, stimulates IL-2 production and T-lymphocyte proliferation (45,46). Thus, it is possible that the aging of the T-cell population is responsible for the decline in the number of fully differentiated macrophages and the loss of IL-2 production, and the T-cell deficiency may be the result of thymic hormone depletion.

Thoman and Weigle (47,48) showed a decreased production of IL-2 in cultures stimulated by concanavalin A (Con A) and alloantigen from aged mice and a restoration of antibody responses to sheep red cells upon supplementation of cultures with IL-2. Both Morgan and Weigle (49) and Miller and Stutman (50) suggest that the lesion in aging is due only to a reduction in production of IL-2, not to inability of old cells to respond to the factor. However, work in rats and humans suggests that both aspects become defective with age (51).

The relationship of IL-1, IL-2, cytolytic T lymphocytes (CTL), and natural killer (NK) activities are also closely interrelated and may be relevant for long-term survival (52). Rodents subjected to dietary restriction without malnutrition live longer and develop spontaneous tumors less often or later in life than unrestricted controls. At all ages the response of restricted mice was less than that of controls. However, after injection of polyinosinic-polycytidylic acid, which increases NK activity, old restricted mice showed NK cytolysis not different from young mice on either diet, and substantially higher responses than old unrestricted mice. In addition, restricted mice showed increased in vitro generation of CTL to YAC-1 and P-815 compared with age-matched controls. In this regard an interesting observation has been made on healthy individuals over 80 years of age who have been monitored for NK activity. In contrast to findings from animal studies, healthy old humans possess higher NK activity than people aged 20–40 years (53). Whether this means that individuals with low NK activity fail to survive into old age is currently unknown, but it poses interesting questions. For example, does a relationship exist between cancer-free human survival and the NK component of the immune system? Or can NK-cell activity be used as a biomarker determinant for longevity?

Natural killer cells from naive spleens of normal mice have been shown to respond directly to TCGF (T-cell growth factor, IL-2) and to clonally replicate without other stimulating agents. The cloned NK cells growing in IL-2 showed potent NK activity against several targets (YAC-1, P-815, and EL-4) without addition of an NK-activating agent, interferon (IFN) (54). Such NK cells proliferating in IL-2 all produced IFN. In the absence of IL-2, neither growth nor IFN production could be detected (55).

Finally, we would like to stress that it is likely that aging of the immune system represents the sum of many mechanisms that are altered at the molecular, cellular, and organ levels. Since it is not possible to study all aspects of immunosenescence simultaneously, we must examine limited numbers of parameters (e.g., IL-2 production and NK activities) that play a role in a number of vitally important functions. It is hoped that through this disciplined approach, the bits and pieces of information that make up the entire fabric of immunity in aging will be eventually assembled.

IV. THYMIC HORMONES IN LONGITUDINAL AND CROSS-SECTIONAL STUDIES

Over the past several years, we have carried out a methodical characterization of TM4, TP5, FTS, and thymosin fraction V on specific and less specific immune functions. These studies included both longitudinal (life time) and cross-sectional assessments. In the cross-sectional studies different age groups were treated 5 times per week for 3 weeks with the different hormone preparations, and animals were then assessed for various immune parameters. The studies were done in three strains of mice: CFW, C57BL/6, and A/He. The parameters measured were peripheral blood lymphocytes (PBL) and spleen mitogen responses, Coombs' autoantibodies (IgG_1, IgG_2, IgG_3, IgA, and IgM classes) to mouse red blood cells, hemolytic IgM autoantibodies to erythrocytes treated with bromelain enzyme (HB antigens), antinuclear antibodies, and thymic and splenic autorosettes. CTL responses to P-815 targets also were assayed by chromium release assays. Weight of animals, hematocrit, PBL counts, and spleen and thymus cell counts were also made throughout the study. All assessments were done on individual animals.

Parallel studies were carried out in longitudinal fashion on the three strains as well. The hormone doses and schedule used for animals in the longitudinal study are shown in Table 1. The specific tasks performed on mice in the longitudinal studies are shown in Table 2. Mice were monitored every 3 months.

Our major observation was that none of the hormones were toxic over long-term treatment, but some accelerated autoimmune antibodies in the strains used. Of all the thymic hormones used, only TM4 showed a specific median life span extension in CFW mice. Life span studies in the C57BL/6 mice could not be completed because of failure of heating equipment during the winter, which occurred during the second year of the study when the C57 mice were 16

Table 1 Thymic Hormones, Dose, and Schedule for the Longitudinal Study[a]

Treatment group[b]	Hormone[c] or control substance	Dose/ mouse	Schedule (times/week)	Provider
A or 1	FTS	1 μg	3	Dr. J.-F. Bach
B or 2	FTS	10 ng	3	
C or 3	TP5	1 μg	1	Dr. G. Goldstein
D or 4	TP5	10 ng	3	
E or 5	TM4	1 ng	1	Dr. G. Goldstein
F or 6	TH	10 μg	1	Dr. A. Goldstein
G or 7	TH	1 μg	1	
H or 8	Saline	0.1 ml	1	UAB Pharmacy

[a]Studies were started in September 1979 with the C57BL/6 strain, followed by CFW in October 1979 and A/He mice in March 1980. Thymic hormone supplementation was started when the mice were approximately 2 months of age. The mice were followed for a number of immunological functions at the inception and every 3 months thereafter.
[b]Each of 25 animals in each group was identified by ear mark individually. At each time of assay the same 15 animals from each group were monitored individually until replacement due to mortality. There were 8 groups for each mouse strain, 200 animals per strain.
[c]FTS = facteur thymique serique, the thymic humoral factor (Glu-Ala-Lys-Ser-Gln-Gly-Gly-Ser-Asn-OH); TP5 = thymopoietin (Arg-Lys-Asp-Val-Tyr); TM4 = an enzyme-resistant variant of FTS (Sar-Lys-Sar-Gln-NH_2); TH = thymosin fraction V.

Table 2 Study I: Longitudinal Studies on Hormone-treated Mice and Untreated Mice

Animal groups and treatment	Number of animals[a]	Measurements performed on 15 mice per group every 3 months
C57Bl (25 mice/hormone), 7 hormones (groups 1–7)	175	Weight Hematocrit
C57Bl, not treated (group 8)	25	Peripheral blood lymphocyte counts
CFW mice, 7 hormones (groups 1–7)	175	Peripheral blood lymphocyte response:
CFW, not treated (group 8)	25	a. Phytohemagglutinin (PHA)
A/He (25 mice/hormone), 7 hormones (groups 1–7)	175	b. Concanavalin A (Con A) c. Lipopolysaccharide (LPS)
A/He, not treated (group 8)	25	Coombs' assay for autoantierythrocyte antibodies of classes IgG_1, IgG_2, IgG_3, IgA, and IgM
		Antierythrocyte antibodies (hemolytic IgM to bromelain-treated erythrocytes)
		Antinuclear antibodies
		Physical appearance
		Life span
		Autopsy of mice found dead during the study (all mice)

[a]Total number of mice = 600.

months old. The results of this trial are included here to show the severe loss that can result from a drop in temperature for a period of 24 h. Although animals did not die immediately during or after the exposure, they never recovered from the effects of hypothermia. The resulting loss of many of the old animals invalidated the life span studies. Survival curves and tables showing the median survival of C57BL/6, CFW, and A/He mice appear in Figures 1-3 and Tables 3-5.

It is clear that there was shortening of maximum life span in the C57BL/6 group of mice (Figure 1). Maximum survival was only 32 months for group 5 (Table 3). The outbred CFW strain showed that group 5 mice treated with TM4 had a median survival time (MST) of 31 months and a 6-month increase in MST over controls. Maximum life span, however, was not increased (Table 4). The theoretical curve of death due to aging for a population would be rectangular. Figure 2 shows that the group 5 mice constituted a more homogeneous population dying because of aging as compared to group 8. There was no survival advantage in treating the A/He strain with the TM4 thymic hormone (Figure 3, Table 5). It would be crucial to confirm the survival results seen for the outbred CFW strain, and to test additional outbred strains for effects of TM4 on life span.

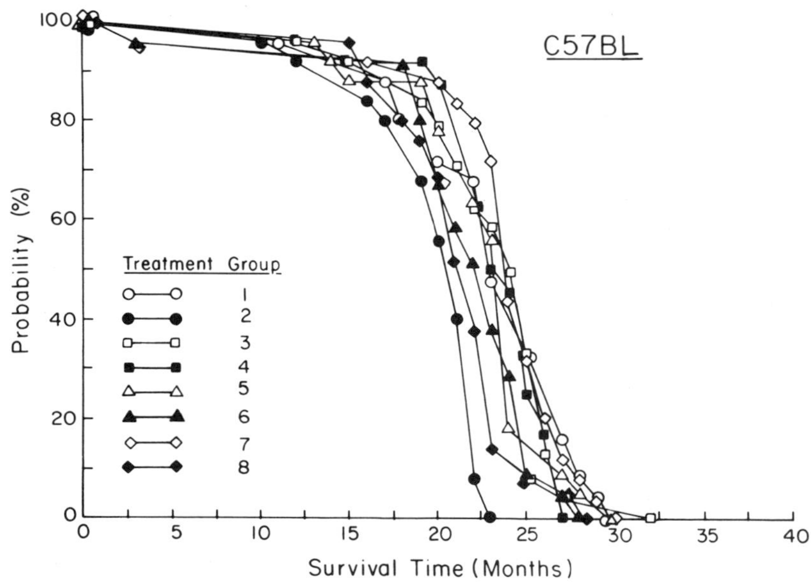

Figure 1 Probability of survival versus survival time of C57BL/6 mice treated with thymic hormone preparations.

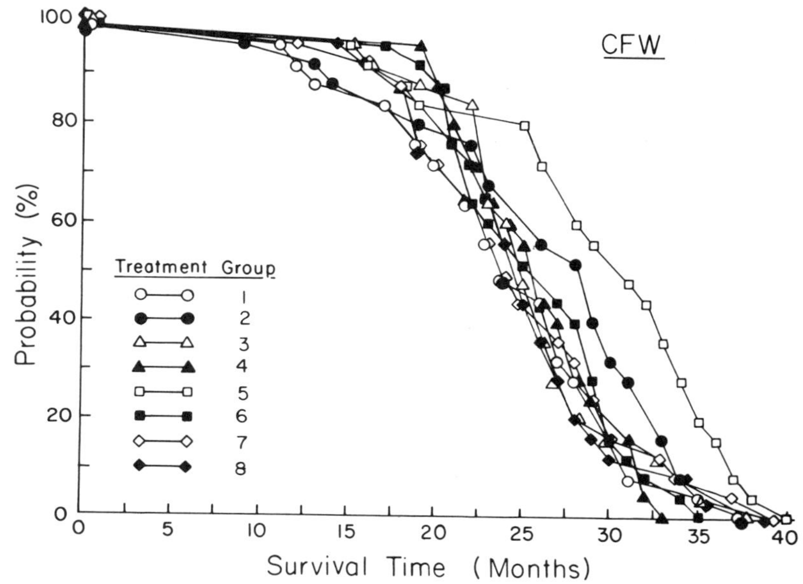

Figure 2 Probability of survival versus survival time of CFW mice treated with thymic hormoné preparations.

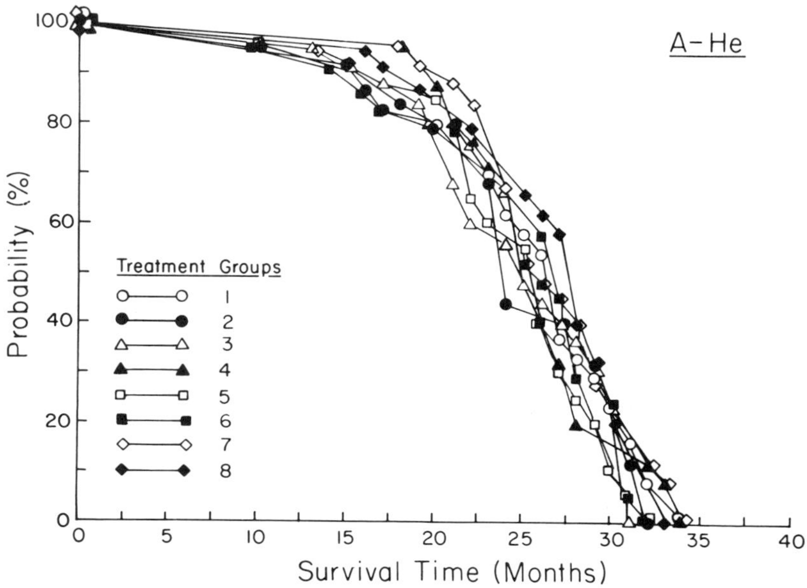

Figure 3 Probability of survival versus survival time of A/He mice treated with thymic hormone preparations.

Table 3 Analysis of Survival of C57BL/6 Mice Treated with Thymic Hormones

Treatment group	Median survival time (months)	% Surviving > 25 months	Maximum survival time (months)	p^a
1	23	32	30	.08
2	20	0	23	.14
3	23	16	30	.07
4	22	8	28	.35
5	24	32	32	.05
6	23	24	27	.02
7	24	32	30	.03
8 (control)	21	8	28	–

[a]Compare with group 8 (control) according to the *overall* survival based on the generalized Wilcoxon test.

We found that mice on long-term hormone treatment (longitudinal studies) produced a greater number of hormone-related changes than mice on short-term treatment (cross-sectional studies). Table 6 shows statistically significant hormone-related enhancement or suppression for changes in weight, PBL numbers, PBL Con-A response, PBL lipopolysaccharide (LPS) response, and antinuclear antibodies (ANA) for C57 mice treated longitudinally as compared to only suppression of hematocrit (Hct) in the short-term treated mice. Therefore, to demonstrate the effects of hormone treatment, longitudinal studies rather than cross-sectional studies should be done.

We have also investigated changes in certain biomarkers with age. Cross-sectional studies showed CTL activity to allogeneic target cells (P-815) declined

Table 4 Analysis of Survival of CFW Mice Treated with Thymic Hormones

Treatment group	Median survival time (months)	% Surviving > 30 months	Maximum survival time (months)	p^a
1	24	16	38	.82
2	28	32	38	.20
3	25	16	38	.65
4	26	24	33	.59
5	31	56	40	.01
6	26	16	35	.63
7	24	24	39	.95
8 (control)	24	12	39	–

[a]Compare with group 8 (control) according to the *overall* survival based on the generalized Wilcoxon test.

Table 5 Analysis of Survival of A/He Mice Treated with Thymic Hormones

Treatment group	Median survival time (months)	% Surviving > 30 months	Maximum survival time (months)	p^a
1	26	28	34	.56
2	24	24	32	.51
3	25	20	31	.35
4	25	20	34	.46
5	25	10	32	.17
6	26	12	32	.42
7	26	24	34	.97
8 (control)	28	20	32	–

[a]Compare with group 8 (control) according to the overall survival based on the generalized Wilcoxon test.

with age, but we found in all three strains (longitudinal studies) that changes in weight, hematocrit, autoantibody levels, PBL count, and phytohemagglutinin (PHA) responses also correlate with aging in all these strains. None of these parameters requires sacrifice of the animals, and the monitoring of these changes, which can serve as biomarkers of aging in mice, provides, perhaps a more uniform way of comparing cohorts of different ages. Figures 4-6 show changes in weight and Figures 7-9 show decline in hematocrit with age in three strains of mice given the different hormone treatments 1-7. Group 8 represents the saline control group. Lines have been connected for group 8. Only values showing a trend of being elevated or depressed repeatedly over time were considered important for inclusion in Table 6. For example, there were distinct effects of thymic hormone on different parameters in different strains of mice. Figure 4 indicates that thymosin-treated C57BL/6 mice (group 6) showed an increased tendency to be heavier than the other hormone-treated groups, whereas mice treated with FTS (groups 1 and 2) and TP5 (group 4) tended to exhibit weight suppression between 52 and 88 weeks. In like manner, thymosin and FTS (groups 6 and 7 and groups 1 and 2, respectively) treatment of A/He mice showed the same tendencies reflected in their weights (Figure 6). The overall appearance of the curve for weight for all three strains was an initial increase, and for CFW and A/He strains, an age-related decrease occurred over time.

The treatment of the different strains with hormone also produced distinctly different effects in the different strains (Figures 7-9 and Table 6). In the CFW mice, TM4 treatment had a tendency to increase hematocrit levels. The overall appearance of the curve for hematocrit declined with age in all three strains.

To explain the long median survival in CFW mice treated with TM4, we considered several alternative explanations. These were: (a) TM4 treatment

Table 6 Similarities and Differences Between Short-Term and Long-Term Treatment for Each Strain

		Strain[b]		
Measurement	Study[a]	C57	CFW	A/He
Weight	L	+ (6) - (1, 2, 4)	0	+ (6) - (1, 2)
	C	0	0	0
Hematocrit	L	0	+ (5)	- (2, 3, 5-7)
	C	- (6)	+ (1, 2)	0
PBL	L	- (1-4, 6, 7)	- (1-6)	0
	C	0	0	- (5)
PBL (unstimulated)	L	0	0	0
	C	0	0	0
PBL, PHA	L	0	- (3)	+ (3)
	C	0	0	0
PBL, PHA, stimulation index	L	0	0	0
	C	0	0	0
PBL, Con A	L	- (1-7)	- (1-6)	+ (1-4)
	C	0	0	+ (4)
PBL, Con A, stimulation index	L	0	- (1-5)	0
	C	0	0	0
PBL, LPS	L	- (1-5)	- (3)	0
	C	0	0	0
PBL, LPS, stimulation index	L	0	- (1-3)	0
	C	0	0	0
Coombs' assay	L	0	0	- (1-3)
	C	0	0	- (1-4, 7)
IgM autoantibody	L	0	0	+ (6)
	C	0	0	0
ANA	L	+ (6)	0	+ (1-6)
	C	0	0	

[a]L = longitudinal studies (long-term treatment), C = cross-sectional studies (short-term treatment).

[b]Key: + = enhanced activity, - = depressed activity, and 0 = no effect. Hormone treatment group numbers given in parenthesis.

extended survival by maintaining immune reactivity over the long term, (b) TM4 caused animals to reduce their caloric intake, which in turn increased the MST, and (c) TM4 treatment reduced the number of malignancies in the CFW strain and thus permitted more animals to live longer. We found that the activities of the different immune parameters that we measured did not correlate with survival of the TM4-treated group. Although caloric restriction and low body weight are known to extend life span, we found that TM4 injections did not

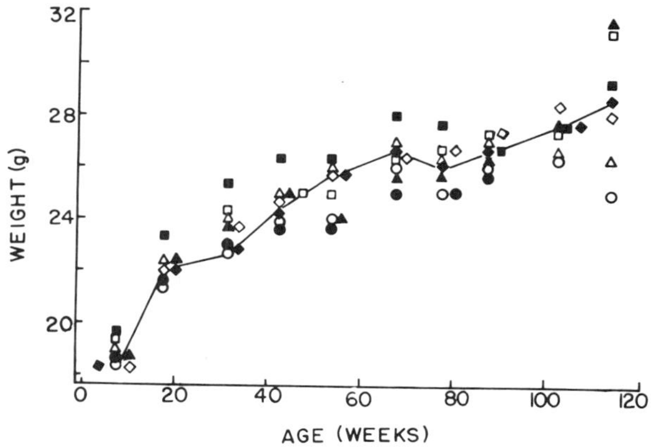

Figure 4 Average body weight per mouse versus age of C57BL/6 mice treated with thymic hormone preparations. The mice were followed every 2-3 months.

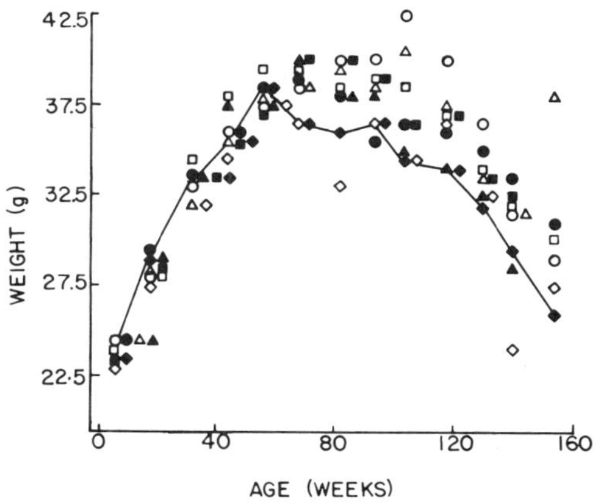

Figure 5 Average body weight per mouse versus age of CFW mice treated with thymic hormone preparations. The mice were followed every 2-3 months.

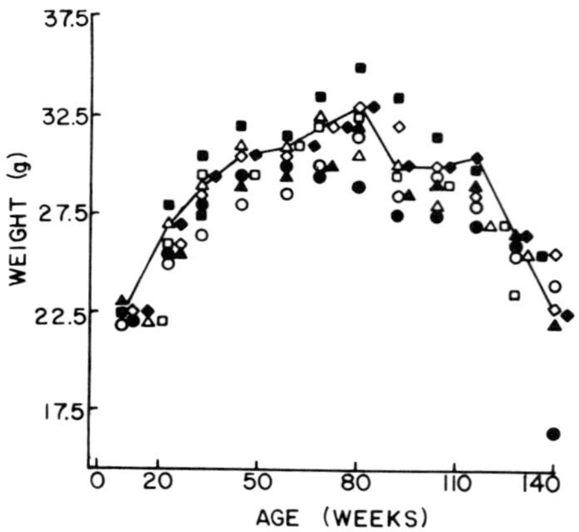

Figure 6 Average body weight per mouse versus age of A/He mice treated with thymic hormone preparations. The mice were followed every 2–3 months.

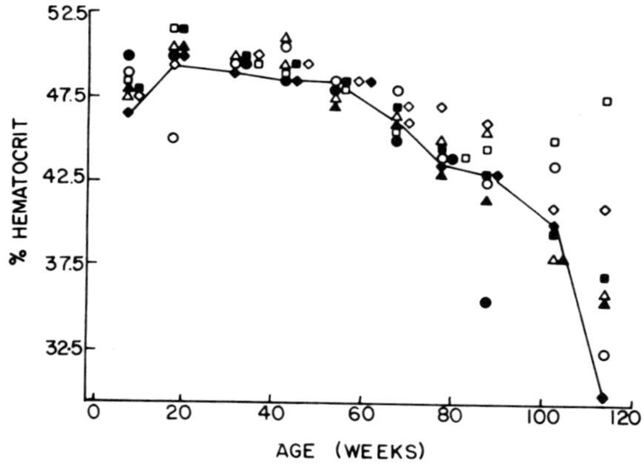

Figure 7 Average percent hematocrit per mouse versus age of C57BL/6 mice treated with thymic hormone preparations. The animals were followed every 2–3 months at the time weight and other functions were monitored.

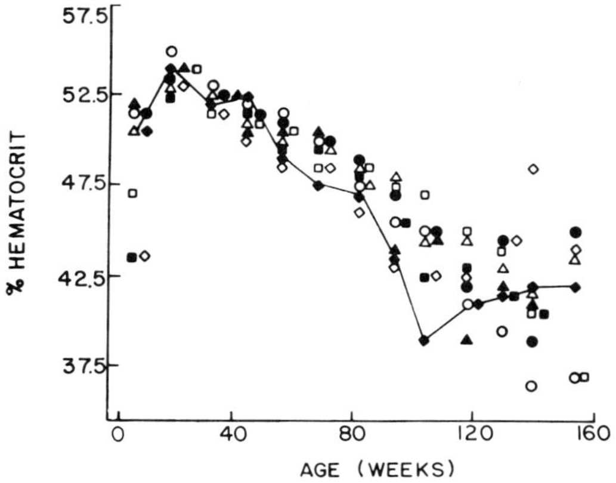

Figure 8 Average percent hematocrit per mouse versus age of CFW mice treated with thymic hormone preparations. The mice were followed every 2-3 months, at the time weight and other functions were monitored.

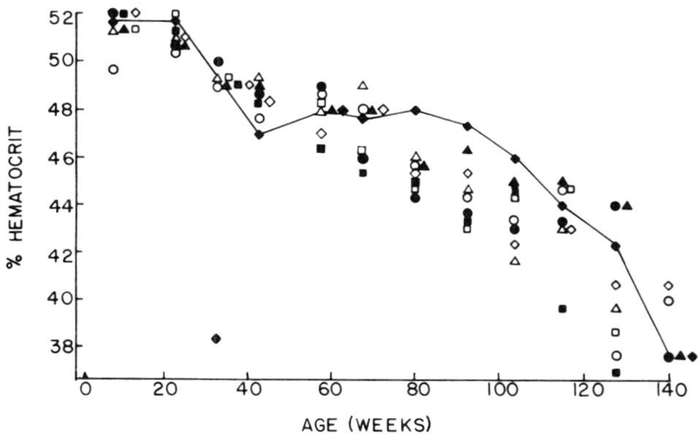

Figure 9 Average percent hematocrit per mouse versus age of A/He mice treated with thymic hormone preparations. The mice were followed every 2-3 months, at the time weight and other functions were monitored.

induce mice to reduce their intake of food. Comparisons of the weights of long-term survivors showed that the TM4-treated animals were heavier than the control group.

If the TM4-treated mice were protected from developing histologically detectable malignancies, such an effect could explain the longer survival for this group. The gross pathology at autopsy (Table 7) appears to support this view in that the TM4 treatment group (5) showed that 44% of the animals had no abnormalities at death whereas group 8 (control) mice had only 24% without gross abnormalities; that is, 76% of the control mice showed abnormalities at autopsy. However, group 1 also had low abnormalities (48%), but the differences were not statistically significant. Histopathological assessment was made on various tissue for three groups: 1, 5, and 8. Group 1 (FTS), whose MST was similar to the saline control group, was included as an additional hormone-treated control for the histopathology studies. No statistically significant differences in types of tumor or number of tumors between groups 1, 5, and 8 were discerned, but the histological examination showed that group 5 mice had no amyloid in their tissues (Table 8). To assess whether amyloid was important in survival, group 1 and 8 animals that had amyloid in their tissues were compared against those that had none. No significant difference in survival could be shown. Therefore, the reason for long-term survival in CFW mice treated with TM4 is still not known.

Amyloid, a proteinaceous substance with a fibrillar structure, is deposited in extracellular tissues in certain diseases and in aging. Amyloid deposits increase in number with age as senile plaques in many tissues, as well as in the brain and are said to be the best single indicator of the aging process. They are found in abundance in senile dementia of the Alzheimer type. Amyloidosis is not a single disease. It can be produced from a variety of proteins, but these have as a common characteristic a β-pleated protein conformation. Scheinberg et al. (56) showed that the administration of thymosin V to mice receiving casein injections preserved T-cell function and exhibited reduced incidence and severity of experimental amyloidosis. The depression of T-cell function observed in experimentally induced amyloidosis and the disordered B-cell function, which is generally seen, imply that aberration of the immune regulatory function may be related to amyloid deposition. Therefore, aside from the possibility of life span extension, treatment with TM4 may have other therapeutic values. The complete absence of amyloid in the TM4-treated group is a most significant observation and requires further study. It may be that long survival is not related to any single parameter but to changes in a number of different parameters. It is interesting to note that group 5 animals showed not only longer survival and no amyloid, but also a tendency to have higher hematocrits between 55 and 117 weeks (Table 8).

Table 7 Histological Findings at Autopsy of CFW Mice That Died from Disease or from Old Age

Treatment group	N	Liver mass	Liver enlarged	Spleen mass	Spleen enlarged	Lung mass	Thymus, mediastinal mass	Lymph node enlarged	Lymph node mass	Edema	Kidney	Reproductive system	Heart	Pancreas	Brain	Adrenal gland	Pituitary gland	Anemia	None
1	25	1 (4%)	1 (4%)		3 (12%)	4 (16%)		6 (24%)	3 (12%)	1 (4%)		3 (12%)							12 (48%)
2	25	1 (4%)	3 (12%)		4 (16%)	7 (28%)		6 (24%)	2 (8%)	1 (4%)		3 (12%)					1 (4%)	3 (12%)	11 (44%)
3	25	3 (12%)	1 (4%)		1 (4%)	4 (16%)		7 (28%)	3 (12%)	2 (8%)		2 (8%)					1 (4%)	1 (4%)	13[a] (52%)
4	25	2 (8%)	1 (4%)		1 (4%)	5 (20%)	3 (12%)	4 (16%)	2 (8%)	1 (4%)	1 (4%)	1 (4%)		2 (8%)	1 (4%)	2 (8%)	1 (4%)	1 (4%)	11 (44%)
5	25	1 (4%)	2 (8%)		1 (4%)	8 (32%)		5 (20%)	3 (12%)	1 (4%)		1 (4%)							11 (44%)
6	25			1 (4%)	1 (4%)	9 (36%)		1 (4%)	3 (12%)	2 (8%)	1 (4%)							2 (8%)	10 (40%)
7	25	2 (8%)		1 (4%)	1 (4%)	6 (24%)	1 (4%)	3 (12%)	3 (12%)	3 (12%)		1 (4%)							14[a] (56%)
8	25	2 (8%)	3 (12%)	1 (4%)	2 (8%)	7 (28%)		11 (44%)	1 (4%)	1 (4%)		1 (4%)				2 (8%)		2 (8%)	6 (24%)
Total	200	12 (6%)	11 (6%)	3 (2%)	14 (7%)	50 (25%)	4 (2%)	43 (22%)	20 (10%)	12 (6%)	2 (1%)	12 (6%)		2 (1%)	1 (1%)	4 (2%)	3 (2%)	9 (5%)	88 (44%)

[a]Significantly different from the group 8 (control), $p < .05$.

Table 8 Comparison of Median Survival and Presence of Amyloid in Three Treatment Groups of CFW Strain

Treatment group	Median survival time (months)	Amyloid (% positive)	Hematocrit
1	24	9/19 (47%)[a]	
5	31	0/16 (0%)	Increased (55–117) weeks
8 (control)	24	9/19 (47%)[a]	

[a]The percentage of mice with amyloid is significant at $p = .001$ when compared with group 5 (TM4).

V. IS THERE A BASIS FOR IMMUNOGERONTOLOGY?

It would be presumptuous to believe that the decline in the function of the thymus gland is the only cause of the general aging process that takes place in animals. It is possible, however, that the thymus is the biological clock that controls the aging of the immune system and that the immune system as it ages plays an important role in influencing the general process of aging of an animal. The maximum life span of each species is predetermined. Therefore, it would be particularly important to identify the gene complex that fixes the limits of the life span of a given animal species. This notion has acquired more precise meaning from the studies of Walford (57). A correlation between the major histocompatibility complex (MHC) haplotype and maximum life span in mice has been found. The mechanisms by which the MHC influences life span are largely unknown, and may or may not involve the immune system. However, since the control of the immune responses is one of the major functions of the MHC, the possible relevance of these studies to immunogerontology should not be neglected.

Segre (58) suggests two major goals to consider: (a) to experimentally test the hypothesis that the deterioration of the immune system is a primary cause of aging, and (b) to find a means to delay the age-related decline of the immune potential. He states, "A demonstration of the primary role of the immune system in aging will require the experimental prolongation of life span by immunologic interventions shown to maintain the integrity of the immune system over time." If this can be accomplished, the second goal will have been fulfilled, as well. In this regard, it is not likely that any intervention used to increase life span, whether by dietary or immunological means, could change the maximum life span of the species, which is genetically predetermined. It is likely that the median life span can be extended.

VI. CONCLUSIONS

We have shown that the immune system may play an important role in aging. The experimental prolongation of the median life span by immunological intervention using TM4 in the outbred CFW strain has been accomplished in mice treated from 2 months of age continuously for life. By selectively testing for changes in key lymphokine pathways and by monitoring selected effector functions, we may be able to establish the basis for the prolongation of life in the CFW strain. Additional studies must be done to determine whether, by hormone treatment, integrity of the immune system is actually being maintained. To further test this concept, it would be important to show whether TM4 treatment will extend MST in other strains of mice. In addition, it would be crucial to determine whether MST can be extended if treatment is started later in the life of the animals (i.e., at 6 and 12 months of age).

ACKNOWLEDGMENT

This work was supported by the National Institute on Aging, National Institute of Health contract NO1 AG-9-2100.

REFERENCES

1. Weksler, M. E. 1979. Age-associated changes in the immune response. *J. Am. Geriatr. Soc.* 30:718.
2. Meredith, P. J., and R. L. Walford. 1979. Autoimmunity, histocompatibility, and aging. *Mech. Ageing Dev.* 9:61.
3. Roberts-Thomson, I. C., S. Wittingham, U. Youngchaiyud, and I. R. MacKay. 1974. Aging immune response and mortality. *Lancet.* 2:368.
4. Goodwin, J. S., R. P. Searles, and S. K. Tung. 1982. Immunologic responses of a healthy elderly population. *Clin. Exp. Immunol.* 48:403.
5. Makinodan, T., and W. H. Adler. 1975. Effects of aging on the differentiation and proliferation potentials of cells of the immune system. *Fed. Proc.* 34:153.
6. Walters, C. S., and H. N. Claman. 1975. Age-related changes in cell-mediated immunity in Balb/c mice. *J. Immunol.* 115:1438.
7. Inkeles, B., J. B. Innes, M. M. Kuntz, A. D. Kadish, and M. E. Weksler. 1977. Immunological studies of aging. III. Cytokinetic basis for the impaired response of lymphocytes from aged humans to plant lectins. *J. Exp. Med.* 145:1176.
8. Hallgren, H. M., J. H. Kersey, D. P. Dubuey, and E. J. Yunis. 1978. Lymphocyte subsets and integrated immune function in aging humans. *Clin. Immunol. Immunopathol.* 10:65.
9. Merhav, S., and H. Gershon. 1977. The mixed lymphocyte response of senescent mice: Sensitivity to antigen and cell replication time. *Cell Immunol.* 34:354.

10. Shigemoto, S., S. Kishimoto, and Y. Yamamura. 1975. T-helper activity and an increase in T-suppressor functions. *J. Immunol.* 115:307.
11. Goidl, E. A., J. B. Innes, and M. E. Weksler. 1976. Immunological studies of aging. II. Loss of IgG and high avidity plaque-forming cells and increased suppressor cell activity in aging mice. *J. Exp. Med.* 144:1037.
12. Doria, G., G. D'Agostaro, and M. Garavini. 1980. Age-dependent changes of B-cell reactivity and T cell–T cell interactions in the in vitro antibody response. *Cell. Immunol.* 53:195.
13. Kishimoto, S., S. Tomino, H. Mitsuya, and H. Nishimura. 1982. Age-related decrease in frequencies of B-cell precursors and specific helper T cells involved in the IgG anti-tetanus toxoid antibody production in humans. *Clin. Immunol. Immunopathol.* 25:1.
14. Mascart-Lemone, F., G. Delespesse, G. Servais, and M. Kunstler. 1982. Characterization of immunoregulatory T-lymphocytes during aging by monoclonal antibodies. *Clin. Exp. Immunol.* 48:148.
15. Adler, S. J., A. A. Morley, and R. S. Seshadri. 1982. Reduced lymphocyte colony formation with age. *Clin. Exp. Immunol.* 49:129.
16. Kishimoto, S., S. Tomino, K. Inomata, S. Kotegawa, T. Saito, M. Kuroki, J. Mitsuya, and S. Hisawitsu. 1978. Age-related changes in subsets and functions of human T-lymphocytes. *J. Immunol.* 121:1773.
17. Girard, J. P., M. Paychere, M. Cueves, and F. Fernandez. 1977. Cell-mediated immunity in an aging population. *Clin. Exp. Immunol.* 27:85.
18. Sohnle, P. G., C. Collins-Loch, and K. E. Huhta. 1983. Kinetics of lymphokine production by lymphocytes from elderly humans. *Gerontology.* 29:169.
19. Gillis, S., R. Kozak, M. Durante, and M. E. Weksler. 1981. Immunological studies of aging. *J. Clin. Invest.* 67:937.
20. Gupta, S. 1984. Autologous mixed lymphocyte reaction in man. *Scand. J. Immunol.* 19:187.
21. Hicks, M. A., J. F. Jones, A. C. Thies, K. A. Weigle, and L. L. Mimumich. 1983. Age-related changes in mitogen-induced lymphocyte function from birth to old age. *Am. J. Clin. Pathol.* 80:159.
22. Otte, R. B., S. Wormsley, and J. W. Hollingsworth. 1983. Cytofluorographic analysis of pokeweed mitogen-stimulated human peripheral blood cells in culture: Age-related characteristics. *J. Am. Geriatr. Soc.* 31:49.
23. Lokhorst, H. M., J. A. Van der Linden, H. F. Schuurman, G.F.H.J. Meyling, E.J.E.G. Bast, and G. C. deGast. 1983. Immune function during aging in man: Relation between serological abnormalities and cellular immune status. *Eur. J. Clin. Invest.* 13:209.
24. Dworsky, R., A. Paganini-Hill, M. Authur, and J. Parker. 1983. Immune responses of healthy humans 83–104 years of age. *J. Natl. Cancer Inst.* 71:265.
25. Goidl, E. A., J. W. Choy, J. J. Gibbons, M. E. Weksler, G. J. Thorbecke, and G. W. Siskind. 1983. Production of anti-antiidiotype antibody during the normal immune response. *J. Exp. Med.* 157:1635.

26. Walford, R. L. 1974. Immunological theory of aging: Current status. *Fed. Proc.* 33:2020.
27. Burnet, M. 1970. An immunological approach to aging. *Lancet.* 2:358.
28. Bach, J. F., M. Dardenne, J. Pleau, and M. Bach. 1975. Isolation and biochemical characteristics, and biological activity of a circulating thymic hormone in the mouse and in the human. *Ann. N.Y. Acad. Sci.* 249:186.
29. Lewis, V. M., J. J. Twomey, P. Bealmear, G. Goldstein, and R. A. Good. 1978. Age, thymic involution, and circulating thymic hormone activity. *J. Clin. Endocrinol. Metab.* 47:145.
30. Trainin, N. 1974. Thymic hormones and the immune response. *Physiol. Rev.* 54:272.
31. Wara, D., A. L. Goldstein, N. Doyle, and A. Ammann. 1975. Thymosin activity in patients with cellular immunodeficiency. *N. Engl. J. Med.* 292: 70.
32. Wara, D. W., D. J. Barrett, A. J. Ammann, and M. J. Cowan. 1979. In vitro and in vivo enhancement of mixed lymphocyte culture reactivity by thymosin in patients with primary immunodeficiency disease. *Ann. N.Y. Acad. Sci.* 332:128.
33. Costanzi, J., J. Daniels, G. Thurman, A. Goldstein, and J. Hokanson. 1979. Clinical trials with thymosin. *Ann. N.Y. Acad. Sci.* 332:148.
34. Chretien, P. B., S. D. Lipson, R. W. Makuch, and D. E. Kenady. 1979. Effects of thymosin in vitro in cancer patients and correlation with clinical course after thymosin therapy. *Ann. N.Y. Acad. Sci.* 332:135.
35. Wara, W. M., A. J. Ammann, and D. W. Wara. 1978. Effect of thymosin and irradiation on immune modulation in head and neck and esophageal cancer patients. *Cancer Treat. Rep.* 62:1775.
36. Simpson, E., and P. Beverley. 1977. T-cell subpopulations. *In* Progress in Immunology, Vol. III. T. E. Mandel et al., editors. Academic Press, New York. 206.
37. Marshall, G. D., T. L. Low, G. B. Thurman, and A. L. Goldstein. 1978. Recent advances in thymosin research. *In* Human Lymphocyte Differentiation: Its Application to Cancer. B. Serron and C. Rosenfield, editors. Elsevier/North Holland, Biomedical Press, Amsterdam. 271.
38. Stutman, O. 1977. Two main features of T-cell development: Thymus traffic and postthymic maturation. *Contemp. Top. Immunobiol.* 7:1.
39. Siskind, G. W. 1979. Ontogeny of B-cell function: A role for the thymus in regulating the maturation of the B-cell population. *In* Aging and Immunity. S. K. Singhal, N. R. Sinclair, and C. K. Stiller, editors. Elsevier/ North Holland, New York. 35.
40. Reimann, J., and T. Diamantstein. 1981. Interleukin-2 allows in vivo induction of anti-erythrocyte autoantibody production in nude mice associated with the injection of rat erythrocytes. *Clin. Exp. Immunol.* 43:641.
41. Knop, J. 1980. Influence of various macrophage populations on Con A induced T-cell proliferation. *Immunology.* 411:379.
42. Beller, D. I., J. M. Kiely, and E. R. Unanue. 1980. Regulation of macro-

phage populations. I. Preferential induction of Ia-rich peritoneal exudates by immunologic stimuli. *J. Immunol.* 124:1426.
43. Scher, M. G., D. I. Beller, and E. R. Unanue. 1980. Demonstration of a soluble mediator that induces exudates rich in Ia-positive macrophages. *J. Exp. Med.* 152:1684.
44. Lu, C. Y., E. Peters, and E. R. Unanue. 1981. Ia-bearing macrophages in athymic mice: Antigen presentation and regulation. *J. Immunol.* 126: 2496.
45. Larsson, E., A. Coutino, and C. Martinez-A. 1980. A suggested mechanism for T lymphocyte activation: Implications on acquisition of functional reactivities. *Immunol. Rev.* 51:61.
46. Larsson, E. L. 1982. Functional heterogeneity of helper T cells: Two distinct helper T cells are required for the production of T-cell growth factor. *J. Immunol.* 128:742.
47. Thoman, M. L., and W. O. Weigle. 1981. Lymphokine and aging: Interleukin-2 production and activity in aged animals. *J. Immunol.* 127:2102.
48. Thoman, M. L., and W. O. Weigle. 1982. Cell-mediated immunity in aged mice: An underlying lesion in IL-2 synthesis. *J. Immunol.* 128:2358.
49. Morgan, E. L., and W. O. Weigle. 1982. The immune response in aged C57BL/6 mice. II. Characterization and reversal of a defect in the ability of aged spleen cells to respond to the adjuvant properties of Fc fragment. *J. Immunol.* 129:36.
50. Miller, R. A., and O. Stutman. 1981. Decline, in aging mice, of the anti-2,4,6-trinitrophenyl (TNP) cytotoxic T-cell response attributable to loss of Lyt-2, interleukin 2-producing helper cell function. *Eur. J. Immunol.* 11:751.
51. Gilman, S. C., J. S. Rosenberg, and J. D. Feldman. 1982. T lymphocytes of young and aged rats. II. Functional defects and the role of interleukin-2. *J. Immunol.* 128:644.
52. Weindruch, R., B. H. Devens, H. V. Raff, and R. L. Walford. 1981. Influence of dietary restriction and aging on natural killer cell activity in mice. *J. Immunol.* 130:993.
53. Krishnaraj, R., and G. Blandford. 1984. Quantitative and qualitative differences in natural killer cell activity in aging. *Gerontologist.* 24:162 (special issue).
54. Suzuki, R., K. Handa, K. Itoh, and K. Kumagai. 1983. Natural killer (NK) cells as a responder to interleukin 2 (IL2) I. Proliferative response and establishment of cloned cells. *J. Immunol.* 130:981.
55. Handa, K., R. Suzuki, H. Matsui, Y. Shimizu, and K. Kumagai. 1983. Natural killer (NK) cells as a responder to interleukin 2 (IL2). II. IL2-induced interferon production. *J. Immunol.* 130:988.
56. Scheinberg, M. A., A. L. Goldstein, and E. S. Cathcart. 1976. Thymosin restores T-cell function and reduces the incidence of amyloid disease in casein-treated mice. *J. Immunol.* 116:156.
57. Walford, R. L. 1980. Immunology and aging. *Am. J. Clin. Pathol.* 74:247.
58. Segre, D. 1982. Experimental immunogerontology: A perspective. *In* Immunology and Aging. N. Fabris, editor. Martinus Nijhoff, Hingham, Mass. 71.

10

Age-Associated Changes in the Synthesis and Function of Cytokines

Marilyn L. Thoman and William O. Weigle

Scripps Clinic and Research Foundation
La Jolla, California

I. INTRODUCTION

The initiation and maintenance of most, if not all, cellular and humoral immune responses requires a series of consecutive signals delivered by antigen and a variety of products of activated lymphocytes and macrophages. Once antigen-specific lymphocytes have been recruited by interaction with antigen, amplification and further differentiation of the recruited lymphocytes is mediated by a cascade of cellular interactions and lymphokines (1). Thus regulation of the synthesis of these factors, or their receptors, has widespread impact on the full spectrum of immunological responses. Indeed, an impairment in the production or activity of several lymphokines is associated with the aging process, as well as various autoimmune disorders, immunodeficiency syndromes, and neoplasms. This chapter outlines the role of several cytokines in maintaining normal immune function and alterations in their production or functions that occur as a consequence of the aging process.

A. Interleukin 1

Also known as endogenous pyrogen and leukocytic endogenous mediator, interleukin 1 (IL-1) is a product of mononuclear phagocytes, corneal epithelial cells, epidermal keratinocytes, and glial cells. The production of IL-1 is induced by a variety of agents including plant lectins, microbial products, antigens, and

Table 1 Interleukin-1 Activity

Function or process	Target cell	Ref.
Proliferation	Thymocytes	30,31
	B cells	12
Prostaglandin synthesis	Hypothalamus	2
Fever induction	Preoptic anterior hypothalamus	26
Collagenase synthesis	Synovial cells	20,21,24
Plasma zinc, copper, and iron concentration regulation	Liver and neutrophils	27,28
Synthesis of acute-phase reactants	Liver	23,29
Protein degradation	Skeletal muscle	25

inflammatory agents (reviewed in Refs. 2,3). IL-1 has numerous biological activities, summarized in Table 1, among which are the abilities to induce fever, to induce the release of acute phase reactants, and to activate B and T lymphocytes.

The mature IL-1 protein is 15,000 Mr, but is synthesized as a high molecular weight precursor form (4). Active subfragments of the 15,000-Mr molecule that have been identified in the serum of less than 5000 Mr retain pyrogenic activity and may represent the physiologically significant form of the protein (5,6). Human IL-1 has an isoelectric point of 6.8–7.0 (7,8), while the murine protein has a *p*I of 5.0–5.4 (9). No evidence suggests that this protein is glycosylated, since neuraminidase treatment has no effect on the isoelectric point or on biological activity (2), and newly synthesized IL-1 is not labeled by inclusion of $[^{14}C]$glucosamine in the culture media (10). Structure-function studies reveal further that no intrachain disulfide linkage is necessary for maintaining IL-1 activity; however, biological function is lost by treatment with the arginine-modifying agent phenylglyoxal (11).

Immunopotentiating properties of IL-1 include the activation of T cells for interleukin-2 (IL-2) production and a B-cell stimulatory activity. As described in detail in Section II.B, IL-2-producing cells require an activation signal delivered via IL-1 to initiate lymphokine synthesis. Originally IL-1 was described as having mitogenic activity for murine thymocytes. However, it is currently believed that the ability of IL-1 to induce T-cell proliferation is secondary to its role in the induction of the T-cell growth factor, IL-2.

In addition to its effects on T cells, IL-1 acts synergistically with other factors to promote B-lymphocyte proliferation. IL-1 is required as a second trigger, apparently late in the G_1 phase of the cell cycle, to facilitate progress of the cells into S phase (12).

The mechanism of IL-1 activity has not been fully elucidated, but it is postulated that a major function is to promote the "maturation" of T and B cells. Incubation of cortical thymocytes with IL-1 causes a decrease in the expression of Thy and Lyt-2 surface markers (13); furthermore, IL-1 incubation increases the expression of antigen receptors (14–16) on murine T cells and markedly increases the frequency of stable E-rosette receptor sites on human peripheral blood T lymphocytes (17), thought to reflect T-cell activation. B-cell maturation may also be influenced by IL-1, since bone marrow cells incubated with IL-1 show an increase in surface Ig, Ia, and complement receptors (18). These data suggest that IL-1 may act on resting B and T cells, and Simic (19) has presented data that IL-1 does in fact interact with thymocytes in the G_0 stage of the cell cycle.

The activation of arachidonic acid metabolism may be important for mediating IL-1 action (20–22). Stimulation of the cyclooxygenase pathway of arachidonic acid breakdown in fibroblasts, in synovial cells, and in the hypothalamus occurs as a consequence of IL-1 interaction with these cells. The activity of the lipoxygenase pathway of arachidonic acid metabolism is essential for thymocyte activation by IL-1, and inhibition of this pathway completely suppresses this response (22).

B. Interleukin 2

Perhaps the best characterized lymphokine is the T-cell growth factor, interleukin 2. The biological activities of this factor are as follows:

Supports long-term T-cell growth
Induces T-cell proliferation
Supports growth of natural killer cells
Required for cytolytic T-cell differentiation
Proliferation cofactor for B cells

Human IL-2 is composed of a single polypeptide chain 133 amino acids long. A single intramolecular disulfide bridge linking residues 58 and 105 is essential for maintaining the biologically active configuration of this protein (30,31). The protein can be variably glycosylated, giving rise to multiple isoelectric species, but apparently the carbohydrate is not required for activity (32,33).

IL-2 is the product of activated T cells, primarily of the helper–inducer subset (34), Lyt-1^+ in the mouse, although production of this factor by T cells of other phenotypes has also been reported (35). Initiation of IL-2 synthesis requires activation of the producer cells by antigen (or mitogen) and a macrophage-derived factor, interleukin 1 (36). Encoding of IL-2 by messenger RNA (mRNA) is found in the activated cells within 2 h after stimulation, and maximal factor activity is found in the culture supernatant at 12–16 h (33,37).

IL-2 synthesis can be regulated at several points (Figure 1). Macrophage control of IL-2 production involves the release of both IL-1 (the necessary cofactor) and suppressive compounds. Prostaglandins of the E series, produced by

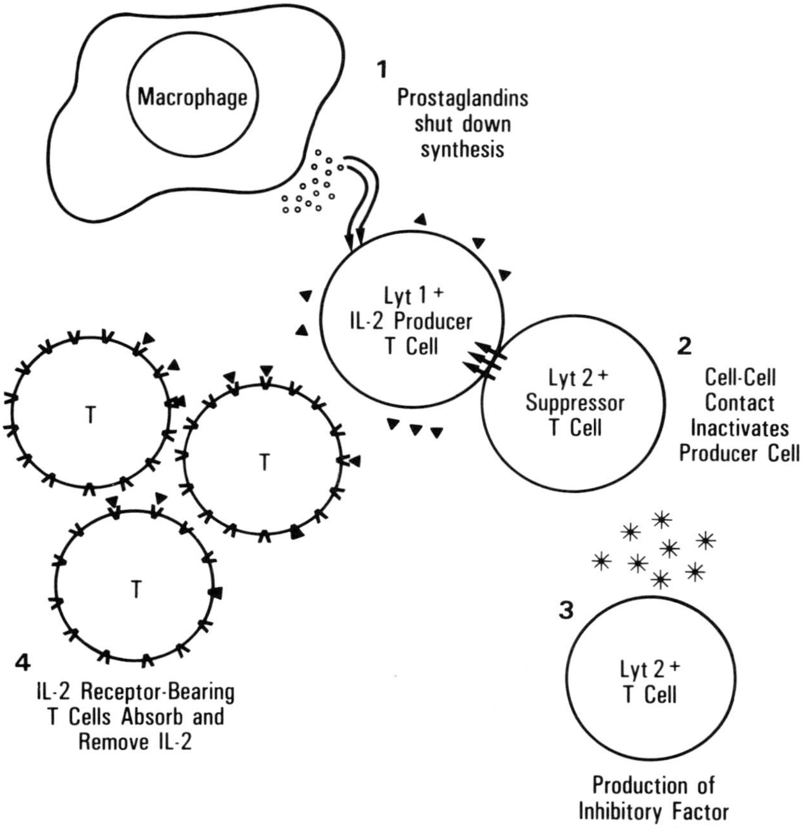

Figure 1 Mechanisms regulating IL-2 synthesis and availability.

activated macrophages, are potent inhibitors of IL-2 synthesis (38–41). Suppressor T cells have also been identified that inactivate IL-2 producer cells (42), absorb IL-2 (43,44), or produce a circulating, inhibitory factor (45) that blocks IL-2 activity. At least four mechanisms have been described that lower the available amount of IL-2, thus limiting the effective range of IL-2 in the microenvironment.

Interleukin 2 activity is dependent on the expression of a cell membrane receptor, originally described as present only on activated T cells (46,47). Recently, IL-2 receptors have also been identified on activated B lymphocytes (48). The human IL-2 receptor is a glycoprotein of 47,000–53,000 Mr. Some evidence suggests that the 47,000-Mr molecule is noncovalently associated with at least two other polypeptides of 113,000 and 180,000 Mr, respectively, forming a receptor complex. The development of monoclonal antibodies reactive to the IL-2 receptor has made possible more detailed biochemical analyses of the synthesis of the receptor, since these antibodies also recognize a 33,000-Mr precursor form of the receptor. This 33,000-Mr polypeptide is glycosylated with both N- and O-linked sugars and sialic acid, and may be further sulfated and phosphorylated before transport of the mature protein to the membrane (47).

Early studies of the IL-2 receptor, using radiolabeled IL-2, identified on activated T cells 4000–10,000 receptors with a Kd of 10^{-12}M (46). No such binding sites could be identified on B cells. However, estimates of the number of IL-2 receptors made using anti-IL-2 receptor antibodies are much higher, between 60,000 and 200,000, since the antibody recognizes a second class of receptor present in large numbers on activated lymphocytes, but having 1000–2000 less binding affinity for IL-2 (47,49). Activated B cells possess this class of low-affinity IL-2 receptor, and thus bind the anti-IL-2 receptor antibody.

Interleukin-2-driven T-cell proliferation requires the acquisition of the receptor on activated T cells, which occurs during the early G_1-G_{1a} phase of the cell cycle. IL-2 receptors can be identified within 2–4 h of cellular activation, and maximum expression is reached by 24 h. Interaction of IL-2 with its receptor initiates a burst of RNA synthesis (G_{1b}) and ultimately DNA synthesis. Although IL-2 originally was felt to be the sole lymphokine necessary for triggering DNA synthesis in T cells, more recent studies suggest a requirement for the binding of transferrin for progress from G_{1b} into S phase (50). If IL-2 is continuously present, cells completing mitosis will initiate a second round of proliferation; with subsequent cell cycles, however, expression of the IL-2 receptor diminishes and ultimately the cells become refractory to IL-2, requiring reactivation by mitogen or antigen. The "reactivated" cells display IL-2 receptors more rapidly and to a higher level than naive cells and are therefore considered to possess some "memory" of their previous expression of this receptor (51,52). The expression of the IL-2 receptor requires new RNA and protein synthesis, and activation of protein kinase appears to be involved. IL-2 itself up-regulates the expression of its own receptor, apparently increasing IL-2 receptor mRNA synthesis (53–55).

The role of the IL-2 receptor on activated B cells is not clear. Binding studies indicate that this receptor is of the low-affinity class, and present in far fewer numbers than on activated T cells. Recently several investigations have probed the effect of IL-2 on B-cell growth and differentiation. Utilizing highly purified tonsillar B cells, preactivated by exposure to *Staphylococcus aureus* Cowan I, Muraguchi et al. (48) demonstrated that IL-2 was able to augment both B-cell growth and differentiation to immunoglobulin synthesis.

In vitro studies have defined the role of IL-2 in initiating and driving B- and T-cell proliferation. However, the in vivo function of this lymphokine has not been completely elucidated. Deficiencies in the production and response to

IL-2 are found associated with several disease conditions, including autoimmune and immunodeficiency syndromes (56,57), suggesting that perturbation in lymphokine function might be involved in the pathogenesis of these conditions. For example, T lymphocytes from acquired immune deficiency syndrome patients not only produce little IL-2, but may also overproduce suppressive factors that block IL-2 function (56).

IL-2 has been shown to induce T-cell markers and to function on splenic lymphocytes when administered intraperitoneally to athymic nude mice. Cytolytic and helper T-cell activity can be generated in nude mice in response to specific antigen or alloantigenic stimulation when IL-2-containing lymphokine preparations are concurrently administered (57–59). Given alone, IL-2 has no T-cell generative effect. Furthermore, administration of IL-2 to normal adult animals can enhance natural killer cell activity and the generation of cytolytic T cells (60). These effects are generally weak (increasing activity approximately twofold), but they clearly demonstrate an effect of this lymphokine on the generation of T-cell responses. By using very large quantitites of recombinant IL-2, Rosenberg et al. (61) enhanced the in vivo generation of cytolytic T cells in adult mice by five- to sevenfold. IL-2 has been shown to prolong the in vivo survival of cytolytic T cells, activated in vitro to a specific antigen (62). The in vivo half-life of IL-2 is quite short, approximately 2 min when administered intravenously and 2 h when given intraperitoneally (63). These results suggest that in vivo IL-2 acts at very short range, influencing cell activity within a local microenvironment, rather than systemically.

C. B-Cell Growth and Differentiation Factors

The activation of B lymphocytes to proliferation and ultimately to immunoglobulin production is a multistep process that may require the action of several growth-promoting and differentiation-inducing factors. At least four distinct lymphokines that are involved in B-cell proliferation have been identified, including B-cell growth factors I and II (BCGF), IL-1, and IL-2. It is not clear, however, whether these factors all trigger the same B-lymphocyte subsets (64–70). Furthermore, two differentiation factors, BCDF I and BCDF II, have been defined which are involved in driving cycling B cells to antibody secretion. The hypothesized sequence of action of these factors is illustrated in Figure 2; Table 2 summarizes the physiochemical properties of these factors.

Although it is assumed that specific cell surface receptors exist for these factors, only two have been identified, the IL-2 receptor (discussed in Section I.B) and the murine BCDF I receptor. The identification and purification of the BCDF I receptor was made feasible by the generation of an antireceptor antibody utilizing the DBA/2Ha mouse strain whose B cells lack the receptor for BCDF I. This antiserum reacts with a 120,000-Mr protein that upon reduction,

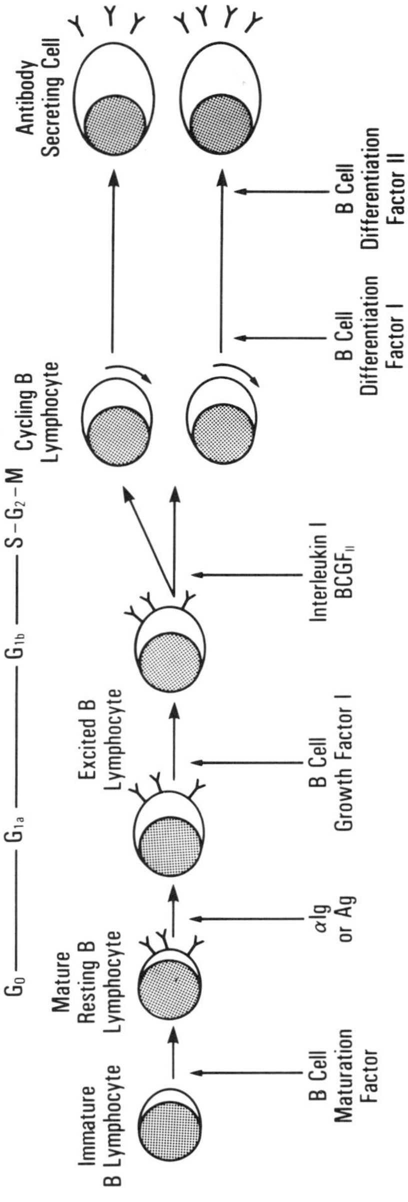

Figure 2 B-cell activation and differentiation: proposed sites of lymphokine action.

Table 2 Physiochemical Properties of Several B-Cell-Active Lymphokines

Factor[a]	Species	Mr ($\times 10^3$)	Isoelectric point	Other properties
BCGF I (BSF-p1)	Murine	15–20	6.4–6.6 7.4–7.6	Weakly hydrophobic
BCGF I (BSF-p1)	Human	15–20	6.5–6.9	
BCGF II (EL-BCGF-swa)	Murine	50–60	4.6 5.4 6.0	Hydrophilic
BCGF II	Human	50		
BCDF I (B15-BCDF-nak, B15-TRF)	Human	45–60	4.9–5.1	
BCDF II (EL-BCDF-nak, EL-TRF)	Murine	30–40	4.5	Moderately hydrophobic
BMF	Murine	50–55	5–6	Highly hydrophobic

[a]BCGF = B-cell growth factor, BCDF = B-cell differentiation factor, TRF = T-cell replacing factor, and BMF = B-cell maturation factor; alternative nomenclature in parentheses.

becomes 60,000 Mr and is present on activated normal murine B cells and on the B-cell leukemia line, BCL_1 (71).

III. SYNTHESIS AND FUNCTION OF LYMPHOKINES IN THE AGED

A. Interleukin 1

Few studies have been made on the synthesis and activity of IL-1 in the aged, but in Table 3 summarizes available findings. Some species differences are found related to the ability to generate or respond to this factor, as is also seen with other lymphokines. Peritoneal macrophages from aged rats, when stimulated with bacterial lipopolysaccharide (LPS), release IL-1 in quantities equal to or greater than the amounts generated in similar cultures containing peritoneal macrophages from young animals (72,73). In contrast, the production of IL-1 by macrophages of aged mice is low (74,75a). Both the spontaneous release (75a) and LPS-stimulated release of IL-1 (74) by murine peritoneal adherent cells is reduced by approximately 50% compared to that produced by young murine macrophages. In these studies, the IL-1 activity was assessed by its lymphostimulatory properties.

A single report exists examining the ability of human peripheral blood monocytes from aged and young individuals to produce endogenous pyrogen (EP). No significant difference in the ability to produce EP was found; un-

Table 3 Effect of Age on Interleukin-1 Synthesis and Receptor Expression

IL-1 activity	Species	Effect
Synthesis	Human	Variable: low to normal
	Rat	Normal
	Mouse	Low
Receptor expression	Mouse	Slightly lower

fortunately, however, the results were not expressed individually, but were averaged over the entire group of aged or young persons. The authors suggest that certain aged individuals displayed impaired EP production (75b). The contention that the synthesis or activity of endogenous pyrogen in aged humans is faulty is supported by the lack of a febrile response in the aged to infectious disease, or other conditions that invoke fever in the young (2). More work is needed to pinpoint the explanation for this observation and to understand how it relates to IL-1 synthesis.

IL-1 receptors on aged murine T cells were quantitated by the ability to absorb this lymphokine. T-cell blasts from aged and young animals, activated by phytohemagglutinin (PHA), were incubated with IL-1-containing media for 2 h, after which the remaining IL-1 activity was quantitated. Young blast cells inactivated approximately 10% more IL-1 than did aged cells, thus suggesting that the number of receptors is slightly higher on young cells (74). One important consideration, however, for interpreting these data is that the "absorption" was performed at 37°C and therefore is more accurately a measurement of utilization or inactivation, rather than absorption. Higher metabolic activity of the young cells could therefore account for the differences seen, even if both populations possessed the same number of lymphokine receptors. Furthermore, IL-1 receptors may be more easily quantitated on resting thymocytes, since the target of this monokine appears to be a cell in G_0 (19).

Attempts to improve immune activity in the aged with IL-1 have met with little success. Exogenous IL-1 does not improve mixed lymphocyte responses or cytotoxic T-cell generation by aged murine spleen cells (74). However, as discussed in Section II.A, IL-1 has numerous nonlymphoid target cells, triggering many and varied responses, only one aspect of which, the lymphostimulatory property, has been examined in the aged. Therefore, more investigations are necessary before the physiological significance of the age-associated reduction in IL-1 synthesis can be fully elucidated.

B. Interleukin 2

The synthesis and the activity of IL-2 in aged humans and experimental animals have been examined. Not unexpectedly, both processes are defective in the elderly (76–80). IL-2 synthesis by aged mice is approximately 50–75% reduced compared to levels generated by cells from young adult animals (76,77). Lymphokine synthesis in response to both mitogenic and allogeneic stimulation is low, indicating that the inability of the aged to produce IL-2 is not merely due to a loss of receptors for plant lectins.

As indicated in Table 4, some species differences in IL-2 synthesis have been identified. Although IL-2 production in response to alloantigenic stimulus in the rat is low, the activation of aged rat spleen cells with the plant lectin concanavalin A results in a normal, high quantity of IL-2 production (78). In contrast, neither human nor murine lymphocytes can be triggered to high levels of lymphokine release with plant lectins.

As outlined in Section II.B, the synthesis of IL-2 is a multistep process that is known to be regulated at several sites. Producer T cells require two activation signals to initiate lymphokine production: the mitogen or antigen, and IL-1, the macrophage-derived factor. As detailed in Section III.A, the production of IL-1 by LPS-activated peritoneal macrophages of aged mice is low. However, this defect does not appear to be responsible for limiting IL-2 synthesis, since macrophages from aged animals are able to support IL-2 synthesis by young adult T cells (74,77,81). Furthermore, young adult macrophages are unable to restore lymphokine production by aged T cells.

Several investigators have failed to identify suppressor cells that might limit IL-2 synthesis in the aged, either in cell mixing experiments or by depletion of putative inhibitory populations. One such experiment, outlined in Table 5, tested the effect on the production of IL-2 of the removal of various classes of suppressor cells, including populations bearing the Lyt-2 surface marker, the histamine type-2 receptor (82,83), or those agglutinable with peanut agglutinin (84). The depletion of either the Lyt-2$^+$ or the histamine-receptor-positive cells results in an increase in IL-2 production by both the aged and young spleen cells. However, the quantity of IL-2 generated by the aged population even after suppressor cell removal does not approach that produced by the young adult population. Depletion of the peanut-agglutinin-positive cells lowers the IL-2 synthesizing capacity of both young and aged spleen cells.

Table 4 Interleukin-2 Synthesis in the Aged

Species	Stimulus[a]	IL-2 production[b]
Human	Mitogen	Low
Rat	Mitogen	High
	Alloantigen	Low
Mouse	Mitogen	Low
	Alloantigen	Low

[a]Agent used to trigger lymphokine production.
[b]Relative to amounts produced by young adult cells under identical conditions.

Table 5 Effect on Interleukin-2 Synthesis of Suppressor Cell Removal in Young and Aged Mice[a]

Suppressor cell type	Animal	Amount of IL-2 (U/ml) Intact	Depleted
Lyt-2$^+$	Young	100	266.7
	Aged	6.7	30
H-2 (histamine receptor), positive	Young	100	167.5
	Aged	12.8	36.5
Peanut agglutinin positive	Young	100	49.4
	Aged	4.7	3.3

[a]Spleen cells from aged or young adult animals were depleted of the various putative suppressors and cultured with concanavalin A for 24 h. The amount of IL-2 in the culture fluid was quantitated in a T-cell growth factor assay.

The producer T-cell population itself is apparently the defective element in the aged animal. Limiting dilution analysis indicates a three- to fivefold decrease in the precursor frequency of IL-2 producer cells in aged mice (85). Despite the decline in the frequency of producer cells, the quantity of IL-2 produced per cell is not altered by the aging process. Using a complementary DNA probe, Cheung et al. (86) have demonstrated that activated aged spleen cells, as a population, contain half the number of mRNA copies for IL-2 as do similarly stimulated young spleen cells. In conjunction with the limiting dilution analysis, this would indicate that the loss of IL-2 synthetic capacity is not due to a block in the translation process allowing an accumulation of IL-2 mRNA without the production of the protein product; rather, it seems to occur at a step preceding message synthesis.

The mechanisms that result in a lack of IL-2 producer cells in the aged are unidentified, but may be related to the involution and loss of endocrine function of the thymus. Although the pluripotent stem cells resident in the bone marrow of aged mice are fully able to reconstitute the immune system of irradiated young adult host animals, T-cell maturation in aged animals is markedly impaired (87,88). Circulating thymic hormones undoubtedly play an important role in this process, and their loss during aging (89) may significantly affect peripheral T-cell maturation and function. Thymic hormones have been used to improve immune responsiveness in both humans and experimental animals (91-97). Furthermore, thymic hormones specifically influence the activity of lymphokine-producing cells as illustrated by the capacity of such to enhance IL-2 production by human peripheral blood lymphocytes (PBL) and murine spleen cells, as well as to induce IL-2-producing cells from spleen cells of the athymic nude mouse (Table 6) (98–100). Hormone treatment of spleen cells

Table 6 Effect of Thymic Hormones on Interleukin-2 Synthesis

Hormone	Target cell	% Increase in units of IL-2 per milliliter after hormone treatment
Thymulin	Spleen cells, nude mice	500–900
Thymosin	Human peripheral blood lymphocytes	20–350
Thymus humoral factor	Murine spleen cells, aged animals	0–784
Thymus humoral factor	Murine spleen cells, young animals	10–100

from immunodeficient aged mice also improved their ability to produce IL-2, although this was not consistently observed (100).

The ability to respond to IL-2 is apparently also impaired in aged individuals. The expression of the IL-2 receptor is reduced in aged human and rat lymphocytes, as inferred by the low capacity of these cells to absorb and remove IL-2 activity from solution (Table 7) (78,79). The direct binding of radiolabeled lymphokine to aged lymphocytes has not been investigated; however, fluorescence studies using antireceptor antibodies indicate that fewer receptors are found on activated aged human and murine lymphocytes than on their younger counterparts (50). However, as discussed earlier, the antireceptor antibody identifies both high- and low-affinity receptors present on both activated B and T cells, and the physiological significance of the low-affinity receptors has not been defined. Therefore, it is not yet known whether the lack of receptors on aged cells is due to a reduction in both high- and low-affinity receptors, or of only one of these populations.

Functional studies utilizing purified IL-2 to reconstitute immunological responses in the aged has met with varied success (Table 8). Two studies using human PBL report conflicting results regarding the ability of exogenous IL-2 to restore PHA-induced proliferation. Gillis et al. (79) reported that the addition of IL-2 had either no effect or an inhibitory effect on the amount of ^{3}H[thymidine] incorporated by aged PBL cocultured with PHA. In contrast, Kennes et al. (80) reported that exogenous IL-2 increased DNA synthesis to levels found in cultures of young adult PBL stimulated by PHA but without extra IL-2. In animal studies, the ability of IL-2 to improve lymphoproliferative responses also appears to vary (72,101–104). However, other immune responses are markedly enhanced by exogenous IL-2 reaching levels equal or near those generated by young adult cells. As shown in Table 8, the generation of cytotoxic, suppressor T cells and helper T-cell responses can be enhanced by exogenous IL-2. Table 9

Table 7 Interleukin-2 Receptor Expression on Aged Lymphocytes

Species	Method of measurement	Receptor expression (compared to adult)
Human	Absorption	Low
	Proliferation	Low–normal
	Binding of antireceptor (αTac) antibody	Low
Rat	Absorption	Low
	Proliferation	Low
Mouse	α-IL-2 receptor binding	Low
	Proliferation	Normal–slightly lower

illustrates that in our hands, aged responses are usually restored by lymphokine to levels equal to those in young unsupplemented cultures.

Exogenous IL-2 is able to markedly enhance both humoral and cellular secondary responses in cultures of aged lymphocytes. These findings are of particular significance because they indicate that antigen sensitization occurs in the aged, and that the loss of the secondary response is due primarily to the limited expansion of the activated T-cell clones. The generation of a secondary response can be divided into a sensitization phase and an expansion phase. Which of these phases is adversely affected by aging can be distinguished through use of IL-2. That is, if sensitization does not occur normally in the aged environment, even adequate clonal proliferation induced by the IL-2 will not reconstitute the response to levels near that displayed by young adult animals. On the other hand,

Table 8 Effect of Interleukin-2 on in Vitro Immune Responses

Species	Immune response	Effect of IL-2	Ref.
Human	Mitogen-induced proliferation	None	79
		Enhancement	80
Rat	Mitogen-induced proliferation	None	73, 78
Mouse	Mitogen-induced proliferation	None–slight enhancement	105
	Alloantigen-induced proliferation	Enhancement	101
	Cytotoxic T-lymphocyte generation	Enhancement	74, 101, 103, 104
	Suppressor T-cell generation	Enhancement	102

Table 9 Magnitude of Interleukin-2 Effect on in Vitro Responses of Young Adult and Aged Mice

Response	Source of responder cells	% Normal response	
		-IL-1	+IL-2
1° Antibody	Young	100	140
	Aged	24	87
2° Antibody	Young	100	90
	Aged	20	79
Mixed lymphocyte reaction	Young	100	117
	Aged	23	108
Cell-mediated lympholysis	Young	100	102
	Aged	17	93
Suppressor cells	Young	100	102
	Aged	10.6	98

Source: Ref. 81.

should sensitization occur normally, but clonal proliferation be limited, addition of IL-2 should fully reconstitute this response, as is demonstrated to occur in aged mice. Thus, the addition of IL-2 is able to promote T-cell proliferation, enabling an adequate secondary response.

IL-2 can reconstitute immune responsiveness in vivo as well as in vitro in aged mice (105). The effect of IL-2 on the in vivo generation of cytolytic T cells and a T-dependent humoral response was assessed, administering the lymphokine in multiple doses over the course of several days, as depicted in Figure 3. The IL-2 used for these studies was either partially purified murine lymphokine or a highly purified human IL-2, prepared by recombinant DNA technology. Table 10 summarizes the results of the experiments analyzing the generation of either primary or secondary cytolytic T-cell responses or primary humoral responses in the presence or absence of IL-2. Both IL-2 preparations were able to markedly enhance the generation of cytotoxic cells in aged animals. The cytolytic activity of both splenocytes and peritoneal cells was enhanced in the presence of the lymphokine, raising the response to levels found in young adult animals. Similarly, the plaque-forming cell (PFC) response to sheep red blood cells (SRBC) was improved by IL-2 administration. These data indicate that the administration of lymphokines has a major impact on in vitro and in vivo immune responsiveness of aged mice.

C. Other Lymphokines

The synthesis of only two other lymphokines has been investigated in the aged, a murine B-cell-activating factor (106) and human leukocytic migration inhibitory

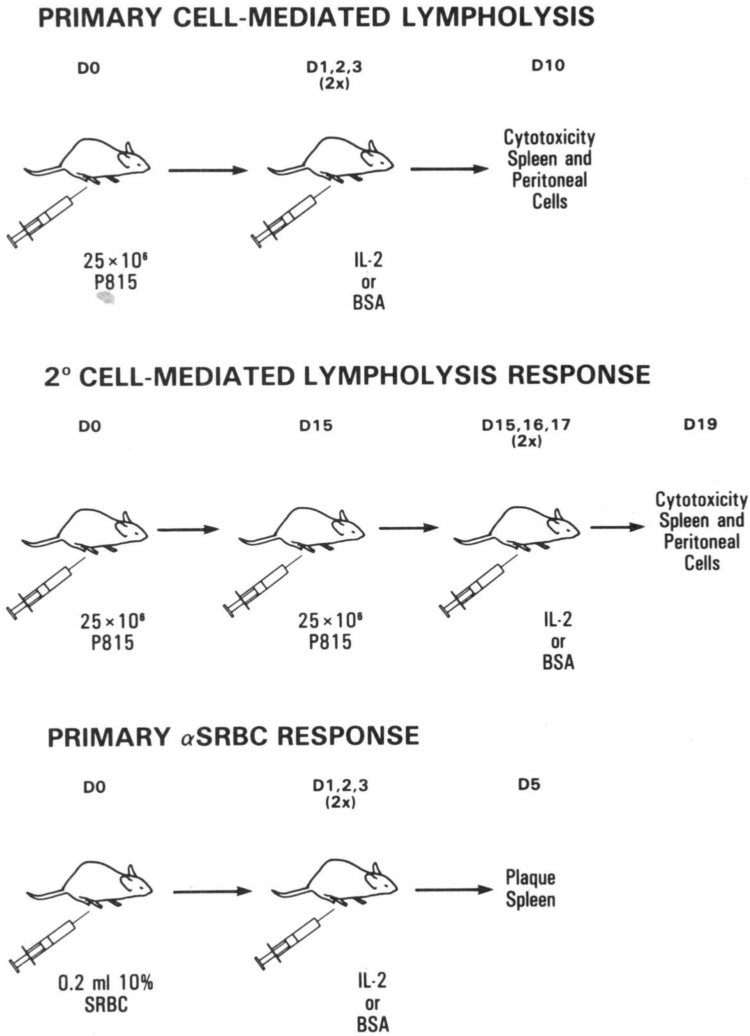

Figure 3 Injection protocols for the generation of in vivo immune responses (SRBC = sheep red blood cells; BSA = bovine serum albumin).

Table 10 Restoration of Immune Responses by in Vivo Administration of Interleukin-2

	Age of mice	IL-2 source		Responses
		Conventional	Recombinant	
				Cytolytic (%)[a]
Primary cytolytic T-cell generation	Young	–	–	83.5
		–	+	76.5
	Aged	–	–	17.3
Secondary cytolytic T-cell generation	Young	–	–	80.4
		–	+	90.3
		+	–	65.4
	Aged	–	–	11.1
		–	+	80.0
		+	–	59.1
				PFC (direct plaques/10^6 input cells)[b]
Primary SRBC PFC response	Young	–	–	833
		–	+	631
	Aged	–	–	36
		–	+	198

[a]Normalized % specific release.
[b]Normalized specific release.
Source: Ref. 105.

factor (LMIF) (107,108). The B-cell-activating factor (BCAF) affects B-lymphocyte differentiation, replacing T-cell function for the induction of a polyclonal antibody response, and enhancing antigen-specific humoral responses (109). Aged mice are unable to generate the polyclonal response, partly because of the lack of BCAF synthesis, which is reduced by approximately 75% in the aged (106, Figure 4). No further characterization of the mechanisms underlying the diminution in BCAF production has been undertaken.

The production of LMIF by PBL from aged humans in response to a variety of recall antigens has also been shown to be defective (Table 11). Interestingly, no defect in the synthesis of this factor can be demonstrated if the PBL are maximally activated by mitogens such as PHA or concanavalin A, suggesting that the activation process is impaired in the aged, rather than the ability to synthesize this lymphokine (107,108).

Although the ability of the aged to synthesize immunologically active lymphokines such as interferon and B-cell growth and differentiation factors has not been investigated, it is likely that these processes too will be impaired. The synthesis of many of these factors appears linked or interdependent. IL-2 has been shown to be important for the induction of γ-interferon, for example

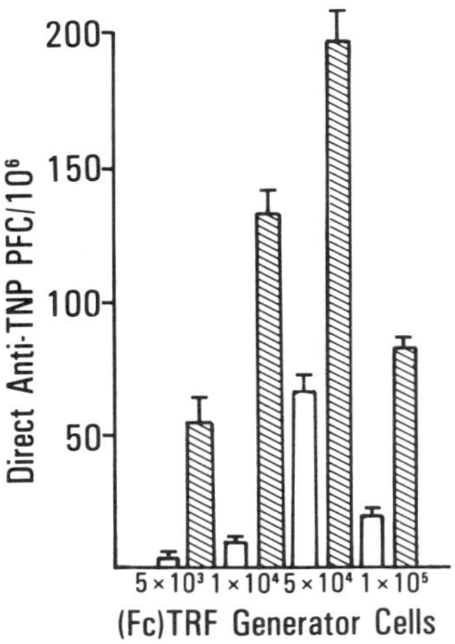

Figure 4 Comparison of the ability of aged (open bars) and adult (hatched bars) spleen cells to produce B-cell activating factor (BCAF). BCAF was generated by stimulating spleen cells with Fc fragments prepared from human immunogen for 24 h (TRF = T-cell replacing factor). BCAF activity was detected by its ability to replace T-cell function in the generation of a polyclonal antibody response (TNP = trinitrophenyl). (From Ref. 109.)

Table 11 Production of Leukocyte Migration Inhibitory Factor by Human Peripheral Blood Lymphocytes

Stimulatory agent	Number of positive subjects	
	Young	Aged
Purified protein derivative	40/42	5/54
Candida	52/53	8/64
Streptokinase streptodornase	9/10	2/10
Tetanus	5/9	1/9
Concanavalin A	10/10	9/10
Phytohemagglutinin	46/49	38/54

Source: Refs. 107 and 108.

(110), and several BCGFs, colony-stimulating factors, and IL-2 appear to be produced by the same T-cell population (111-113). Therefore, if such a population is diminished during the aging process, the production of several lymphokines would be adversely affected. Understanding the processes contributing to the loss of lymphokine-synthesizing capability will be the experimental challenge of the next few years, with the ultimate goal of preventing the deterioration of this function and preserving immunological vigor of the aged.

REFERENCES

1. Farrar, J. J., W. R. Benjamin, M. L. Hilfiker, M. Howard, W. L. Farrar, and J. Fuller-Farrar. 1982. The biochemistry, biology, and role of interleukin 2 in the induction of cytotoxic T cell and antibody-forming cell responses. *Immunol. Rev.* 63:129.
2. Dinarello, C. A. 1984. Interleukin-1. *Rev. Infect. Dis.* 6:51.
3. Dinarello, C. A. 1982. Leukocytic pyrogen. *In* Lymphokines. E. Pick and M. Landy, editors. Academic Press, Orlando, Fla. 24.
4. Mizel, S., and D. Rosenstreich. 1979. Regulation of lymphocyte-activating factor (LAF) production and secretion in $P388D_1$ cells: Identification of high molecular weight precursors of LAF. *J. Immunol.* 122:2173.
5. Gordon, A., and I. Parker. 1980. A pyrogen derived from human white cells which is active in mice. *Br. J. Exp. Pathol.* 61:534.
6. Clowes, G., B. George, C. Villee, and C. Saravis. 1983. Muscle proteolysis induced by a circulating peptide in patients with sepsis or trauma. *N. Engl. J. Med.* 308:545.
7. Blyden, G., and R. E. Handschumacher. 1977. Purification and properties of human lymphocyte-activating factor (LAF). *J. Immunol.* 118:1631.
8. Lachman, L. B., M. P. Hacker, and R. E. Handschumacher. 1977. Partial purification of human lymphocyte-activating factor (LAF) by ultrafiltration and electrophoretic techniques. *J. Immunol.* 119:2019.

9. Mizel, S. B. 1979. Physicochemical characterization of lymphocyte-activating factor (LAF). *J. Immunol.* 122:2167.
10. Murphy, P., T. Cebula, and B. Windle. 1981. Heterogeneity of rabbit endogenous pyrogens is not attributable to glycosylated variants of a single peptide chain. *Infect. Immun.* 34:184.
11. Mizel, S. B. 1980. Studies on the purification and structure–function relationships of murine lymphocyte activating factor (interleukin 1). *Mol. Immunol.* 17:571.
12. Falkoff, R.J.M., A. Muraguchi, J.-X. Hong, J. L. Butler, C. A. Dinarello, and A. S. Fauci. 1983. The effects of interleukin 1 on human B cell activation and proliferation. *J. Immunol.* 131:801.
13. Beller, D. I., and E. R. Unanue. 1977. Thymic maturation in vitro by a secretory product from macrophages. *J. Immunol.* 118:1780.
14. Puri, J., M. Shinitzky, and P. Lonai. 1980. Concomitant increase in antigen binding and in T cell membrane lipid viscosity induced by the lymphocyte-activating factor, LAF. *J. Immunol.* 124:1937.
15. Rosenwasser, L. J., C. A. Dinarello, and A. S. Rosenthal. 1979. Adherent cell function in murine T-lymphocyte antigen recognition. IV. Enhancement of murine T-cell antigen recognition by human leukocytic pyrogen. *J. Exp. Med.* 150:709.
16. Lonai, P., and L. Steinman. 1977. Physiological regulation of antigen binding to T cells: Role of a soluble macrophage factor and of interferon. *Proc. Natl. Acad. Sci. USA.* 74:5662.
17. Ben-Zvi, A., S. B. Mizel, and J. J. Oppenheim. 1981. Generation of human peripheral blood stable E-rosette-forming T cells by interleukin 1. *Clin. Immunol. Immunopathol.* 19:330.
18. Hoffman, M., S. Koenig, R. Mittler, H. Oettgen, P. Ralph, C. Galanos, and U. Hammerling. 1979. Macrophage factor controlling differentiation of B cells. *J. Immunol.* 122:497.
19. Simic, M. M. 1983. Sensitivity of T cells to interleukin 1 (IL-1) in relation to the cell cycle. *In* Interleukins, Lymphokines, and Cytokines. J. J. Oppenheim and S. Cohen, editors. Academic Press, Orlando, Fla. 481.
20. Dayer, J.-M., J. Breard, L. Chess, and S. M. Krane. 1979. Participation of monocyte-macrophages and lymphocytes in the production of a factor that stimulates collagenase and prostaglandin release in rheumatoid synovial cells. *J. Clin. Invest.* 64:1386.
21. Mizel, S. B., J.-M. Dayer, S. M. Krane, and S. E. Mergenhagen. 1981. Stimulation of rheumatoid synovial cell collagenase and prostaglandin production by partially purified lymphocyte-activating factor (interleukin 1). *Proc. Natl. Acad. Sci. USA.* 78:2474.
22. Dinarello, C. A., S. O. Marnoy, and L. J. Rosenwasser. 1983. Role of arachidonate metabolism in the immunoregulatory function of human leukocyte pyrogen/lymphocyte activating factor/interleukin-1. *In* Interleukins, Lymphokines, and Cytokines. J. J. Oppenheim and S. Cohn, editors. Academic Press, Orlando, Fla. 495.
23. Sztein, M. B., S. N. Vogel, J. D. Sipe, P. A. Murphy, S. B. Mizel, J. J. Oppen-

heim, and D. L. Rosenstreich. 1981. The role of macrophages in the acute-phase response: SAA inducer is closely related to lymphocyte activating factor and endogenous pyrogen. *Cell. Immunol.* 63:164.
24. Postlethwaite, A. E., L. B. Lachman, C. L. Mainardi, and A. H. Kang. 1983. Interleukin 1 stimulation of collagenase production by cultured fibroblasts. *J. Exp. Med.* 157:801.
25. Baracos, V., H. Rodemann, C. Dinarello, and A. Goldberg. 1983. Stimulation of muscle protein degration and prostaglandin E_2 release by leukocyte pyrogen (interleukin 1). A mechanism for the increased degradation of muscle proteins during fever. *N. Engl. J. Med.* 308:553.
26. Kampschmidt, R. 1981. Leukocytic endogenous mediator/endogenous pyrogen. *In* The Physiologic and Metabolic Responses of the Host. M. Powanda and P. Canonico, editors. Elsevier/North Holland, Amsterdam. 55.
27. Kampschmidt, R., and L. Pulliam. 1978. Effect of human monocyte pyrogen on plasma iron, plasma zinc, and blood neutrophils in rabbits and rats. *Proc. Soc. Exp. Biol. Med.* 158:32.
28. Kampschmidt, R., H. Upchurch, and M. Worthington. 1983. Further comparisons of endogenous pyrogens and leukocytic endogenous mediators. *Infect. Immun.* 41:6.
29. Turchik, J., and D. Bronstein. 1980. Role of the central nervous system in acute-phase responses to leukocytic pyrogen. *Infect. Immun.* 30:439.
30. Gery, I., R. Gershon, and B. Waksman. 1971. Potentiation of cultured mouse thymocyte responses by factors released by peripheral leukocytes. *J. Immunol.* 107:1778.
31. Rosenwasser, L., and C. Dinarello. 1981. Ability of human leukocytic pyrogen to enhance phytohemagglutin induced murine thymocyte proliferation. *Cell. Immunol.* 63:134.
32. Robb, R. J., and K. A. Smith. 1981. Heterogeneity of human T-cell growth factor(s) due to variable glycosylation. *Mol. Immunol.* 18:1087.
33. Paetkau, V., R. C. Bleackley, D. Riendeau, D. G. Harnish, and E. W. Holowachuk. 1985. Toward the molecular biology of IL-2. *In* Contemporary Topics in Molecular Immunology. S. Gillis and F. P. Inman, editors. Plenum Press, New York. Vol. 10. 35.
34. Pickel, K., U. Hammerling, and M. K. Hoffmann. 1976. Ly phenotype of T-cells releasing T-cell replacing factor. *Nature.* 264:72.
35. Andrus, L., S. J. Prowse, and K. J. Lafferty. 1981. Interleukin 2 production by both $Lyt2^+$ and $Lyt2^-$ T-cell subsets. *Scand. J. Immunol.* 13:297.
36. Smith, K. A., L. B. Lachman, J. J. Oppenheim, and M. F. Favata. 1980. The functional relationship of the interleukins. *J. Exp. Med.* 151:1551.
37. Bleackley, R. C., B. Caplan, C. Havele, R. G. Ritzel, T. R. Mosmann, J. J. Farrar, and V. Paetkau. 1981. Translation of lymphocyte mRNA into biologically active interleukin 2 in oocytes. *J. Immunol.* 127:2432.
38. Chouab, S., and D. Fradelizi. 1982. The mechanism of inhibition of human IL-2 production. *J. Immunol.* 129:2463.
39. Tilden, A., and C. Balch. 1982. A comparison of PGE_2 effects on human suppressor cell function and on interleukin 2 function. *J. Immunol.* 129:2469.

40. Rappaport, R., and G. Dodge. 1982. Prostaglandin E inhibits the production of human interleukin 2. *J. Exp. Med.* 155:943.
41. Baker, P. E., J. V. Fahey, and A. Munck. 1981. Prostaglandin inhibition of T-cell proliferation is mediated at two levels. *Cell. Immunol.* 61:52.
42. Gullberg, M., F. Ivars, A. Coutinho, and E.-L. Larsson. 1981. Regulation of T cell growth factor production: Arrest of TCGF production after 18 h in normal lectin-stimulated mouse spleen cell cultures. *J. Immunol.* 127: 407.
43. Palacios, R., and G. Moller. 1981. T cell growth factor abrogates concanavalin A-induced suppressor cell function. *J. Exp. Med.* 153:1360.
44. Thoman, M. L., and W. O. Weigle. 1984. Interleukin 2 induction of antigen-nonspecific suppressor cells. *Cell. Immunol.* 85:215.
45. Hardt, C., M. Rollinghoff, K., Pfizenmaier, H. Mosmann, and H. Wagner. 1981. Lyt-2,3$^+$ cyclophosphamide-sensitive T cells regulate the activity of an interleukin 2 inhibitor in vivo. *J. Exp. Med.* 154:262.
46. Robb, R. J., A. Munck, and K. A. Smith. 1981. T cell growth factor receptors. *J. Exp. Med.* 154:1455.
47. Greene, W. C., and R. J. Robb. 1985. Receptor for T-cell growth factor: Structure, function and expression on normal and neoplastic cells. *In* Contemporary Topics in Molecular Immunology. S. Gillis and F. P. Inman, editors. Plenum Press, New York. Vol. 10. 1.
48. Muraguchi, A., J. H. Kehrl, D. L. Longo, D. J. Volkman, K. A. Smith, and A. S. Fauci. 1985. Interleukin 2 receptors on human B cells. *J. Exp. Med.* 161:181.
49. Rusk, C. M., and R. J. Robb. 1985. High and low affinity IL-2 receptors. *Fed. Proc.* 44:575.
50. de Weck, A. L., F. Kristensen, F. Joncourt, F. Bettens, C. Walker, and Y. Wang. 1984. Lymphocyte proliferation, lymphokine production, and lymphokine receptors in ageing and various clinical conditions. *Springer Semin. Immunopathol.* 7:273.
51. Cantrell, D. A., and K. A. Smith. 1983. Transient expression of interleukin 2 receptors: Consequences for T cell growth. *J. Exp. Med.* 158: 1895.
52. Cantrell, D. A., and K. A. Smith. 1984. The interleukin-2 T-cell system: A new cell growth model. *Science.* 224:1312.
53. Reem, G. H., and N.-H. Yeh. 1985. Regulation by interleukin 2 of interleukin 2 receptors and γ-interferon synthesis by human thymocytes: Augmentation of interleukin 2 receptors by interleukin 2. *J. Immunol.* 134:953.
54. Havran, W. L., D.-K. Kim, R. L. Moldwin, D. W. Lancki, and F. W. Fitch. 1985. IL-2 causes increased expression of IL-2 receptors on cloned murine T cells. *Fed. Proc.* 44:950.
55. Nabholz, M., F. Erard, R. Sekali, J. Lowenthal, P. Corthesy, M.-C. Combe, and H. R. MacDonald. 1985. Regulation of IL-2 receptors expression by IL-2 and IL-1. *Fed. Proc.* 44:1304.
56. Rook, A. H., H. Masur, H. C. Lane, W. Frederick, T. Kasahara, A. M. Macher, J. Y. Djeu, J. F. Manichewitz, L. Jackson, A. S. Fauci, and G. V.

Quinnan, Jr. 1983. Interleukin-2 enhances the depressed natural killer and cytomegalovirus-specific cytotoxic activities of lymphocytes from patients with the acquired immune deficiency syndrome. *J. Clin. Invest.* 72:398.
57. Wagner, H., C. Hardt, K. Heeg, M. Rollinghoff, and K. Pfizenmaier. 1980. T-cell-derived helper factor allows in vivo induction of cytotoxic T cells in nu/nu mice. *Nature.* 284:278.
58. Gillis, S., and J. Watson. 1981. Interleukin-2 induction of hapten-specific cytolytic T cells in nude mice. *J. Immunol.* 126:1245.
59. Dennert, G., and R. Hyman. 1980. Functional Thy-1$^+$ cells in cultures of spleen cells and from nu/nu mice. *Eur. J. Immunol.* 10:583.
60. Hefeneider, S. H., P. J. Conlon, C. S. Henney, and S. Gillis. 1983. In vivo interleukin 2 administration augments the generation of alloreactive cytolytic T lymphocytes and resident natural killer cells. *J. Immunol.* 130:222.
61. Rosenberg, S., E. Grimm, M. McGrogan, M. Doyle, E. Kawasaki, K. Koths, and D. Mark. 1984. Biological activity of recombinant human interleukin 2 produced in *Escherichia coli. Science.* 223:1412.
62. Cheever, M. A., and P. D. Greenberg. 1985. In vivo administration of interleukin-2. *In* Contemporary Topics in Molecular Immunology. S. Gillis and F. P. Inman, editors. Plenum Press, New York. Vol. 10. 263.
63. Donohue, J., and S. Rosenberg. 1983. The fate of interleukin-2 after in vivo administration. *J. Immunol.* 130:2203.
64. Howard, M., K. Nakanishi, and W. E. Paul. 1984. B cell growth and differentiation factors. *Immunol. Rev.* 78:185.
65. Yoshizaki, K., T. Nakagawa, K. Fukunaga, T. Kaieda, S. Maruyama, S. Kishimoto, Y. Yamamura, and T. Kishimoto. 1983. Characterization of human B cell growth factor (BCGF) from cloned T cells or mitogen-stimulated T cells. *J. Immunol.* 130:1241.
66. Dutton, R. W., G. D. Wetzel, and S. L. Swain. 1984. Partial purification and characterization of a BCGF II from EL4 culture supernatants. *J. Immunol.* 132:2451.
67. Paige, C. J., M. H. Schreier, and C. L. Sidman. 1982. Mediators from cloned T helper cell lines affect immunoglobulin expression by B cells. *Proc. Natl. Acad. Sci. USA.* 79:1982.
68. Muraguchi, A., J. L. Butler, J. H. Kehrl, and A. S. Fauci. 1983. Differential sensitivity of human B cell subsets to activation signals delivered by anti-μ antibody and proliferative signals delivered by a monoclonal B cell growth factor. *J. Exp. Med.* 157:530.
69. Okada, M., N. Sakaguchi, N. Yoshimura, H. Hara, K. Shimizu, N. Yoshida, K. Yoshizaki, S. Kishimoto, Y. Yamamura, and T. Kishimoto. 1983. B cell growth factors and B cell differentiation factor from human T hybridomas. *J. Exp. Med.* 157:583.
70. Farrar, J. J., M. Howard, J. Fuller-Farrar, and W. E. Paul. 1983. Biochemical and physicochemical characterization of mouse B cell growth factor: A lymphokine distinct from interleukin 2. *J. Immunol.* 131:1838.
71. Hamaoka, T. 1985. T-cell-replacing factor and its acceptor site on B cells: Molecular properties and immunogenic aspects. *In* Contemporary Topics

in Molecular Immunology. S. Gillis and F. P. Inman, editors. Plenum Press, New York. Vol. 10. 231.

72. Rosenberg, J. S., S. C. Gilman, and J. D. Feldman. 1983. Effects of aging on cell cooperation and lymphocyte responsiveness to cytokines. *J. Immunol.* 130:1754.
73. Gilman, S. C. 1984. Lymphokines in immunological aging. *Lymphokine Res.* 3:119.
74. Bruley-Rosset, M., and I. Vergnon. 1984. Interleukin-1 synthesis and activity in aged mice. *Mech. Ageing Dev.* 24:247.

75a. Gorczynski, R. M., M.-P. Chang, M. Kennedy, S. MacRae, K. Benzing, and G. B. Price. 1984. Alterations in lymphocyte recognition repertoire during aging. I. Analysis of changes in immune response potential of B lymphocytes from non-immunized aged mice, and the role of accessory cells in the expression of that potential. *Immunopharmacology.* 7:179.

75b. Jones, P., C. Kauffman, and M. Kluger. 1983. Endogenous pyrogen production by monocytes from elderly persons. *Clin. Res.* 31:366A.

76. Thoman, M. L., and W. O. Weigle. 1981. Lymphokines and aging: Interleukin-2 production and activity in aged animals. *J. Immunol.* 127:2102.
77. Chang, M.-P., T. Makinodan, W. J. Peterson, and B. L. Strehler. 1982. Role of T cells and adherent cells in age-related decline in murine interleukin 2 production. *J. Immunol.* 129:2426.
78. Gilman, S., J. Rosenberg, and J. Feldman. 1982. T lymphocytes of young and aged rats. II. Function defects and the role of interleukin 2. *J. Immunol.* 128:644.
79. Gillis, S., R. Kozak, M. Durante, and M. E. Weksler. 1981. Immunological studies of aging. *J. Clin. Invest.* 67:937.
80. Kennes, B., D. Brohee, and P. Neve. 1983. Lymphocyte activation in human ageing. V. Acquisition of response to T cell growth factor and production of growth factors by mitogen-stimulated lymphocytes. *Mech. Ageing Dev.* 23:103.
81. Thoman, M. L., and W. O. Weigle. 1985. Interleukin-2 reconstitution of aged immune function. *Cancer Treat. Symp.* 1:83.
82. Plaut, M., L. Lichtenstein, and C. Henney. 1975. Properties of a subpopulation of T cells bearing histamine receptors. *J. Clin. Invest.* 55:856.
83. Shearer, G., Y. Weinstein, and K. Melman. 1974. Enhancement of immune response potential of mouse lymphoid cells fractionated over insolubilized conjugated histamine columns. *J. Immunol.* 113:597.
84. Globerson, A., L. Abel, and T. Umiel. 1981. Immune reactivity during ageing. III. Removal of peanut-agglutinin binding cells from ageing mouse spleen cells leads to increased reactivity to mitogens. *Mech. Ageing Dev.* 16:275.
85. Miller, R. 1984. Age-associated decline in precursor frequency for different T cell-mediated reactions, with preservation of helper or cytotoxic effect per precursor cell. *J. Immunol.* 132:63.
86. Cheung, H. T., W. T. Wu, M. Pahlavani, and A. Richardson. 1985. Effect of age on the interleukin 2 messenger RNA level. *Fed. Proc.* 44:573.

87. Harrison, D. E., C. M. Astle, and J. W. Doubleday. 1977. Stem cell lines from old immunodeficient donors give normal responses in young recipients. *J. Immunol.* 118:1223.
88. Astle, C. M., and D. E. Harrison. 1984. Effects of marrow donor and recipient age on immune responses. *J. Immunol.* 132:673.
89. Lewis, V., J. Twomey, P. Bealmear, G. Goldstein, and R. Good. 1978. Age, thymic involution, and circulating thymic hormone activity. *J. Clin. Endocrinol. Metab.* 47:145.
90. Goldstein, A. L., T.L.K. Low, G. B. Thurman, M. M. Zatz, N. Hall, J. Chen, S.-K. Hu, P. B. Naylor, and J. E. McClure. 1981. Current status of thymosin and other hormones of the thymus gland. *Rec. Prog. Hormone Res.* 37:369.
91. D'Agostaro, G., D. Frasca, M. Garavini, and G. Doria. 1980. Immunorestoration of old mice by injection of thymus extract: Enhancement of T cell–T cell cooperation in the in vitro antibody response. *Cell. Immunol.* 53:207.
92. Weksler, M. E., J. B. Innes, and G. Goldstein. 1978. Immunological studies of aging. IV. The contribution of thymic involution to the immune deficiencies of aging mice and reversal with thymopoietin$_{32-36}$. *J. Exp. Med.* 148:1978.
93. Goldberg, E. H., G. Goldstein, E. A. Boyse, and M. P. Scheid. 1981. Effect of the TP5 analogue of thymopoietin on the rejection of male skin by aged and thymectomized female mice. *Immunogenetics.* 13:201.
94. Cowan, M. J., P. Fujiwara, D. W. Wara, and A. J. Ammann. 1981. Effect of thymosin on cellular immunity in old age. *Mech. Ageing Dev.* 15:29.
95. Verhaegen, H., W. DeCock, J. DeCree, and G. Goldstein. 1981. Restoration of the impaired lymphocyte stimulation in old people by thymopoietin pentapeptide. *J. Clin. Lab. Immunol.* 6:103.
96. Ghanta, V. K., P. J. Noble, M. E. Brown, P. J. Cox, N. S. Hiramoto, and R. N. Hiramoto. 1983. Alloreactivity. I. Effects of age and thymic hormone treatment on cell-mediated immunity in C57BL/6NNia mice. *Mech. Ageing Dev.* 22:309.
97. Ershler, W. B., A. L. Moore, M. P. Hacker, J. Ninomiya, P. Naylor, and A. L. Goldstein. 1984. Specific antibody synthesis in vitro. II. Age-associated thymosin enhancement of antitetanus antibody synthesis. *Immunopharmacology.* 8:69.
98. Palacios, R., C. Fernandez, and P. Sideras. 1982. Development and continuous growth in culture of interleukin 2-producer lymphocytes from athymic nu/nu mice. *Eur. J. Immunol.* 12:777.
99. Zatz, M. M., J. Oliver, C. Samuels, A. B. Skotnicki, M. B. Sztein, and A. L. Goldstein. Thymosin increases production of T-cell growth factor by normal human peripheral blood lymphocytes. *Proc. Natl. Acad. Sci. USA.* 81:2882.
100. Grinblat, J., K. Schauenstein, E. Saltz, N. Trainin, and A. Globerson. 1983. Regulatory effects of thymus humoral factor on T cell growth factor in aging mice. *Mech. Ageing Dev.* 22:209.

101. Thoman, M. L., and W. O. Weigle. 1982. Cell-mediated immunity in aged mice: An underlying lesion in IL-2 synthesis. *J. Immunol.* 128:2358.
102. Thoman, M. L., and W. O. Weigle. 1983. Deficiency in suppressor T cell activity in aged animals. *J. Exp. Med.* 157:2184.
103. Miller, R. A., and O. Stutman. 1981. Decline, in aging mice, of the anti-2,4,6-trinitrophenyl (TNP) cytotoxic T cell response attributable to loss of Lyt-2^{-}, interleukin 2-producing helper cell function. *Eur. J. Immunol.* 11:751.
104. Zharhary, D., Y. Segev, and H. E. Gershon. 1984. T-cell cytotoxicity and aging: Differing causes of reduced response in individual mice. *Mech. Ageing Dev.* 25:129.
105. Thoman, M. L., and W. O. Weigle. 1985. Reconstitution of in vivo cell-mediated lympholysis responses in aged mice with interleukin 2. *J. Immunol.* 134:949.
106. Morgan, E. L., M. L. Thoman, and W. O. Weigle. 1981. The immune response in aged C57BL/6 mice. I. Assessment of lesions in the B-cell and T-cell compartments of aged mice utilizing the Fc fragment-mediated polyclonal antibody response. *Cell. Immunol.* 63:16.
107. Girard, J. P., Paychere, M., M. Cuevas, and B. Fernandes. 1977. Cell-mediated immunity in an ageing population. *Clin. Exp. Immunol.* 27:85.
108. Sohnle, P. G., S. E. Larson, C. Collins-Lech, and A. R. Guansing. 1980. Failure of lymphokine-producing lymphocytes from aged humans to undergo activation by recall antigens. *J. Immunol.* 124:2169.
109. Thoman, M. L., and W. O. Weigle. 1982. Preliminary chemical and biologic characterization of (Fc)TRF: An Fc fragment-induced T cell-replacing factor. *J. Immunol.* 128:590.
110. Reem, G., and N. Yeh. 1984. Interleukin 2 regulates the expression of its receptor and the synthesis of gamma interferon by human T cells. *Science.* 225:429.
111. Schrader, J. W., I. Clark-Lewis, and P. F. Bartlett. 1982. T-cell hybridoma-derived lymphokines: Biology and biochemistry of factors regulating hemopoietic and lymphoid cells. *In* Lymphokines, Vol. 5. M. Feldmann and M. H. Schreier, editors. Academic Press, New York. 291.
112. Hilfiker, M. L., R. N. Moore, and J. J. Farrar. 1981. Biologic properties of chromatographically separated murine thyoma-derived interleukin 2 and colony-stimulating factor. *J. Immunol.* 127:183.
113. Nakanishi, K., T. R. Malek, K. A. Smith, T. Hamaoka, E. M. Shevach, and W. E. Paul. 1984. Both interleukin 2 and a second T cell-derived factor in EL-4 supernatant have activity as differentiation factors in IgM synthesis. *J. Exp. Med.* 160:1605.

11

Influence of Nutrition on Autoimmune Disease

Gabriel Fernandes

The University of Texas Health Science Center at San Antonio
San Antonio, Texas

I. INTRODUCTION

Several autoimmune disorders including systemic lupus erythematosus (SLE) comprise an important group of degenerative diseases in humans. Their study has been facilitated by the availability of short-lived strains of mice that are highly prone to develop autoimmune rheumatic and SLE diseases including severe renal disease (1). Within the past several years, several investigators using NZB, (NXB × NZW) F_1 (B/W), and MRL/lpr mice, as well as normal strains of mice, have found that nutrition not only can profoundly affect the development of autoimmune disease but also can affect immune function and survival rate of mice either susceptible or resistant to autoimmune disease.

More than 50 years ago McCay et al. (2) demonstrated that restriction of total food intake increases the life span of rats. Since then several studies have noted that possible mechanisms of this effect of caloric or total food restriction on life span may occur by inhibiting the appearance of tumors as well as renal diseases. Many studies in rodents have established that restricting food intake may also have profound effects on the physiological and immunological parameters during the aging process (3-5).

In this chapter we will summarize nutritional studies undertaken in autoimmune-prone mice that compared changes in immune function and the disease process itself; these may eventually lead to new nutritional strategies for preventing and/or inhibiting the severity of the autoimmune diseases such as SLE and rheumatoid arthritis.

II. DIET AND AUTOIMMUNITY

In the course of studying the influence of dietary nutrition on immunological function, we began to investigate the utility of NZB mice and their F_1 hybrid as models of genetic propensity to develop autoimmunity. First, we studied the influence of diet on reproduction, litter size, and expression of autoimmunity, especially in NZB mice (6). Initial experiments revealed that mice given a diet high in protein and relatively low in fat reproduced less well but lived significantly longer than did mice fed a diet high in fat and lower in protein. These responses to different diets were accompanied by very different expressions of autoimmune hemolytic anemia, and different effects on thymic size and immunological functions. Animals fed the lower protein, higher fat diet showed early thymic involution, more extensive splenomegaly, and earlier and greater manifestations of autoimmunity than did mice fed the ration higher in protein and lower in fat. Although mice fed the protein-restricted diet showed profound immunological involution, they did not live significantly longer than mice fed a diet higher in protein. These fascinating influences of diet on the development of autoimmune hemolytic anemia led us to the next set of investigations, which demonstrated striking effects of diet on longevity, autoimmunity, and renal and vascular disease in several strains of inbred mice prone to develop autoimmunity and renal disease.

III. PROTEIN RESTRICTION AND AUTOIMMUNITY

The changes caused by levels of dietary fat in a commercial laboratory chow diet were then pursued in NZB and later in B/W mice using more precisely defined diets. Initially, we studied the influence of diets of restricted protein composition in NZB mice in which protein (casein) was the only component of the diet that was varied (7). Mice fed a low-protein diet (6% vs. 22% casein) showed delayed onset of autoimmunity, delayed and reduced rate of thymic involution, inhibition of the development of splenomegaly, a slower rate of development of autoimmunities, slower and less involution of the lymphoid system, and reduced levels of immunodeficiencies of, e.g., T killer cell, with aging. However, since food was given isocalorically, no change in survival rate was observed in NZB mice. Thus, as a next step we decided to study restriction of caloric intake in autoimmune-prone mice.

IV. CALORIE RESTRICTION AND AUTOIMMUNITY

We studied the influence of restriction (up to 50%) of all semipurified dietary components (except vitamin and mineral intake, which remained equal) on length of life, immunological regression with aging, thymic involution, formation of circulating immune complexes with aging, and development of autoantibodies and renal disease in mice of the $(B/W)F_1$ hybrid strain (8). Early in life mice of this strain show a profound involution of immunological function, development of numerous autoantibodies, and progressive renal disease based on immune complex deposition in glomeruli. This entire complex of immunological events is dramatically delayed and inhibited by reduction of total calorie intake from the time of weaning. Furthermore, the regular progressive reduction in the ability to develop the plaque-forming cell response against sheep red blood cells in aging B/W mice was prevented in mice fed the calorie-restricted diet. B/W mice fed a low-calorie diet from weaning lived at least twice as long as B/W mice fed a putatively normal intake of calories. Indeed, several male mice treated by calorie restriction from weaning lived three times as long as any of the mice in the normal dietary intake group. Ability of the mice to produce antinuclear antibodies and anti-DNA antibodies was considerably reduced, but not eliminated.

Several studies by Dixon's group found that immune complexes composed of complement, the antigen–antibody complex for GP70, and the gross virus develop in the blood of B/W mice. Furthermore, the development and disposition of these complexes in the glomeruli correlate well with the development of progressive renal disease in these mice (9). In collaboration with Izui et al. (10), we found that mice fed a low-calorie diet from weaning fail to develop both autoantibodies and immune complexes and do not have deposits of the complexes in the glomeruli. The GP70 is a glycoprotein coded for by the genome of a virus produced by nonmalignant cells (e.g., liver cells) in the B/W mice that bear the virus. Gardner et al. (11) also found that dietary manipulation prevents the development of the renal disease in B/W mice, but that this dietary manipulation does not inhibit the expression of the xenotrophic virus in these animals. In our studies with Izui et al. (10), we noted that caloric restriction in B/W mice, which inhibits almost entirely the expression of GP70 antigen and anti-GP70 antibody, does not inhibit production of albumin. This regimen, however, does inhibit production of another glycoprotein, haptoglobin, which is also produced by liver cells. The increase in the level of circulating immune complexes is strikingly depressed at 6 and 9 months but not so much in mice 12 and 14 months of age.

An important question that arose from these experiments with dietary prevention of autoimmunity, immune complex formation, lupuslike renal disease, and inflammatory vascular disease in the B/W mice was whether a delay in dietary restriction until after the onset of autoimmunity and renal disease might still exert a beneficial influence. This question was clearly answered in the affirmative by the experiments of Friend et al. (12). In these studies, we showed that when dietary restriction was delayed to 4–5 months, clear inhibition of immunological abnormalities as well as inhibition of progression of renal disease and survival occurred.

Whereas caloric restriction inhibited immunological involution, as well as development of autoimmunity, immune complex, and renal disease in B/W mice, no such dramatic influence was observed when protein was restricted in these mice. Fat, however, proved to be a critical variable, and restriction of dietary fat, when coupled with caloric restriction, led to changes in immune function and autoimmunity in these mice.

V. DIETARY FATS AND AUTOIMMUNITY

More recently, several investigators have studied the influence of fat on B/W mice by utilizing isocaloric semipurified diets differing only in qualitative and quantitative fat content. Several studies have examined the effects of saturated versus polyunsaturated fats (PUFA) on the progression of autoimmune disease. These studies showed that low-fat diets significantly prolonged survival and delayed the onset of disease, while high-fat diets (regardless of the type of fatty acid content) enhanced immune complex nephritis and promoted the early death of B/W animals (13). Dietary fats seemed to alter autoantibody production according to the degree of saturation of fat. Mice receiving a diet high in saturated fat exhibited enhanced titers of natural thymocytotoxic antibody, an IgM autoantibody, whereas mice given a diet high in unsaturated fat had increased levels of anti-DNA IgG autoantibodies. This observation suggests that the type of dietary fat can alternatively affect different populations of antibody-producing B cells and the function of helper or suppressor T cells. Also, high-fat diets appear to have deleterious effects on several cellular immunological functions, including natural killer cell activity and macrophage phagocytosis (14).

In addition to serological alterations, histopathological examinations have shown specific effects of high-fat diets on tissues of B/W mice. Yumura et al. (15) recently showed that isocaloric diets containing 10% of either saturated or unsaturated fat led to deposition of immune complexes in the glomeruli of the kidneys, whereas diets of lower fat content showed primarily mesangial deposition. In another group of experiments, Kelley and Izui (16) showed that a very high concentration of saturated fat (50%) in the diet increased lipid deposition in the glomerulus, caused severe vascular injury, and accelerated the development of glomerulonephritis.

VI. DIET AND VASCULITIS

We have discovered that the composition of the diet can profoundly influence the development of atheromatous lesions in the coronary arteries as well as in the aorta and its large branches in B/W mice. The lesions that develop include inflammatory vasculitis and noninflammatory atheromatous lesions, both with and without lipid deposits (17). To develop these lesions, the autoimmune-prone

B/W mice must be fed diets high in calories and fats; a high-lard diet in particular is associated with glomerulosclerosis as well as the occurrence of perivascular lesions at a much higher frequency (Fig. 1). Furthermore, the standard Purina Laboratory Chow ad-libitum-fed diet that is apparently relatively low in fat and high in fiber produces less severe lesions (Fig. 2), whereas food restriction not only protects against renal disease but results in much less vascular disease in B/W mice (Fig. 3).

Although much further study is needed before the pathogenesis of these arteriosclerotic and glomerulosclerotic lesions that develop in B/W mice are understood, it already seems clear that diets high in saturated fats are particularly conducive to developing such lesions. Thus in inbred autoimmune-prone mice, genetic factors, immunological events (particularly immune complex formation), dietary fat, and protein composition all influence the development of althero-sclerotic lesions. Similar manipulations do not generally produce arteriosclerotic lesions in long-lived, autoimmune-resistant mice. These provocative observations, which require further study, suggest, in agreement with observations that poly-unsaturated dietary fats may aid in the prevention of kidney grafts (18) and experimental allergic reactions related to high lipid intake (19), that immunological processes, perhaps including immune complex formation, may predispose to deposition of fatty substances derived from dietary lipids and may play a vital role in the pathogenesis of certain forms of atherosclerosis in the presence of chronic autoimmune disease.

VII. MODULATION OF LYMPHOCYTE SUBSETS BY DIET

Utilizing monoclonal antibodies and the fluorescence-activated cell sorter (FACS), studies were undertaken to analyze the influence of diet on populations of lymphoid cells and their subsets in young (4 months old) and old (8-10 months old) autoimmune-prone B/W mice. The results showed minimal changes in cell subpopulations of young animals (3-5 months) maintained from weaning age on high (20%) and/or low (5%) dietary fat (corn oil) or 50% restricted calorie intake (Thy-1$^+$, 42% to 47%; Lyt-1$^+$, 45% to 52%; Lyt-2$^+$, 15% to 18%; Ig$^+$, 22% to 28%: control vs. calorie-restricted, respectively). However, old mice maintained on a high-fat diet from weaning age displayed significant decreases in the percentage of Thy-1$^+$ (to 29%), Lyt-1$^+$ (to 33%), and Lyt-2$^+$ (to 7%) cells. The effects of diet and age were also seen in ratios of Lyt-1$^+$ to Lyt-2$^+$. Food-restricted mice maintained a nearly equal ratio (young, 3.0; old, 2.9), while mice receiving the low-fat (5%) diet (young, 3.0; old, 4.0) and high-fat diet (young, 2.8; old, 5.1) did not. Cells from aging, high-fat-fed mice produced less interleukin 2 (IL-2), had reduced percentages of Lyt-2$^+$ cells, and had increases in the percentage of Ig$^+$ cells (Fig. 4). In addition, we also observed (unpublished

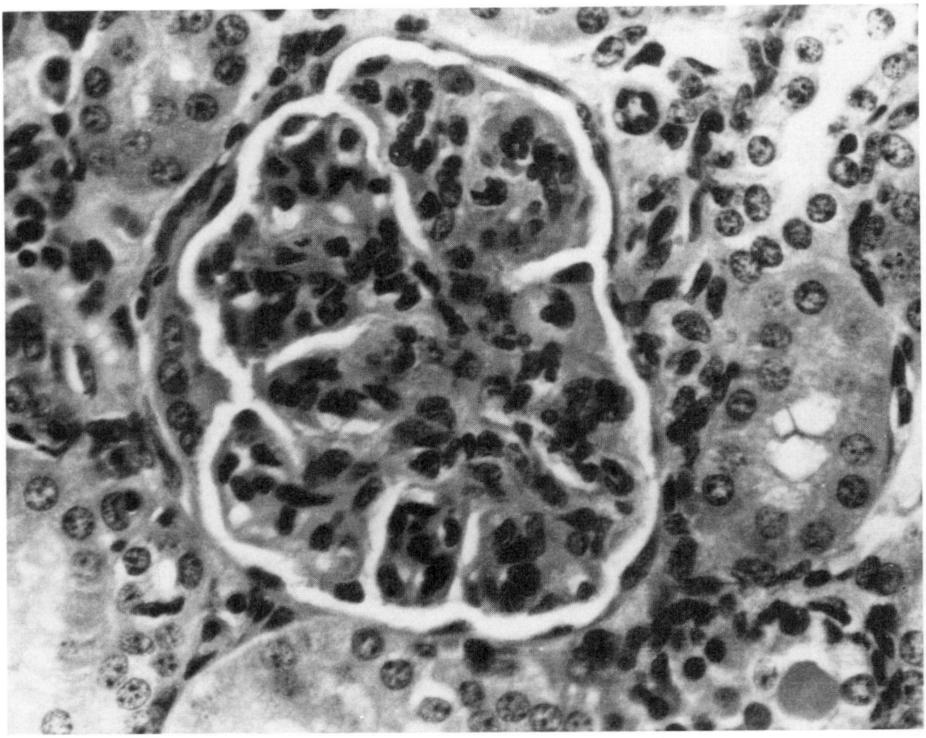

(a)

Figure 1 (*A*) This glomerulus from a lard-fed B/W female mouse displayed marked (3+) increase in mesangial cellularity, accentuated lobular pattern, and increase in mesangial matrix. (676X.) (*B*) This vessel in the kidney of a lard-fed female B/W mouse showed grade 3+/4+ perivascular infiltrates. (280X.)

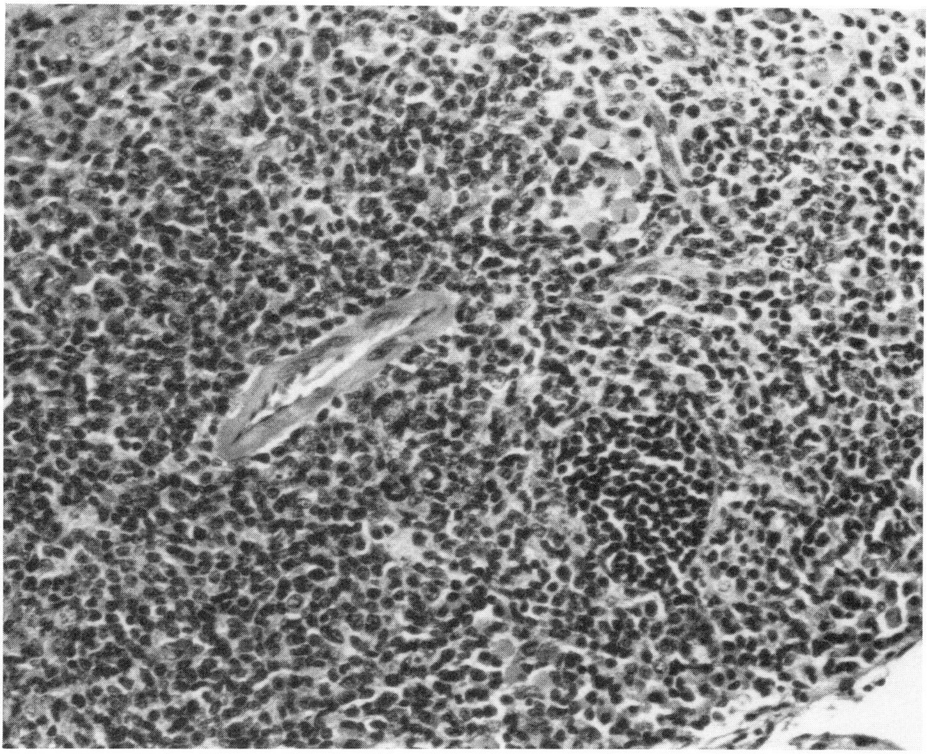

(b)

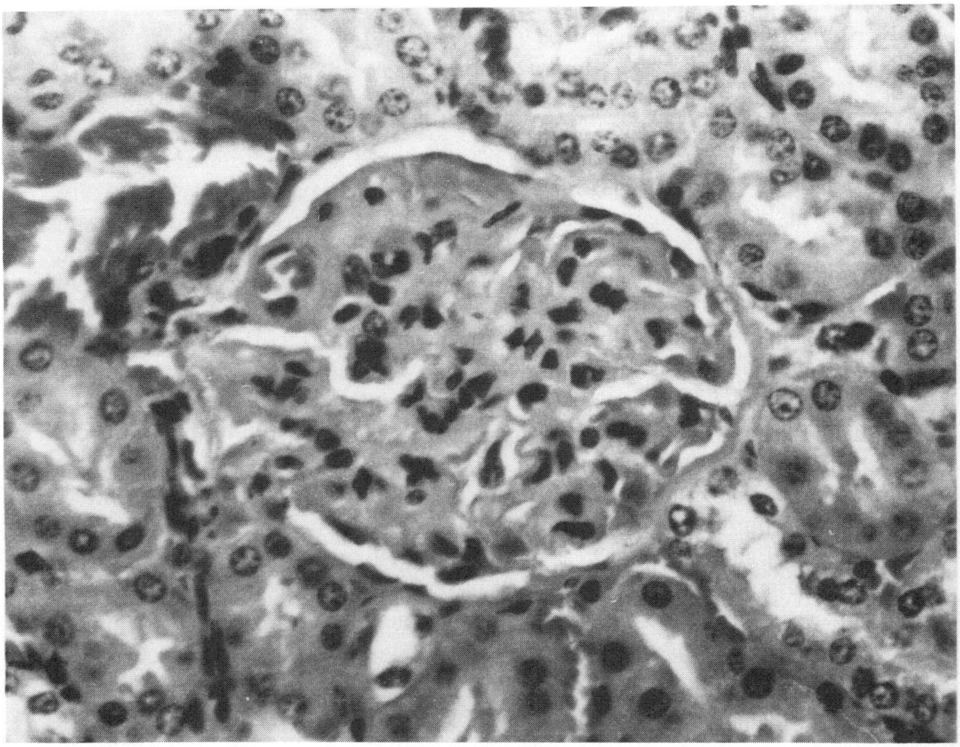

(a)

Figure 2 (*A*) Glomerulus from ad-libitum; lab-chow-fed female B/W mouse 2+/4+; the glomeruli from this animal were slightly enlarged and displayed a modest increase in mesangial matrix and cellularity. (676X.) (*B*) This medium-sized vessel in the kidney of an ad-libitum, lab-chow-fed B/W female mouse showed grade 1–2+/4+ perivascular infiltration. (280X.)

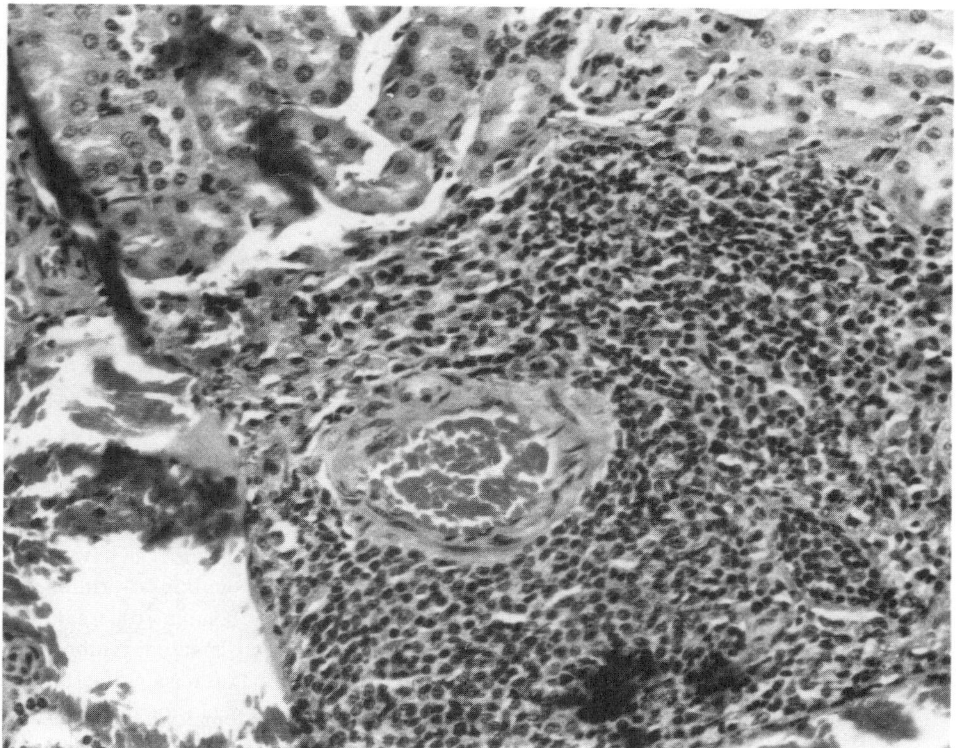

(b)

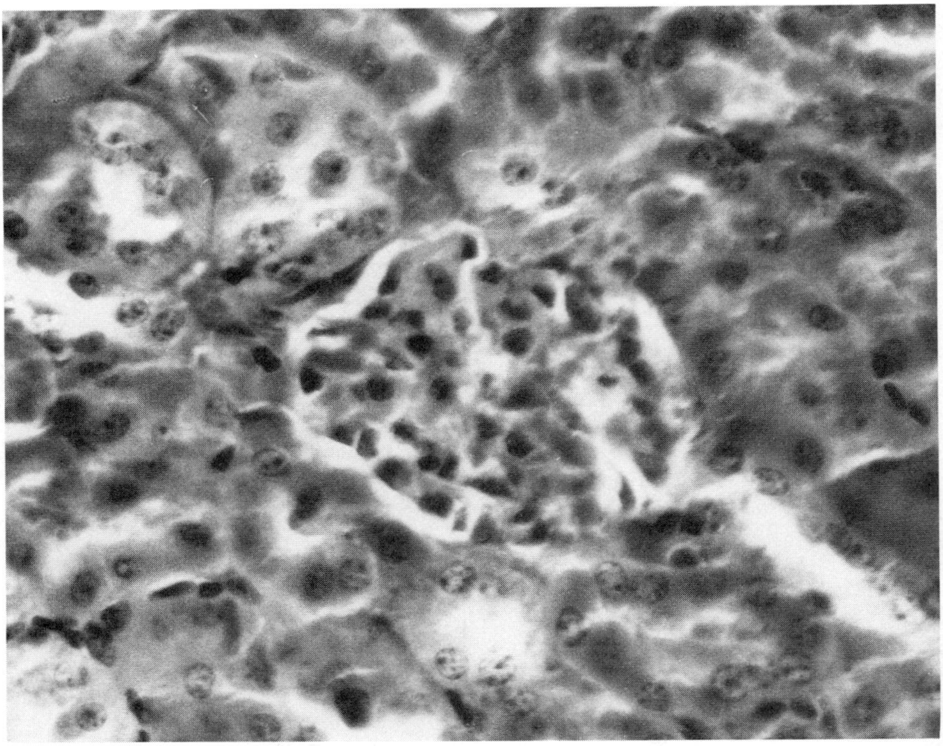

(a)

Figure 3 (*A*) This glomerulus from a calorie-restricted B/W female mouse is graded 0–1+/4+; such glomeruli showed only minimal increases in cellularity and mesangial matrix. (788×.) (*B*) This medium-sized vessel in the kidney of a calorie-restricted B/W female mouse showed minimal lymphocytic perivascular infiltration. (280×.)

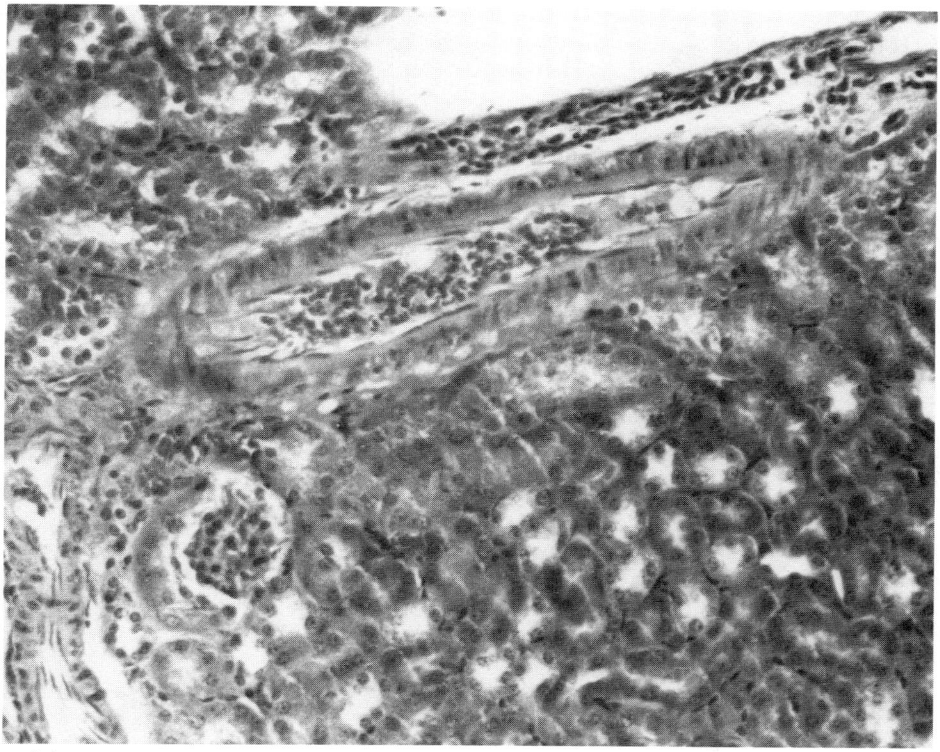

(b)

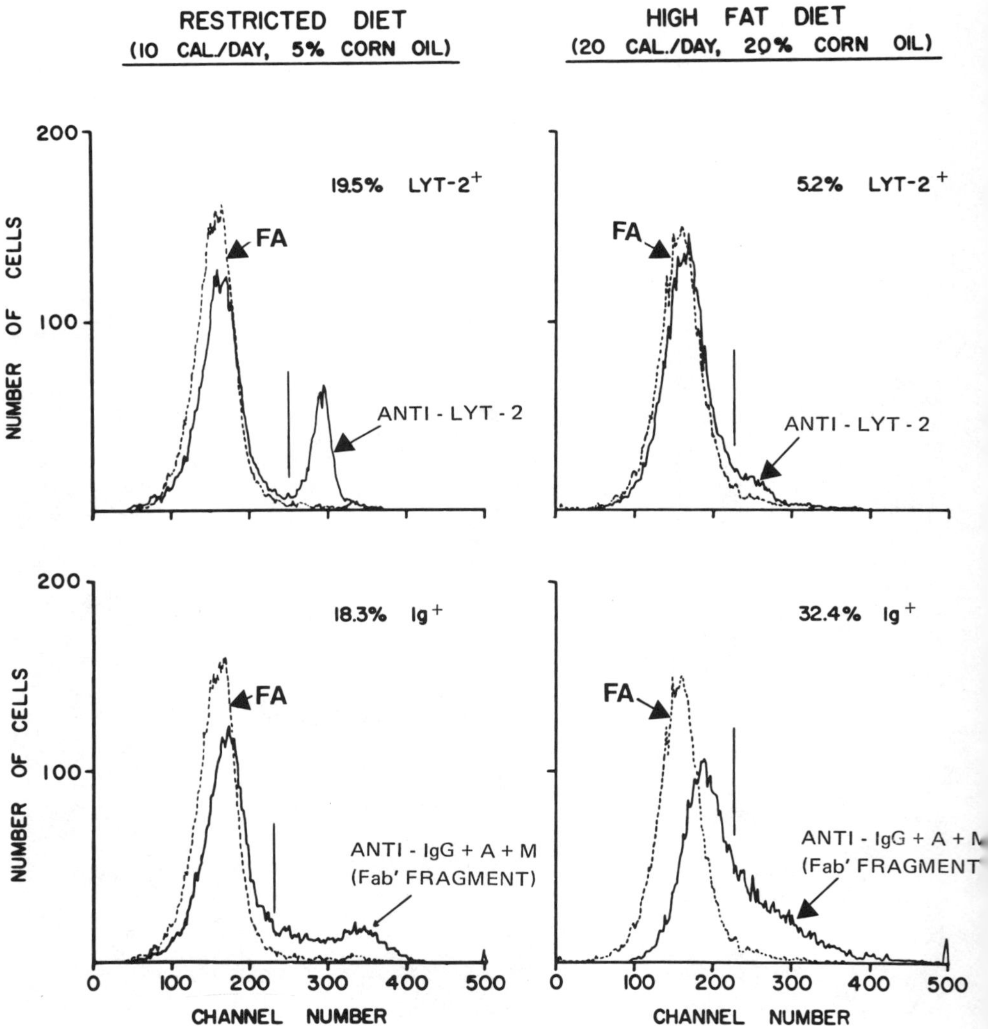

Figure 4 FACS analysis of splenocytes from individual 10-month-old B/W female mice.

data) that a striking alteration in the subpopulation of B cells occurs secondary to calorie restriction. It is known that Ly-1 B cells [B cells that express the Lyt (T-cell) surface determinants] are present in smaller percentages (2-5%) in normal mice than in autoimmune mice (10-25%) (20). Recently we found that in food-restricted B/W mice, Ly-1 B is significantly reduced, compared to ad-libitum-fed mice. These results further suggest that high caloric intake (particularly intake high in lipids) induces alterations in lymphoid cell subsets and thus exacerbates autoimmune renal and cardiovascular disease.

VIII. DIETARY FISH OIL AND AUTOIMMUNITY

More recently, several studies have further established that both saturated (animal) and polyunsaturated (vegetable) fat intake (equal to 35-40% of the total calorie source) have been found to shorten the life span of autoimmune prone mice by concomitantly exacerbating renal and vascular autoimmune disease (21-23) and increasing the levels of cyclooxygenase metabolites such as prostaglandins (PG) and thromboxane, in both tissues and immune cells. In contrast, a similar level of fish oil intake (20%) has been found to suppress inflammatory mediators and protect against autoimmune renal disease and/or lymphoproliferative disease (24-26). Initially, diets rich in linoleic acid were assumed to foster the production of immunostimulatory PG in lupus-prone mice and thereby stimulate the inflammatory process responsible for the progression of the disease. While a diet rich in saturated fat, but deficient in extended fatty acids (EFA), markedly increased survival and reduced all manifestations of the disease in B/W mice, a diet of safflower oil containing 78% linoleic acid did not exacerbate the disease as expected (21-22). The investigators proposed that in addition to the PG effect, EFA-deficient diets may affect the hormonal balance of the animals, which can affect the course and severity of the disease both in B/W mice (27) and in humans (28). Furthermore, B/W mice placed on fish oil diet rich in eicosapentaenoic acid (EPA) were found to have less autoimmune nephritis, and this effect was also observed when the fish oil diet was given even late in life (24). Such results could not be attributed to levels of anti-DNA autoantibodies that were found equal late in the life of the animals, but it appeared that in these animals the EPA-rich diet favored the formation of the immunoinhibitory substances PGE3 and LT5, which suppress the synthesis of inflammatory products of arachidonic acid metabolism (30). A fish oil diet was also able to suppress the autoimmune lymphoproliferative disease in MRL/l mice (26). In this particular study, one group of MRL/lpr male and females 1-2 months old were fed a diet containing safflower oil (20%), a rich source of linoleic acid (18:2n6), which is metabolished to the intermediate arachidonic acid (20:4n6) and eventually is converted to the dienoic prostaglandins (PG2). Another group was fed a diet containing 20% menhaden fish oil, a rich source of EPA (17%) and docosahexaenoic acid (DHA-8%). EPA is the precursor of trienoic prostaglandins (PG3), which are not generally present in tissues. When compared to a safflower-oil-fed group, the fish-oil-fed mice had decreased T-cell lymphoproliferation and expression of Ia antigen on peritoneal macrophages. The fish oil diet was associated with reduced PGE2, thromboxane B2, and prostacyclin levels in the lungs and kidneys, and increased renal PGE3 levels. This diet also prevented the formation of circulating retroviral GP70 immune complexes and delayed the development of immune nephritis in the MRL/1 mice (26).

Although several studies have examined the effect of these dietary fats on inflammation and tissue injury, including levels of autoantibodies, there is as yet no precise information available regarding changes in lymphocyte subsets, functional abilities, and capacity to produce various lymphokines.

We, therefore, recently carried out a detailed study using large numbers of B/W female and male mice by feeding them isocalorically three different lipids in the ration: (a) vegetable oil as corn oil, (b) animal fat as lard, and (c) menhaden fish oil (EPA). Furthermore, since calorie restriction was reported to inhibit autoimmune disease, we also compared two groups: a diet (normal calories) containing a low level of corn oil (5%), a food-restricted group (50% calorie restriction).

Our recent results showed that only the food restriction and the diet containing fish oil extended life spans, and they did so both by maintaining better immune function and by lowering incidence of autoimmune renal disease in female and male mice alike. A diet containing low fat (5%) but a high level of calories, as well as other two diets (e.g., lard and corn oil 20%), caused depressed immune functions and shortened the life span (31).

The mechanism of the protection obtained by food restriction and/or by fish oil intake appears similar in both groups of mice. For example, we found by FACS analysis that both food-restricted and fish-oil-fed mice maintained higher proportions of T helper and T suppressor cell populations and prevented the rise in B cells (Table 1). Furthermore, both diets also prevented the rise in Ly-1 B cells. The Ly-1 B cells are significantly increased in number (four- to fivefold) in autoimmune-prone mice and are known to produce increased levels of IgM autoantibodies in both normal and autoimmune-prone mice (32). In our laboratory, two-color FACS analysis revealed that in both food-restricted and in fish-oil-fed mice Ly-1 B cells remained at the 2–5% level, whereas it showed that in ad-libitum-fed or high-fat-fed mice (lard or corn oil 20%) these cells represented 15–25% of B cells in B/W mice 8–10 months old (unpublished data). Thus, inhibition of autoimmunity by either food restriction or dietary fish oil appears to be due to the maintenance of higher proportion of Lyt-2^+ (suppressor T) cells and by preventing the rise in Ly-1 B cells.

We also observed that food restriction and fish-oil-containing diets maintained: higher T and B cell proliferative responses to mitogens (Table 2); in-

Table 1 Effects of Diets on Lymphocyte Subsets: FACS Analysis of B/W Spleen Cells (8–12 months old) Found Percent Positive

Diet	Thy-1.2$^+$	Ly-1$^+$	$L_3T_4^+$	Lyt-2$^+$	Surface Ig$^+$	*n*
Corn oil 5%	33	43	35	9	38	12
Corn oil 5% (restricted)	47	61	48	14	29	9
Corn oil 20%	38	48	42	9	36	9
Lard 20%	33	34	31	11	35	4
Fish oil 20%	49	56	48	14	24	5

creased IL-2 production, decreased IL-2 production, and decreased autoantibody levels (31).

In contrast, natural killer cell activity (generally correlated with preventing the appearance of tumors) was low in the groups fed fish oil and lard but was high in corn-oil-fed and food-restricted animals. This observation requires further long-term studies in animals to monitor the appearance of any benign or malignant tumors, particularly in liver or lung tissues. Furthermore, we observed that rates of renal and vascular disease were highest in lard-fed animals, followed by fish-oil-fed animals, whereas vascular damage was minimal in food-restricted animals as well as in animals fed normal calorie diets that were low or high in corn oil. In the latter groups of B/W mice, early deaths were mostly due to im-

Table 2 Effects of Dietary Fats on Mitogenic Responses of Spleen Cells from B/W Female Mice

			Response (cpm) to:		
Group	Diet	Age[a]	Phytohemagglutinin	Concanavalin A	Lipopolysaccharides
1.	Corn oil 5%	Y	86,500	105,100	44,000
		O	33,800	46,300	35,700
2.	Corn oil (5%)	Y	97,500	147,000	71,000
	(restricted)	O	69,160	110,500	63,900
3.	Corn oil 20%	Y	45,700	111,500	60,500
		O	29,700	27,100	33,800
4.	Lard 20%	Y	63,100	115,100	71,600
		O	10,300	9,000	9,800
5.	Fish oil 20%	Y	72,900	187,900	79,500
		O	64,800	98,100	46,900

[a]Y(oung) = 4–5 months (8–10 mice/group), O(ld) = 8–12 months (6–8 mice/group).

munological deficiency resulting in pulmonary and/or renal disease. Thus, our ongoing studies further establish that food restriction and/or fish-oil-containing diets have a profound effect on immune cells, which consequently protect against the severity of autoimmune lupus disease in animals.

IX. CONCLUSIONS

All lupus-prone strains of mice show hypergammaglobulinemia, anti-dsDNA, anti-ssDNA, antiretroviral GP70 antibodies, circulating immune complexes, IL-2 deficiency, and glomerulonephritis (1,33). MRL/l mice are also shown to have arteritis, myocardial lesions, anti-Sm antibodies, and more frequently monoclonal γ-globulins of the IgG_1 and IgG_{2a} subclasses (1). This indicates that major defects may arise in the immune regulatory mechanism for regulation of antibody production in lupus mice. There is growing evidence to indicate that lymphocyte activation, proliferation, and differentiation processes are defective in autoimmune mice.

Dixon et al. (34) suggested the murine SLE has two types of abnormality. One is the hypersecretion of T helper factors (e.g., BCDF) as seen in the MRL/l, and the other is the B-cell abnormality as seen in BXSB and NZB/W, resulting in excessive and poorly regulated B-cell activation, proliferation, and differentiation. Our study showed that food restriction in lupus strains retarded B-cell activation and/or proliferation, and maintained better IL-2 production and utilization ability (35), as well as prolonging the life span. However, it is not clear how diets high in saturated and unsaturated fat influence the autoimmune processes by modulating lymphokine production, or T-cell and B-cell responses to antigens in these mice. Our hypothesis is that nutritional factors, particularly specific types of food antigen, act at multiple sites in the immune system mainly by altering growth factors and membrane recognition and/or antigen presentation systems (36,37). Furthermore, the metabolic and membrane lipid bilayer changes induced by dietary fats may activate genes or inhibit synthesis of several key enzymes including cyclooxygenase and lipoxygenase pathways as well as downregulating auto-anti-idiotypes (38), and thus may promote changes in lymphokine production, alter immune functions, and promote autoimmunity. It is important to undertake a systematic study to compare animals fed restricted calories versus animals fed different types of higher dietary fat levels by measuring levels of IL-1, IL-2, BCDF, prostaglandins, and mRNA for growth factors and/or oncogene expressions in lymphoid cells. Recently, expression of a selective abnormal proto-oncogene associated with abnormal cell growth or differentiation of certain subpopulations of lymphocytes has been noted in autoimmune-prone mice (39).

Molecular studies undertaken recently in our laboratory revealed greatly diminished levels of mRNAs for several oncogenes (c-myc, v-myc, v-fos, v-abl, and v-raf) in B6/1pr, C3H/1pr and MRL/1pr mice maintained either on food restriction and/or fish-oil-containing diets. In contrast, spleen as well as lymph node cells from mice fed either low-fat, high-calorie or high-fat, high calorie (corn oil and lard, 20%) showed significantly higher levels of oncogene expression (40).

In summary, studies of the effects of dietary fatty acids on the production of lymphokines in lupus-prone animals, cell–cell interaction studies, as well as measurement of interleukin mRNA levels and oncogene mRNA expression, should provide new information for understanding the development of autoimmunity and arthritis. This will hopefully demonstrate potential for controlling the development of autoimmune disease in humans by manipulation of diet and/or dietary fat intake by reducing chronic stimulation by food antigens.

ACKNOWLEDGMENT

This work was supported in part by National Institute on Aging grant AG-03417.

REFERENCES

1. Theofilopoulos, A. N., and F. J. Dixon. 1981. *Immunol. Rev.* 55:179.
2. McCay, C., M. Crowell, and L. Maynard. 1935. *J. Nutr.* 10:63.
3. Weindruch, R., S.R.S. Gottesman, and R. L. Walford. 1982. *Proc. Natl. Acad. Sci. USA* 79:898.
4. Masoro, E. J., B. D. Yu, and H. A. Bertrand. 1982. *Proc. Natl. Acad. Sci. USA* 79:4239.
5. Fernandes, G. 1984. *Pharmacol. Rev.* 36:123s.
6. Fernandes, G., E. J. Yunis, and R. A. Good. 1976. *Proc. Natl. Acad. Sci. USA* 73:1279.
7. Fernandes, G., E. J. Yunis, and R. A. Good. 1976. *J. Immunol.* 116:782.
8. Fernandes, G., P. Friend, E. J. Yunis, and R. A. Good. 1978. *Proc. Natl. Acad. Sci. USA* 75:1500.
9. Izui, S., P. J. McConahey, A. N. Theofilopoulos, and F. J. Dixon. 1979. *J. Exp. Med.* 149:1099.
10. Izui, S., G. Fernandes, I. Hara, P. J. McConahey, F. C. Jensen, F. J. Dixon, and R. A. Good. 1981. *J. Exp. Med.* 154:1116.
11. Gardner, M. B., J. N. Ihle, R. J. Pillarsetty, N. Talal, B. L. Dubois, and J. A. Levy. 1977. *Nature* 268:341.
12. Friend, P. S., G. Fernandes, R. A. Good, A. F. Micheal, and E. J. Yunis. 1978. *Lab Invest.* 38:629.
13. Levy, J. A., A. B. Ibrahim, T. Shirai, K. Ohta, R. Nagasawa, H. Yoshida, J. Estes, and M. Gardner. 1982. *Proc. Natl. Acad. Sci. USA* 79:1974.
14. Morrow, W.J.W., J. A. Hall, J. Pribnow, S. J. Hirose, T. Shirai, and J. A. Levy. 1985. *J. Immunol.* 175:3857.

15. Yamura, W., S. Hattori, D. C. Mayes, J. A. Levy, and T. Shirai. 1985. *J. Immunol.* 175:3865.
16. Kelley, V. E., and S. Izui. 1985. *Am. J. Pathol. III* 288.
17. Fernandes, G., D. R. Alonso, T. Tanaka, H. T. Thaler, E. J. Yunis, and R. A. Good. 1983. *Proc. Natl. Acad. Sci. USA* 80:876.
18. Uldall, P. R. et al. 1974. *Lancet* 2:514.
19. Mead, C. J., and J. Mertin. 1978. *J. Adv. Lipid Res.* 16:127.
20. Hayakawa, K., R. R. Hardy, and L. A. Herzenberg. 1985. *J. Exp. Med.* 161:1554.
21. Hurd, E. R., J. M. Johnston, J. R. Okita, P. C. MacDonald, M. Ziff, and J. N. Gilliam. 1981. *J. Clin. Invest.* 67:476.
22. Kelly, V. E., and S. Izui. 1983. *Am. J. Pathol. III* 288.
23. Mark, D. A., D. R. Alonso, F. Quimby, H. T. Thaler, Y. T. Kim, G. Fernandes, R. A. Good, and M. C. Weksler. 1984. *Am. J. Pathol.* 117:110.
24. Prickett, J. D., D. R. Robinson, and A. D. Steinberg. 1981. *J. Clin. Invest.* 68:556.
25. Robinson, D. R., J. D. Prickett, R. Polisson, A. D. Steinberg, and L. Levine. 1985. *Prostaglandins* 30:51.
26. Kelley, V. E., A. Ferretti, S. Izui, and T. B. Strom. 1985. *J. Immunol.* 134:1914.
27. Roubinian, J. R., R. Papoian, and N. Talal. 1978. *J. Clin. Invest.* 59:1568.
28. Lahita, R. G., H. L. Bradlow, J. Fishman, and H. G. Kunkel. 1982. *Am. J. Kidney Dis.* 2:206.
29. Morley, K. D., A. Parke, and G.R.V. Hughes. 1982. *Br. Med. J.* 284:1431.
30. Prickett, J. D., D. R. Robinson, and A. D. Steinberg. 1983. *Arthritis Rheum.* 26(2):133.
31. Fernandes, G., L. Sandburg, A. Khare, and D. Troyer. 1986. *Arthritis Rheum.* 29:540.
32. Hayakawa, K., R. R. Hardy, M. Honda, L. A. Hertzenberg, and A. D. Steinberg. 1984. *Proc. Natl. Acad. Sci. USA* 81:2494.
33. Dauphinée, M. D., S. B. Kipper, D. Wofsy, and N. Talal. 1981. *J. Immunol.* 127:2483.
34. Dixon, F. J., A. N. Theofilopoulos, P. McConahey, and G. J. Prud'homme. 1983. *In* Progress in Immunology, Vol. 5. Y. Yamamura and T. Toda, editors. Academic Press, New York, p. 1115.
35. Jung, L.K.L., M. A. Palladino, S. Calvano, D. A. Mark, R. A. Good, and G. Fernandes. 1982. *Clin. Immunol. Immunopathol.* 25:295.
36. Christadoss, P., N. Talal, J. Lindstrom, and G. Fernandes. 1984. *Cell Immunol.* 88:1.
37. Fischbach, M. 1984. *J. Immunol.* 133:2365.
38. Goidl, E. A., R. A. Good, G. W. Siskind, M. E. Weksler, and G. Fernandes. 1986. *Cell Immunol.* (in press).
39. Mountz, J. D., J. F. Mushinski, G. E. Mark, and A. D. Steinberg. 1985. *J. Mol. Cell Immunol.* 2:121.
40. Khare, A., W. Freidrichs, and G. Fernandes. 1986. Paper presented at the International Symposium on Nutritional Regulation of Immunity and Infection, Toronto, Canada, July 3–5 (abstract).

12

Specific and Nonspecific Suppressor Cells in Aged Animals

Susan R. S. Gottesman and G. J. Thorbecke

New York University School of Medicine
New York, New York

Roy L. Walford

University of California at Los Angeles School of Medicine
Los Angeles, California

> After a certain time, as the result of sickness or disease, the effect of accident, or the consequence of old age, sooner or later, the animal dies. The multitudinous operations of this beautiful mechanism flag in their performance, the horse loses its vigour, and after passing through the curious series of changes comprised in its formation and preservation, it finally decays, and ends its life by going back into that inorganic world. . . .
>
> *Thomas H. Huxley, 1898*

I. INTRODUCTION

As an organism ages, its ability to adapt to changes in its internal or external environment becomes impaired. This altered adaptability is obvious in all organ systems in the body—particularly in the neurological, endocrine, cardiac, and respiratory systems, and also in the immune system (1). Part of the complexity and intrigue of the immune system rests with its capacity to respond to virtually any foreign antigen, while at the same time regulating the level of response and preventing attacks on self antigens. This tight control may be achieved through immunoregulatory circuits (2,3). What happens to this precise control with advanced age?

As the organism ages, its ability to respond to foreign antigen decreases (4). The immune system of an aged individual, however, has had a lifetime of experiences with foreign challenges. Therefore, when analyzing the outcome of a foreign challenge in an old animal, one must consider not only the decreasing ability to respond, but also the cumulative effects of past environmental exposures. The organism's ability to maintain control of or to limit its remaining immune capabilities also appears to be altered with age, resulting particularly in the appearance of autoimmune diseases (5).

The end result of these processes is an aged organism with a profound defect in its response to novel antigens, with at least partial maintenance of memory responses, and with an increasing tendency to attack self antigens.

II. SUPPRESSIVE MECHANISMS NORMALLY CONTROLLING THE LEVEL OF THE IMMUNE RESPONSE

The induction and functioning of suppressor cells play a central role in immunoregulatory circuits. Whereas major emphasis in studies of young animals has been placed on antigen-specific suppressor cells in these circuits (2), investigations in aging animals have focused on both antigen-specific and antigen-nonspecific suppressor cells. Current evidence suggests that in antigen-specific systems, several different T suppressor (Ts) subsets may function in a cascade-like manner (6). Several laboratories have concluded that at least two to three distinguishable T-cell types are involved in generating the final suppressive response. The Ts_1 cells or inducer cells ($Ly2^-$) are the first to be activated by antigen. They then either induce Ts_2 cells, which go on to activate Ts_3 cells (the effectors of suppression), or they directly induce effector cells ($Ly2^+$). Each suppressor T cell operates through the production of soluble factors. Each step requires a period of several days for induction of the next cell and is antigen specific. The final suppressor mechanism, although antigen dependent, is nonspecific; thus, under certain circumstances, bystander suppression can occur. Several cascades of suppressor cells may exist, resulting in suppressor effectors with different target cells (i.e., T helper cell, B cell) (6).

"Nonspecific" suppressor cells may be nonspecific in both induction and action or, alternatively, they may reflect the cumulative effects of specific suppressor cells activated in a polyclonal fashion. An example of naturally occurring suppressor cells is presented by Strober (7), who investigated their existence in neonatal animals and in adult mice following total lymphoid irradiation. These large granular lymphocytes belong to the "null" cell population according to their surface markers and may be immature cells not normally operative in the adult mouse. Mitchell and co-workers (8) have also presented evidence for a nonspecific suppressor cell in the macrophage lineage.

Polyclonal activation of cells by concanavalin A (Con A), or by in vitro incubation in medium containing fetal calf serum, leads to the development of suppressor cells that also appear to act nonspecifically (9,10). Since Con A-induced suppressor cells have been characterized as T cells, their apparent nonspecific action could in fact result from activation of multiple clones of specific cells (9). These cells could then be specific in their individual effector functions and could cause nonspecific suppression through the production of inhibitory lymphokines (11,12) or the absorption of stimulatory lymphokines, e.g., interleukin 2 (IL-2) (13).

The generation of specific suppressor cells to a new antigen may reflect the ability of the immune system to respond, while the level of nonspecific suppressor cells may primarily reflect the organism's previous experiences. In the studies reviewed below, the "nonspecific" suppressor cells may be cells that do act nonspecifically. Alternatively, even though polyclonal activation may not be part of the experimental design, in vivo exposures over the organism's lifetime, prior to intentional antigen administration, may have simulated such an effect. This could have resulted in multiple clones of cross-reactive and, possibly, specific suppressor T cells directed against the antigen used in the experiments.

Since changes in the ability to generate specific and nonspecific suppressor cells may exert different degrees of influence in the aged organism, the literature on suppressor cells in aged animals is discussed here with particular emphasis on their division into these two groups. If indeed a difference exists in the effect of aging on specific and nonspecific suppressor cells, this difference may, at least partially, account for the apparent disparity seen in the aged organism's response to challenge with foreign and self antigens. The hypothesis could then be suggested that an increase in nonspecific suppressor cells in the aged diminishes the immune response to foreign challenge, whereas a decline in certain specific suppressor cells allows for the emergence of autoimmune disease.

III. SUPPRESSOR CELLS IN AGING

A. Suppressor Cells from Unimmunized Donors

When cells from unimmunized young and aged donor mice are cotransferred into irradiated recipients, the humoral response to subsequent challenge with antigen is lower than the expected additive result (14-16). Goidl et al. (14) found that this suppressor activity increased with age from 12 to 34 months in the BALB/c strain. Since the suppression was not preferential for high avidity or IgG isotype antibody formation, it could not completely account for the qualitative changes seen in the antibody response of the intact aged animal. Makinodan et al. (15) found that the majority of individually tested aged animals, with histologically normal spleens, demonstrated suppressor cells after cotransfer with cells from young mice. They obtained similar results using an in vitro assay system (15). Callard et al. (16) demonstrated nonspecific suppression of the humoral response of cells from both immunized and unimmunized young mice by spleen cells from unimmunized old CBA mice. Treatment with anti-Thy-1, anti-Ly1, anti-Ly2, or anti-Ia plus complement (C) before transfer eliminated the suppressive activity of spleen cells from aged donors. This activity was restored by mixing equal portions of a population treated with anti-Ly1 plus C and a population treated with anti-Ly2 plus C. It was concluded that two cell types, one $Ly1^+$ and one $Ly2^+$, collaborated in the suppression, and that at least one of these was Ia^+ (16). These investigators further observed that nonspecific suppressor cells of aged mice are most predominantly represented in the bone marrow (16); however, they did not characterize the suppressor cells from this tissue source.

Liu et al. (17) transplanted Millipore diffusion chambers containing cells from unimmunized mice of different ages, cells from immunized young mice, and antigen into the peritoneal cavities of cyclophosphamide-pretreated outbred recipients. After 7–8 days the cells were recovered from the chambers and assayed for plaque-forming cells (PFC). Cells from unimmunized aged donors suppressed the responses of cells from immunized young mice (17). Similar results had been obtained by these investigators using immunized cells from young and aged donors (18) (see Section III. B). Unimmunized mice tested at 26 months of age, following a 1-year in vivo treatment with anti-I-J monoclonal antibody, showed levels of suppression in this system equal to that of saline-treated, age-matched control (19). Unfortunately, the majority of the aged mice used in the latter study had malignant tumors, a problem frequently encountered in aging research. The suppressor activity from untreated mice appeared to have increased rapidly as a function of age until 15 months and then remained at a high level, while helper T-cell activity declined at a constant rate with age. Based on the frequency of defects found in aged animals, the authors hypothesized that initially, suppressor cells increase with age, followed at an older age by a decrease in helper T-cell activity (20).

DeKruyff and co-workers (21), using Mishell Dutton cultures to generate primary antibody responses in vitro to T-independent (dinitrophenyl polyacrylamide: DNP-PAA) and T-dependent (sheep red blood cells: SRBC) antigens, demonstrated suppressor activity in spleen cells from old mice (18 months) of both the LAF_1 and BALB/c strains. The suppressive activity of cells from unimmunized aged donors was apparent when mixed (1:1) with spleen cells from unimmunized young adults. Removal of T cells from the aged donor spleen population eliminated the suppressive effect. The authors (21) concluded that spleen cells from aged mice have significant spontaneous nonspecific T suppressor activity.

Singhal and co-workers (22) found suppressor activity in the bone marrow of young and aged animals, and in the spleens of aged animals. This activity was also demonstrated by assaying antibody responses after incubating the cells in Mishell Dutton cultures with unimmunized spleen cells from young syngeneic animals and SRBC. They, however, characterized the suppressor cell from the bone marrow as a non-T, non-B, nonmacrophage, Fc-receptor-positive, medium-to-large lymphocyte (23). Evidence suggested that the cell was not a pre-T cell (23). The suppressor population in the spleen was also characterized as a non-T cell that was radiation sensitive (22). They hypothesized that a suppressor population in the bone marrow expands with age and migrates to the periphery (22).

Segre and co-workers (24) detected nonspecific suppressor cells in the spleens of mice that had been treated with cyclophosphamide 7 days previously. They used an assay system identical to that described earlier by them (see above) (17). This suppressor population was also not a typical T cell, B cell, or macrophage and worked in an antigen-nonspecific manner to decrease the secondary antibody response to T-dependent antigens. The investigators suggested that cyclophosphamide depletion of the spleen leads to a regeneration that simulates ontogenetic processes normally operative in neonatal spleen to establish tolerance to self antigens. To their surprise, they found an increase with age in these suppressor cells in C57BL/6 mice. In the $BC3F_1$ strain, no age-related changes were detected.

The studies above looked at humoral immune responses, and all demonstrated an increase of suppressor cells in the spleens of unimmunized aged animals. Liu and co-workers (17) point out that although these cells do not appear to be antigen specific, this interpretation is complicated by the fact that antigenic stimulation was part of the assay system. However, particularly in instances in which immunized cells were used as the population to be suppressed, it would seem unlikely that generation of antigen-specific suppressor cells to a novel antigen could occur in sufficient time to inhibit the function of primed T helper cells and primed B cells. Evidence for a cascade of T suppressor cells in antigen-specific systems (6) suggests that at least several days are required to induce the final effector cell. The suppressor cells being measured above were, more likely, already present in the aged spleen, although perhaps in inactive form. These cells could truly be nonspecific. Alternatively, they could be memory suppressor T cells, reactivated when confronted with antigen cross-reactive to a previously experienced environmental antigen, particularly in assays in which the suppressor cells have been characterized as T cells. In systems in which the suppressor population has been characterized as a "null cell" (22–24), the possibility still exists that these cells are precursor cells pushed to maturity during the assay period.

If indeed, during the period of coincubation of young and old cells, antigen-specific suppressor cells are derived from the cells of the unimmunized aged animals, they are then being generated in the presence of cells from young animals. Thus, it is possible that the competent cells from the young donors are providing lymphokines normally deficient in the aged animals, which now allow the generation of suppressor cells. This consideration also applies to findings concerning suppression of cell-mediated immune responses (see below).

In the assay used by Chang et al. (25) to demonstrate suppressor cells in aged mouse spleen, specific antigen was not included in the incubation. The suppressor cells were detected in vitro by stimulating mixtures of spleen cells from young and aged mice with lipopolysaccharide (LPS) to produce a polyclonal antibody response (25). In this system the suppressor cells from the aged mice were most probably acting nonspecifically.

Thoman and Weigle (26) reported a decrease in nonspecific suppressor cells with age in the C57BL/6 strain. These cells were detected after 3-4 days of in vitro incubation of spleen cells without specific antigen, but with fetal calf serum in the medium. The cultured cell population was then treated with anti-Ly1 and C and assayed for suppressive activity by coincubation for 48 h with $Ly2^-$ nylon wool-nonadherent spleen cells from mice primed with SRBC. The cell mixtures were then recollected, treated with anti-Ly2 and C to eliminate the suppressor cells, and assayed for helper cell activity by culturing them with unimmunized B cells and SRBC. Antibody responses were measured 5 days later. Culture-generated suppressor cells from young mice were more effective in inhibiting the production of helper cells than those generated from 30-month-old mice. Addition of IL-2-rich supernatants to the initial culture increased the generation of suppressor cells from aged mice. One of the advantages of their system is that the suppressor cells were generated or expanded without the presence of cells from young mice, which could provide missing lymphokines.

In a cell-mediated immune system, Gerbase-DeLima et al. (27) were able to detect suppression of the mixed lymphocyte culture (MLC) responses of cells from young mice by spleen cells from unimmunized syngeneic aged animals in three of the four strains tested. Spleen cells from aged C57BL/10 mice caused neither synergy nor suppression when added to MLCs of responder cells from young C57BL/10 mice. In our studies we also obtained an additive response when spleen cells from unimmunized young and aged C57BL/6 mice were combined in MLCs using irradiated DBA/2 spleen cells as stimulators (Figure 1). Although cells from aged C57BL/6 mice had a profoundly deficient proliferative response in the MLC, an excess of preexisting suppressor cells could not be demonstrated in this strain by simple mixing experiments. Zharhary and co-workers (28) also found that spleen cells from the majority of aged C57BL/6 mice tested gave additive results when combined with spleen cells from young donors in T-cell-mediated cytotoxic assays.

Chang and co-workers (25) tested the responses of mixtures of spleen cells from young and aged C57BL/6 mice to T- and B-cell mitogens: phytohemagglutinin (PHA), Con A, and LPS, and found no evidence for synergy or suppression in these cultures. Since they did find suppression of LPS-stimulated polyclonal activation of the antibody response, these investigators suggested that the

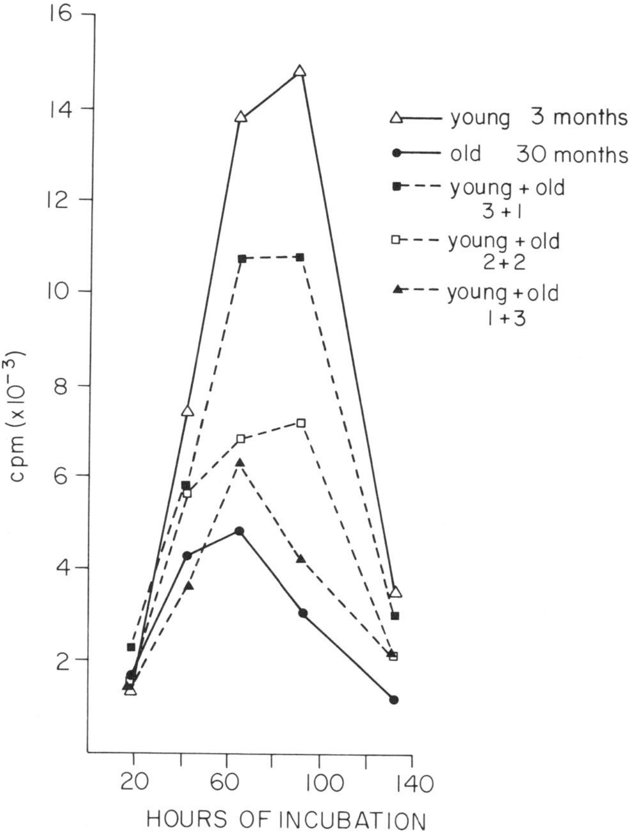

Figure 1 Mixtures of spleen cells from young and aged C57BL/6 mice used as responders in MLC with DBA/2 stimulators. Mixtures were set up with the same total number of responder cells and stimulated with an equal number of irradiated DBA/2 cells. Aliquots were taken every 24 h and labeled with tritiated thymidine for 14 h to establish a kinetics curve. Mixtures gave additive results, therefore demonstrating neither synergy nor suppression when responder cells from young and aged mice were mixed.

regulatory cells in spleens from old mice could inhibit B-cell differentiation but not B- or T-cell proliferation (25).

Bruley-Rosset and co-workers (29) found that if they removed the nylon wool-adherent cell population from spleen cells of middle-aged (DBA/2 × B6)F_1 mice, the response to T-cell mitogens increased. This suggested the presence of non-T natural suppressor cells in the middle-aged animals. Combining spleen cells from young and aged (22 months old) (B6 × BALB/c) F_1 mice, they found however that the nylon wool-nonadherent population, not the plastic-adherent cells, from aged, but not from young mice decreased the mitogen response of spleen cells from young animals (30).

Globerson and co-workers (31), however, found that cells from aged mice caused suppression of responses of cells from young animals of (C3H × C57BL/6) F_1 and (BALB × C57BL/6) F_1 strains. This spontaneous suppression was at a low level unless large numbers of cells were added. These naturally occurring suppressor cells were pretreated with mitomycin C or irradiation and assayed for suppression of Con A, PHA, and MLC responses. They were resistant to anti-Thy-1 and C, although they appeared to have receptors for peanut agglutinin (PNA), a property suggestive of immature T cells (32). More recent studies (33) suggested that the PNA^+ naturally occurring suppressor cells lacked Ly2, but that at least some were $Ly1^+$ and $Ly6^+$. The possibility therefore exists that this nonspecific suppressor population was composed of immature T cells, B cells, or a mixture of both. The nonadherent properties of the cells suggested that macrophages did not form a major component of the population. The authors suggested that the involution of the thymus in aged mice causes the appearance of immature T cells in the periphery (33). These then act as nonspecific suppressor cells. The differences between these results and those discussed above (25,27) using similar assay systems may reflect differences in the mouse strains used. On the other hand, Singhal (22,23), Segre (24), and Globerson (31-33) all described an increase with age in "null" suppressor cells. Globerson proposed that these cells were pre-T cells. It is improbable that Globerson et al. (31-33) and Singhal and co-workers (22,23) are investigating the same suppressor cell population, since the former group found their suppressor activity to be radiation resistant whereas, in Singhal's antibody system, suppression was radiation sensitive. The suppressor cells detected in the spleen after cyclophosphamide treatment by Segre et al. (24) may be a population identical to or overlapping with those found by Globerson and co-workers (31).

When Con A was used by Globerson and co-workers (31) to expand the population of suppressor cells in young and aged (C3H × C57BL/6)F_1 and (BALB × C57BL/6)F_1 mice, the young animals generated more effective suppression than the aged mice. The Con-A-induced suppressor cells were at least partially sensitive to anti-Thy-1 and C treatment (31).

In an autologous system, using peripheral blood lymphocytes (PBL) from sheep, Ellis and Demartini (34) induced suppressor cells by preincubation with Con A, treated them with mitomycin C, and used them to suppress responses to T-cell mitogens. They found an increase in Con-A-induced suppressor cells with age.

Gutowski and Weksler (35) investigated the basis for the decline in the syngeneic mixed lymphocyte reaction (SMLR) with age in the BALB/c strain.

They found that the ability of whole irradiated spleen to function as stimulators decreased by middle age, an age at which the responder T-cell population was still functionally intact. Combining stimulator cells from young and aged donors, the investigators found evidence for a suppressor population among the irradiated spleen cells from aged mice (35).

In experiments in which cells from unimmunized donors of different ages are mixed, the final result has, in most instances, been a lower than expected (additive) response, suggesting suppressor activity. Interpretation of such experiments is difficult because direct comparisons between the suppressor cell populations of donors of different ages are usually not made. The ratio between suppressor and helper cells in each population may also affect the outcome (15). In most of the experimental designs, even when cells from unimmunized donors of different ages are tested on cells from immunized animals, the balance between these two functions (help vs. suppression) can determine the result. Perhaps more accurate assessment could be made by first eliminating the effect of T helper cells, as was done by Thoman and Weigle (26). If possible, in experiments in which the final assay system measures a proliferative response, the contribution of the "suppressor" population to the proliferation should be first eliminated by pretreatment with irradiation or mitomycin C. These reservations also apply to many of the experiments discussed below in which specific suppressor cells are evaluated. Most investigators do agree, however, that cells from unimmunized aged donors lower the humoral response of cells from young animals (14–17,19–22,25). Whether this lowering can be attributed to a preexisting or newly expanded population of suppressor cells is subject to the above-discussed reservations. When tried, elimination of suppressor cells from the population has not led to an increase in the ability of cells from aged mice to respond (33). This suggests that the presence of spontaneous suppressor cells does not fully account for the deficient immunological responses of aged animals. When the ability to generate suppressor cells from young and aged animals is directly compared, disparate results have been obtained (24,26,31-34).

B. Suppressor Cells from Immunized Donors (in vivo or in vitro)

Immunizations frequently lead to a mixture of effector and suppressor cells, with some schedules favoring the development of one over the other. One method of immunization that favors induction of suppressor cells is the intravenous (I.V.) injection of antigen-coupled syngeneic spleen cells. This approach was used by Doria and co-workers (36), who specifically induced suppressor cells to azobenzene arsonate (ABA) by immunizing with ABA-syngeneic spleen cells. They found that using suboptimal conditions, ABA-specific suppressor cells could be more readily induced in aged mice. They also studied the sensitivity to suppression of effector cells from aged animals. Although the responses by aged mice were quite low even in the absence of suppressor cells, within these limitations of the experimental system, they found that cells from aged mice appeared to be more resistant to suppression than cells from young mice.

Callard et al. (16) induced antigen-specific memory suppressor T cells by I.V. injection of deaggregated human γ-globulin into primed animals. These cells were assayed by adoptive transfer, with hapten- and carrier-primed spleen cells, into irradiated recipients. No differences were found in the ability of young and aged animals to generate the antigen-specific suppressor memory cells. In contrast, the same investigators had found an increase in nonspecific suppressor cells with age (16) (Section III.A).

Segre and Segre (18) transferred immunized spleen cells (antigen: DNP–keyhole limpet hemocyamin–bentonite) from young and aged (C57BL × C3H)F_1 mice into diffusion chambers in the peritoneal cavities of young irradiated outbred recipients. Aged donors had had a longer time period between priming and cell transfer (> 25 months) than had the young donors (1–4 months). Spleen cells from the aged donors that gave the lowest antibody responses when tested alone effected the highest levels of suppression when cotransferred with cells from young mice. The immunization schedule used for the induction of suppressor cells, however, was the same as that used to generate immune responsiveness (18).

An additional method that has been used in the evaluation of the functional status of suppressor cells is the determination of the ease with which tolerance to soluble antigen can be induced. Neonatal animals are the most easily tolerized age group, and this ease of induction is lost with progressive maturation of the immune system (37). The mechanism for maintenance of tolerance during the neonatal period may differ from that involved in maintaining tolerance induced during adulthood. The "null" cell suppressors may have an important role in neonatal tolerance (Section III.A). During adult life, tolerance is at least partially maintained by specific suppressor T cells.

Amagai and co-workers (38) and Habicht (39) found that resistance to tolerance induction increased with advancing age in all mouse strains tested. Habicht (39) demonstrated that the age at which tolerance induction was lost was related to the life span of the strain. Amagai et al. (38) divided the strains they tested into three groups, based on when in their life span the ability to become tolerized was lost. In fact, in some strains, what would be a tolerogenic dose of antigen in young mice resulted in sensitization in older mice (38). Amagai and co-workers (38) concluded that a decrease in the generation of specific suppressor cells occurred with age, as demonstrated by a reduced ability to transfer "infectious tolerance," but that this decrease did not fully account for the resistance to tolerance induction. Habicht (39,40) concluded, from cell transfer experiments on the mechanism of B-cell tolerance in mice of various ages, that most of the age-related resistance to tolerance induction was due to an effect of the environment rather than to an intrinsic change in either the stem cells or the peripheral lymphoid cells.

One complication that may arise in suppressor cell experiments was brought out by Hausman and co-workers (41). They induced antigen-specific T-suppressor cells to trinitrophenyl (TNP) by I.V. immunization with TNP-modified syngeneic spleen cells in C57BL/6 mice of various ages. The suppressor cells were assayed by cotransfer of splenic T cells and antigen (TNP-conjugates) into syngeneic animals of various ages. They found that for suppression of antibody formation to be effective, the donors of the T cells containing the suppressor cell population and the recipients had to be age matched. Levels of suppression generated at different ages were not compared. Having also previously shown that sera containing anti-idiotypic antibodies preferentially inhibited plaque-forming cells (PFC) from age-matched donors, suggesting the occurrence of idiotypic changes with age (42), these investigators hypothesized that idiotypic changes result in a nonidentity between cells from syngeneic animals of different ages. This potential complication of these suppressor cell experiments may also apply to systems assaying suppression of cell-mediated immunity (see below).

Flood and co-workers (43) used a system in which they generated suppression of cytotoxic activity to syngeneic UV-induced tumors. This "suppression," in fact, resulted from the action of cytotoxic T lymphocytes (CTL) reactive to the common idiotype (Id) expressed on tumor-specific CTLs. These anti-Id CTLs were generated by immunizing the mice with tumor-specific CTLs. Using the CBA/HeN strain, the investigators found that the ability to generate the anti-Id response decreased during adulthood (9–12 months); however, the appearance of anti-tumor CTLs with the common Id on their surface also decreased (8 months). In vivo rejection of tumor challenge was decreased in 9- to 14-month-old mice and essentially nonexistent in 16- to 22-month-old animals (43). This study illustrates the importance of differentiating between true suppressor cells and other negative influences on immune responses that could mimic suppressor cell activity.

In our own experiments we have attempted to compare the changes with age in the ability of mice to generate proliferative, cytotoxic, and suppressive activity against allogeneic stimulator cells (44–46). We reasoned that studying these T-cell functions would give us an indication of the overall status of the cell-mediated immune system of aged mice, since we could measure these functions from the same cultures and, as such, frequently measured them in the same individual mice.

The proliferative response of spleen cells from C57BL/6 mice to DBA/2 spleen cells decreased by 14 months of age (Figure 2). The cytotoxic response generated in the same cultures to the H-2^d alloantigen did not appear to decline

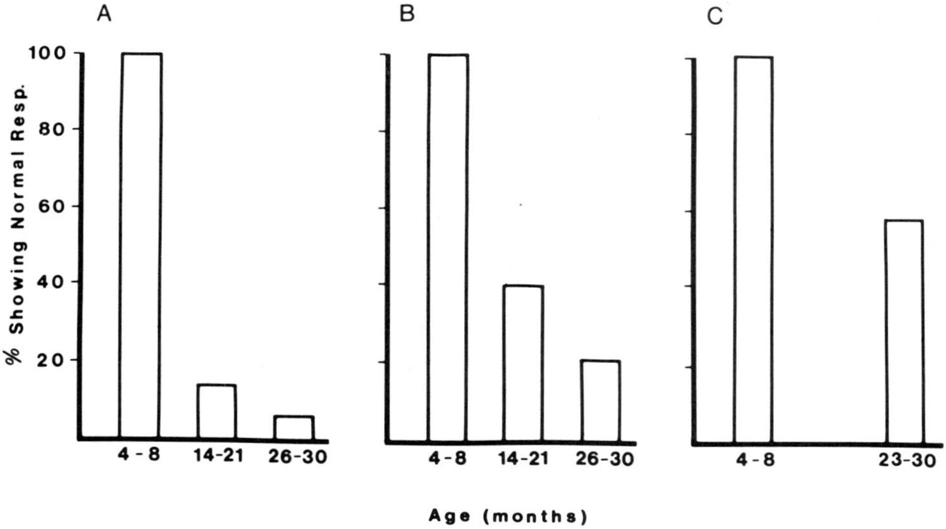

Figure 2 Summary graph of animals assayed. Percent of animals of different ages whose spleen cells showed no significant difference (by two-tailed *t*-test analysis) when compared with cells from young adult mice (4–8 months) assayed simultaneously. Fourteen mice, aged 14–21 months, and 17 mice, aged 26–30 months, were assayed in both MLC (*A*) and cytotoxicity (*B*) assays. Twenty-two mice, aged 23–30 months, were assayed for generation of specific suppressor cell activity along with young controls (*C*). Seven of that aged population were also tested in the MLC (data not shown), and all but one showed a decreased proliferative response. All three assays were against the H-2^d allotype.

in the majority of the individual mice tested until 26 months of age, unless suboptimal tissue culture conditions were used (44). Using the same type of sensitization culture, we tested the generation of specific suppressor cells (45). Once generated, these cells are radiation resistant and they were, therefore, irradiated before transfer to fresh 5-day MLCs between C57BL/6 responders and DBA/2 stimulators. The irradiation eliminated the proliferative cells, which otherwise would have responded to the DBA/2 stimulators with a secondary response. The suppressor cells were sensitive to anti-Thy-1 plus C and specifically suppressed responses to H-2^d. Identity between the stimulators of the suppressor cells and the stimulators in the assay cultures was required only at H-2K and H-2I, and was independent of the M locus.

We directed much effort at ensuring that the "suppressor cells" were not simply cytotoxic cells, killing fresh responder or stimulator cells. Cytotoxic cells to the stimulator cells are simultaneously generated in such cultures and would be expected to function for a period of time in spite of radiation. However, small numbers of suppressor cells were highly effective in reducing the level of response (1 suppressor cell : 20 responder cells : 20 stimulator cells), and this was a strong argument against the possibility that the suppression was due to cytotoxic cells. This number of "cytotoxic" cells and this ratio of "cytotoxic" to target cells (1:20) would not give a detectable level of cytotoxicity in a 4-h assay. In 5-day cultures, only a limited amount of recycling of killer cells was possible, since the cells were first irradiated. Moreover, there was no evidence that suppression could be overcome by additional stimulator cells (Figure 3).

Comparing the ability of young and aged C57BL/6 mice to generate specific suppression, we found that 41% of the 22 aged mice (23–28 months)

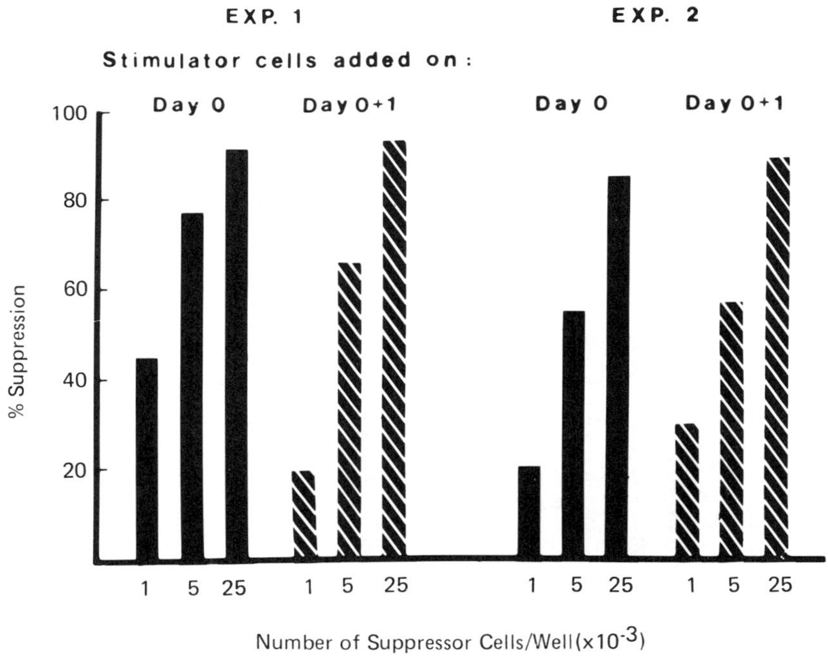

Figure 3 Inability of additional stimulator cells to overcome suppression. C57BL/6 suppressor cells were generated in 5-day MLC against DBA/2 stimulators and were assayed after irradiation by addition of varying doses to fresh MLCs of C57BL/6 responders and DBA/2 stimulators (2×10^5 cells/well). Additional DBA/2 stimulator cells (2×10^5 cells/well) were added on day 1 to compensate for possible lysis of stimulator cells. Cultures without suppressor cells gave 21,000–31,000 cpm.

tested generated significantly less suppression ($p < .01$) than young control mice (3-8 months) examined simultaneously (Figure 2). Figure 4 shows a representative experiment comparing one aged mouse and one young mouse in their ability to generate suppression. For each animal tested, a similar dose-response curve was generated. Table 1 summarizes the data at two suppressor cell doses. The suppressor cell doses chosen for comparison were those that gave between 25 and 85% suppression when suppressor cells from young control animals were used. Over the series of experiments, these suppressor cell doses were found to be consistent.

Figure 2 compares the ability to generate suppressor cells with the ability to generate proliferative and cytotoxic cells. The same aged and young animal populations were used for the proliferative and cytotoxic responses. Seven of the

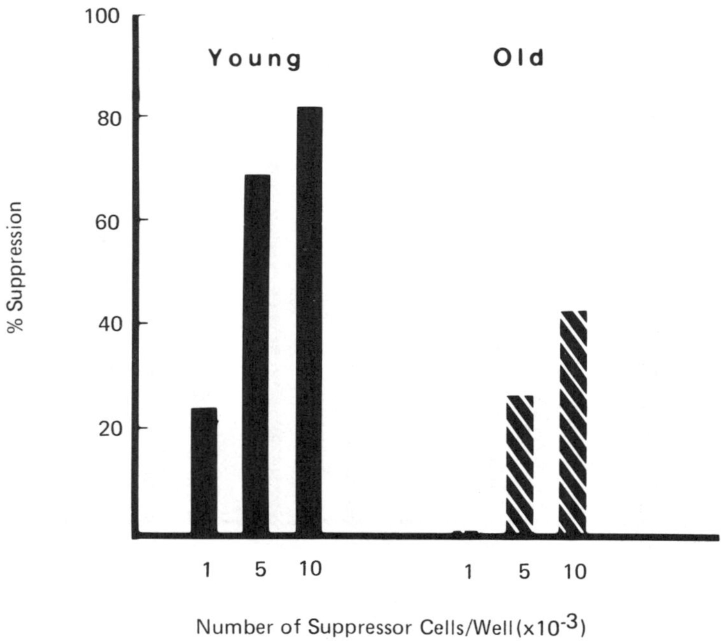

Figure 4 Representative experiment comparing the ability of young and aged C57BL/6 mice to generate suppressor cells in MLC against DBA/2 stimulator cells. Cells were irradiated (1000 R) after generation and added in varying doses to fresh MLC of C57BL/6 responder cells (2×10^5 cells/well) and DBA/2 stimulator cells. Similar results were obtained using responder cell doses of 1×10^5 and 1.5×10^5 cells/well. The young mouse was 4 months old and the aged was 25 months old. Cultures without added suppressor cells gave 42,760 cpm.

Table 1 Efficiency of Specific Suppressor Cell Generation in Population of Aged Mice

Donor of spleen cells for suppression	Mean percent suppression: Suppressor cell dose[a] Single (% ±SE)	Double (% ±SE)
Young mice[b]	54.6 ±5.1	72.3 ±3.5
	(n = 14)	(n = 15)
Aged mice, group I[c]	53.8 ±6.3	70.0 ±5.5
	(n = 12)	(n = 13)
	$p > .5$[d]	$p > .5$[d]
Aged mice, group II[e]	33.7 ±5.9	57.2 ±4.9
	(n = 7)	(n = 8)
	p = .02	p = .02

[a]MLC-generated, C57BL/6 specific suppressor cells were induced by 4- or 5-day incubations with irradiated DBA/2 stimulator cells. The suppressor cells were irradiated (1000 R) before being assayed in fresh MLCs between C57BL/6 responders and DBA/2 stimulator cells. After a 5-day generation a single suppressor cell dose of 5×10^3 cells/well was used and after a 4-day generation the single dose was 2.5×10^3 cells/well. Suppressor cell doses chosen for comparison between young and aged were those that gave 25–85% suppression by the young control populations. Over the entire series of experiments these doses were consistent for a given set of experimental conditions (number of days of incubation).
[b]Young mice that served as controls for suppressor experiments with aged mice, group I, were not significantly different from those that were controls for experiments with aged mice, group II.
[c]Aged mice, group I, were not significantly different from young control mice in their ability to generate suppressor cells.
[d]Two-tailed Student's t test was used to compare each aged group to the young control at the same suppressor cell dose.
[e]Aged mice, group II, generated significantly fewer suppressor cells than young control mice assayed simultaneously.

aged animals tested for suppressor cell generation were also assayed for proliferative response (data not shown). Of these seven aged animals, six had markedly decreased proliferative responses (45). This corresponded with the results on the proliferative responses of the larger series of animals (Figure 2*A*). Whereas the proliferative response shows the earliest decline with age, it seemed that even in the absence of optimal proliferation, the cells were still capable of generating functional effector cells (cytotoxic and suppressor cells).

In light of reports by other investigators showing a decrease in IL-2 production with age (47–51), we tested the ability of exogenous IL-2-rich supernatants to enhance the proliferative and suppressor generating capacity of aged C57BL/6 mice (46). Both responses were improved by the addition of an exogenous source of IL-2. The proliferative response, greatly deficient in the majority of aged C57BL/6 mice, was however not increased to the level of young adult mice. The ability of aged mice to generate specific suppressor cells was restored by the addition of IL-2-rich supernatant to the generation cultures. Overall, the level of suppression generated in the presence of IL-2 increased 16.3% for the five aged animals tested and only 1.8% for the three young mice assayed (46). This average change for the aged animals included mice that had normal suppressor cell generation in the absence of IL-2 and were essentially unaffected by addition of the lymphokine (similar to results with the young adults tested). An example of the effect of IL-2 on suppressor cell generation by spleen cells

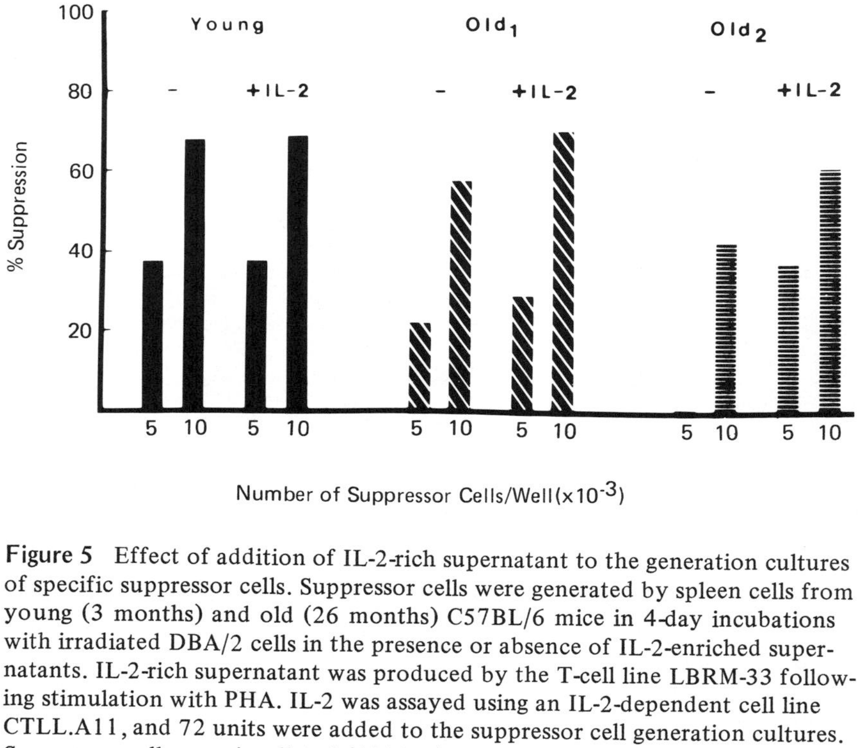

Figure 5 Effect of addition of IL-2-rich supernatant to the generation cultures of specific suppressor cells. Suppressor cells were generated by spleen cells from young (3 months) and old (26 months) C57BL/6 mice in 4-day incubations with irradiated DBA/2 cells in the presence or absence of IL-2-enriched supernatants. IL-2-rich supernatant was produced by the T-cell line LBRM-33 following stimulation with PHA. IL-2 was assayed using an IL-2-dependent cell line CTLL.A11, and 72 units were added to the suppressor cell generation cultures. Suppressor cells were irradiated (1000 R) before being added in varying doses (5 or 10×10^3 cells/well) to fresh assay MLC between young C57BL/6 responders (1.5×10^5 cells/well) and DBA/2 stimulators. Cultures of young responders alone gave 37,960 cpm. Old$_2$ was deficient in suppressor cell generation compared to the young control, whereas old$_1$ was not deficient in suppressor cell generation. IL-2-rich supernatant was effective only on suppressor cell generation by old$_2$.

from three mice (one young and two old) is shown in Figure 5. One aged animal (old_1) had normal suppressor cell generation and was unaffected by addition of IL-2, whereas the defective response of the second aged animal (old_2) was significantly improved. Therefore, it is possible that the defect in the ability to generate specific suppressor cells is primarily due to a relative lack of lymphokine production needed for suppressor cell proliferation. The presence of additional defects, however, such as precursor cell number or responsiveness, which might be overcome by an increase in proliferation with addition of IL-2, cannot be excluded.

To investigate the possibility that idiotypic changes with age led to an inability of suppressor cells generated from aged mice to act on young responder cells in our assay system, we also tested suppression of the MLC response of middle-aged (18 months) animals. We chose the middle-aged group as our responders because the age-related decline in MLC responsiveness was already apparent (44); however the response was not so low as to make suppression difficult to detect. Additionally, the idiotypic changes with age, which have been reported in other systems (41,42), are evident by 18 months (middle age) in the C57BL/6 strain. We found that suppressor cells generated from old mice were equally ineffective in their ability to suppress the MLC response of middle-aged mice and in their ability to suppress the response of cells from young animals (Figure 6). In contrast, the suppressor cells from young animals suppressed both groups of responder cells equally well (Figure 6). This evidence suggests that idiotypic changes with age do not account for the inability of cells from aged mice to suppress responders in our assay system.

Gorczynski and co-workers (52) investigated the development of specific suppressor cells in the spleens of irradiated $(C3B6)F_1$ recipients of C57BL/6 bone marrow taken from mice of different ages. The spleen cells of these bone marrow chimeras were examined 60 days after reconstitution. They were added (5×10^4), unirradiated, to limiting dilution assays of lymph node cells from untreated young C57BL/6 mice. The spleen cells from the chimeras suppressed the development of CTL to $H\text{-}2^k$ stimulators but not to third-party stimulators. This suppressor activity decreased with age of the bone marrow donors. There was, however, a concomitant rise in the ability of spleen cells from the chimeras to themselves develop CTLs against the "forbidden" $H\text{-}2^k$. Whether this development of CTLs represented a deficiency of suppressor cell generation in vivo or defective thymus education to self could be debated. The investigators (52) interpreted their findings as demonstrating a decrease of suppressor cell generation with age. They also used a second system to assay suppressor cells derived from C57BL/6 bone marrow (52). T-cell colonies were grown with PHA in methylcellulose. These cells, although nonspecifically expanded, were used to suppress the CTL response of allogeneic cells against targets of the same H-2 type as that of the T-cell colonies. Again they found a decrease in suppressor cell

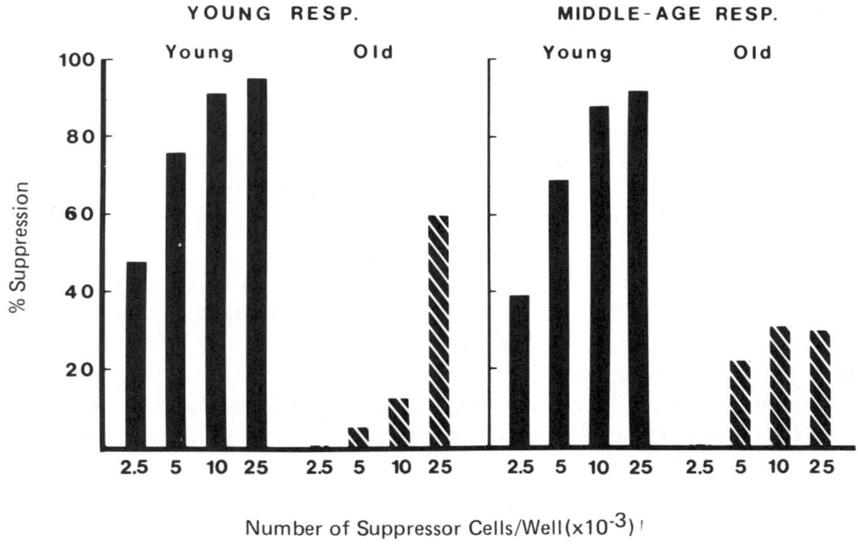

Figure 6 Lack of requirement for age matching between suppressor and responder cells. Suppressor cells were generated by spleen cells from young (3 months) and old (28 months) C57BL/6 mice in 4-day incubations with irradiated DBA/2 cells. These cells were then harvested, irradiated (1000 R), and assayed for their ability to suppress spleen cell responders from (*A*) young (3 months) and (*B*) middle-aged (18 months) C57BL/6 mice in their MLC response to DBA/2 stimulators. Suppressor cells were added in varying doses ($1-25 \times 10^3$ cells/well) to 2×10^5 responder cells/well. Proliferative responses to DBA/2 stimulators for each population alone (2×10^5 cells/well) were: young, 75,700; middle-aged, 30,400; and old, 4800 cpm. Significant levels of suppression were seen using suppressor cells from young mice tested on responder cells from young mice ($p < .01$ for suppressor cell doses 25, 10, 5, and 2.5×10^3 cells/well) and from middle-aged mice ($p < .01$ for suppressor cell doses 25, 10, and 5×10^3 cells/well, $p < .05$ for 2.5×10^3 suppressor cells/well). Cells from aged mice only showed significant suppression ($p < .01$) when tested at 25×10^3 cells/well on responder cells from young mice.

generation with age of the bone marrow donor. No suppressor activity was found in allogeneic MLCs against third-party targets. They proposed that they may have been measuring anti-idiotypic suppressor T cells normally present.

In summary, the few investigations comparing young and aged animals in their ability to generate specific suppressor cells give disparate results (16,18,20, 36,45,46,52). Although no consensus on specific suppressor cells in aging is reached, several important points are raised. The first is the importance of the idiotype–anti-idiotype network in regulating the magnitude of the immune response. This control operates directly among effector T cells in addition to operating at the level of the antibody response. A detailed discussion of idiotype–anti-idiotype regulation is, however, outside the scope of this chapter.

A second point (41,42) is the possibility that because of changes in idiotype expression with age, effector cells generated in aged animals are not functional when asked to collaborate with or act on cells from young mice. This would complicate interpretation of experiments on suppressor cells, including our own, where the read-out is the level of response by cells from young animals. The apparent decrease in suppressor cell activity may be an artifact of an assay system that uses responder cells from young animals. Indeed, for optimal estimation of the presence of suppressor cells, studies using age-matched recipients or cells from age-matched donors may be needed. On the other hand, responses of aged recipients are so low that suppression is difficult to evaluate, creating a complicated experimental dilemma.

A third point, which derives from the work of Flood et al. (43), is that the presence of various levels of interacting cells in the immune response may confound the interpretation of changes observed with age. Their system measured the ability to generate a second level of cytotoxic cells whose action led to an apparent depression of the first-level response being assayed. A decrease in the first level of response would itself have induced a lower response at the second level. Although Flood et al. (43) studied cytotoxic cells, similar considerations would apply to suppressor cell systems in which an immune population is first required to induce the suppressor cells.

IV. SUMMARY AND CONCLUSIONS

In Table 2, which summarizes the literature reviewed in this chapter, investigations of suppression of humoral immunity are grouped and can be compared with those of suppression of T-cell-mediated immunity. A brief description of the induction system used in each case is given. This organization differs from the order in the chapter and thus emphasizes different aspects of the studies.

Whereas a general consensus exists with respect to changes in the humoral and proliferative responses in the aging organism, an overall conclusion is difficult to arrive at for suppressor cell generation (Table 2). Nonspecific suppressor cells have been found to increase with age in most studies, whereas the status of specific suppressor cells appears to be more variable. Attention to the mouse strain used may be of great importance (27). It is not apparent why animals with C57BL background may have fewer suppressor cells with age in comparison to other strains (27). C57BL mice are a particularly long-lived strain, which do not develop a high incidence of autoimmune disease with age, although they do have

Table 2 Summary of Literature Reviewed

Assay system	Induction method	Characterization of suppressor cells	Reported change in function	Ref.
Antibody response in vivo	Mixture of unimmunized cells, young + aged, into irradiated T_x hosts	Nonspecific	↑	14
Antibody response in vivo and in vitro	Mixture of unimmunized cells, young + aged, into irradiated hosts or culture	Nonspecific	↑	15
Antibody response in vivo, T-dependent and T-independent antigens	Mixture of unimmunized cells from aged with immunized or unimmunized cells from young into irradiated hosts	Nonspecific: Thy-1^+, $Ly1^+$ and Thy-1^+, $Ly2^+$	↑	16
Antibody response in vivo	Mixture of unimmunized cells from young or aged + immunized cells from young ± Ag in diffusion chambers in peritoneal cavities of cyclophosphamide-treated hosts	Nonspecific	↑	17,19,20
Antibody response in vivo	Mixture of unimmunized cells from cyclophosphamide-pretreated young or aged + immunized cells from young ± Ag in diffusion chambers in peritoneal cavities of cyclophosphamide-treated hosts	Nonspecific: Thy-1^-, nylon wool-nonadherent spleen cell present in nude and T_x irradiated bone marrow reconstituted mice	↑	24
Antibody response in vitro	Mixture of unimmunized cells, young + aged in Mishell-Dutton cultures	Nonspecific: T cells	↑	21
Antibody response in vitro	Mixture of unimmunized cells, young + aged in Mishell-Dutton cultures	Nonspecific: spleen (non-T cells radiation sensitive), bone marrow (FcR^+ null cells)	↑	22,23

Antibody response in vitro, polyclonal LPS stimulated	Mixture of unimmunized cells, young + aged	Nonspecific	↑	25
Antibody response in vivo	Mixture of immunized cells from young or aged + immunized young + Ag in diffusion chambers in peritoneal cavities of cyclophosphamide-treated hosts	Specific	↑	18
Antibody response in vitro, assayed with carrier-primed T cells	Immunization in vivo of young or aged mice with ABA-syngeneic cells	Specific	↑	36
Antibody response in vivo	In vivo-induced (deaggregated Ag) specific suppressor cells from young or aged + primed cells from young into irradiated hosts	Specific	=	16
Antibody response in vitro assaying T helper cell function with primed B cells	In vitro culture-generated suppressor cells, young or aged then added to young primed T helper cells	Nonspecific	↓	26
Antibody response in vivo	Ability to be tolerized in vivo	Specific	↓	38
Antibody response in vivo	Ability to transfer tolerance with thymus cells or spleen when given with unimmunized young cells to irradiated hosts	Specific	↓	38
MLC response in vitro	Mixture of unimmunized cells, young + aged	Nonspecific	↑	27
MLC, PHA, Con A responses	Mixture of unimmunized cells, young + aged	Nonspecific: $Ly1^+$, $Ly2^-$, $Ly6^+$, PNA^+, $Thy\text{-}1^-$ nonadherent cells; radiation resistant	↑	31–33
Con A response in sheep	Mixture of Con A-pretreated cells, young or aged + untreated autologous cells	Nonspecific	↑	34
PHA, Con A responses	Removal of nylon wool-adherent cells from resp. populations, young or aged	Nonspecific: non-T	↑	29

Table 2 (Continued)

Assay system	Induction method	Characterization of suppressor cells	Reported change in function	Ref.
PHA, Con A responses	Mixture of unimmunized cells, young + young or young + aged	Nonspecific: nylon wool nonadherent	↑	30
SMLR response	Mixture of irradiated whole spleen cells, young + aged, as stimulator cells with young resp.	Nonspecific	↑	35
T- and B-cell mitogen response in vitro	Mixture of unimmunized cells, young + aged	Nonspecific	=	25
MLC response in vitro	Mixture of unimmunized C57BL/10 cells, young + aged	Nonspecific	=	27
CML response in vitro	Mixture of unimmunized C57BL/6 cells, young + aged	Nonspecific	=	28
MLC, PHA, Con A responses	Mixture of Con A-pretreated cells, young or aged + untreated young cells	Nonspecific: Thy-1$^+$ cells	↓	31,32
MLC response	MLC-generated suppressor cells from young or aged	Specific: T cells; radiation resistant	↓	45
CTL development in vitro by P_1 cells against P_2 targets, suppressed by spleen cells from chimeras	Parental bone marrow (P_1) from young or aged used to reconstitute irradiated P_1 recipients	Specific	↓	52

autoreactive antibodies (1). When the issue of suppressor cell generation is considered, individual assay systems may have to be carefully analyzed. For example, specific systems may activate different populations of cells (i.e., distinct suppressor cell populations: specific vs. nonspecific, T vs. non-T cells) or may result in changes in the ratios among helper, suppressor, and effector cells. An obvious difference between animal and human studies is that investigations in humans have utilized peripheral blood lymphocytes, whereas most animal experiments have used spleen or lymph node cells. Few comparisons have been done on changes in suppressor cell activity in the different peripheral lymphoid compartments.

The aged individual shows a decreased ability to respond to foreign challenge. Elegant studies by Zharhary and Klinman (53) have demonstrated the relative lack of effect of aging on the B-cell compartment before emergence from the bone marrow. Earlier studies by Harrison and co-workers (54), using serial transplantation, suggested that the stem cells, including the prethymic cells, were also intact in the aging animal. Bone marrow from aged animals could reconstitute the T-cell compartment of irradiated young mice. What happens in the periphery, therefore, to cause defects in effector function and in cell communication? There are numerous influences from the periphery on the ability of cells to function. The results of Goidl et al. (55) and Kim et al. (56) suggested an important influence of the idiotype network in the periphery, which includes both T and B cells, on the functional activity of the emerging B cells. Since suppressor activity, whether specific or nonspecific, is by definition a measure of the outcome of an interaction between at least two cells, idiotypic interactions are also likely to be of great importance in influencing suppressor activity. In addition to considerations of idiotypic changes with age, any difficulty cells from aged individuals have in producing and responding to soluble mediators, both stimulatory and inhibitory, will be reflected in their effector cell functions, including suppressor cell activity. Soluble mediators play a major role in communications between different cell subsets. Changes in the rigidity of the cell membrane, such as have been described in lymphoid and nonlymphoid cells (57), may lead to a state of decreased responsiveness to signals in general. The T-cell compartment, which includes suppressor cells, may be particularly affected by the environment. The relative contribution of newly formed T cells by the thymus to the T-cell repertoire is smaller in aged than in young animals. Much of the variability among individual old animals of an inbred strain may reflect the cumulative influences of the peripheral environment acting on the long-lived T-cell component. What these environmental factors are, how they can be distinguished from intrinsic aging, and how their detrimental effects can be overcome are questions to be examined in the future.

ACKNOWLEDGMENTS

We thank Dr. R. Coico and H. Gottesman for their constructive criticism in the preparation of the manuscript and A. Clark-Fanelli and Elizabeth Kane for secretarial assistance. This work was supported by U.S. Public Health Service grant AG-04860 from the National Institute on Aging.

REFERENCES

1. Walford, R. L. 1969. The Immunologic Theory of Aging. Munksgaard, Copenhagen.
2. Eardley, D. D., and R. K. Gershon. 1975. Feedback induction of suppressor T cell activity. *J. Exp. Med.* 142:524.
3. Jerne, N.-K. 1974. Towards a network theory of the immune system. *Ann. Immunol.* 125C:373.
4. Makinodan, T. 1977. Immunity and aging. *In* Handbook of the Biology of Aging. C. E. Finch and L. Hayflick, editors. Von Nostrand Reinhold Co., New York. 379.
5. Gottesman, S.R.S., and R. L. Walford. 1981. Autoimmunity and aging. *In* Methods in Aging Research. R. C. Adelman and G. S. Roth, editors. CRC Press, Boca Raton, Fla. XIV:233.
6. Dorf, M. E., and B. Benacerraf. 1984. Suppressor cells and immunoregulation. *Annu. Rev. Immunol.* 2:127.
7. Strober, S. 1984. Natural suppressor cells, neonatal tolerance and total lymphoid irradiation: Exploring obscure relationships. *Annu. Rev. Immunol.* 2:219.
8. Bennett, J. A., V. S. Rao, and M. S. Mitchell. 1978. Systemic *Bacillus Calmette-Guerin* (BCG) activates natural suppressor cells. *Proc. Natl. Acad. Sci. USA.* 75:5142.
9. Rich, R., and C. Pierce. 1973. Biological expressions of lymphocyte activation. II. Generation of a population of thymus derived suppressor lymphocytes. *J. Exp. Med.* 137:649.
10. Rollwagen, F. M., and O. Stutman. 1981. Culture generated suppressor cells: Evidence for an adherent cell component. *Cell. Immunol.* 64:371.
11. Aune, T. M., and C. W. Pierce. 1981. Identification and initial characterization of a nonspecific suppressor factor (Mϕ-SF) produced by soluble immune response suppressor (SIRS)-treated macrophages. *J. Immunol.* 127:1828.
12. Irons, R. D., R. W. Pfeifer, T. M. Aune, and C. W. Pierce. 1984. Soluble immune response suppressor (SIRS) inhibits microtubule function in vivo and microtubule assembly in vitro. *J. Immunol.* 133:2032.
13. Gunther, J., W. Hass, and H. G. Von Boehmer. 1982. Suppression of T cell responses through competition for T cell growth factor (interleukin 2). *Eur. J. Immunol.* 12:247.
14. Goidl, E. A., J. B. Innes, and M. E. Weksler. 1976. Immunological studies of aging. II. Loss of IgG and high avidity plaque-forming cells and increased suppressor cell activity in aging mice. *J. Exp. Med.* 144:1037.

15. Makinodan, T., J. W. Albright, P. I. Good, C. P. Peter, and M. L. Heidrick. 1976. Reduced humoral immune activity in long-lived old mice: An approach to elucidating its mechanisms. *Immunology.* 31:903.
16. Callard, R. E., B. De St. Groth, A. Basten, and I.F.C. McKenzie. 1980. Immune function in aged mice. V. Role of suppressor cells. *J. Immunol.* 124:52.
17. Liu, J. J., M. Segre, and D. Segre. 1982. Changes in suppressor, helper and B-cell functions in aging mice. *Cell. Immunol.* 66:372.
18. Segre, D., and M. Segre. 1976. Humoral immunity in aged mice. II. Increased suppressor T cell activity in immunologically deficient old mice. *J. Immunol.* 116:735.
19. Liu, J. J., D. Segre, H. B. Gelberg, H. H. Fudenberg, K. Y. Tsang, N. Khansari, C. R. Waltenbaugh, and M. Segre. 1984. Effects of long-term treatment of mice with anti-I-J monoclonal antibody and dialyzable leukocyte extract on immune function and lifespan. *Mech. Ageing Dev.* 27:359.
20. Segre, D., and M. Segre. 1977. Age-related changes in B and T lymphocytes and decline of humoral immune responsiveness in aged mice. *Mech. Ageing Dev.* 6:115.
21. DeKruyff, R. H., Y. T. Kim, G. W. Siskind, and M. E. Weksler. 1980. Age related changes in the in vitro immune response: Increased suppressor activity in immature and aged mice. *J. Immunol.* 125:142.
22. Roder, J. D., A. K. Duwe, D. A. Bell, and S. K. Singhal. 1978. Immunological senescence. I. The role of suppressor cells. *Immunology.* 35:837.
23. Duwe, A. K., and S. K. Singhal. 1979. The immunoregulatory role of bone marrow. II. Characterization of a suppressor cell inhibiting the in vitro antibody response. *Cell. Immunol.* 43:372.
24. Segre, D., E. H. Greeley, and M. Segre. 1981. Cyclophosphamide induction of non-T suppressor cells and their possible role in self-tolerance. *In* Immunological Aspects of Aging. D. Segre and L. Smith, editors. Marcel Dekker, New York. 151.
25. Chang, M.-P., J. L. Tanaka, S. Stosic-Grujicic, E. K. Yamamoto, E. H. Perkins, B. L. Strehler, and T. Makinodan. 1982. Restoration of impaired immune functions in aging animals. VI. Differential potentiating effect of 2-mercaptoethanol on young and old murine spleen cells. *Int. J. Immunopharmacol.* 4:429.
26. Thoman, M. L., and W. O. Weigle. 1983. Deficiency in suppressor T cell activity in aged animals. Reconstitution of this activity by interleukin 2. *J. Exp. Med.* 157:2184.
27. Gerbase-DeLima, M., P. Meredith, and R. L. Walford. 1975. Age-related changes, including synergy and suppression, in the mixed lymphocyte reaction in long-lived mice. *Fed. Proc.* 34:159.
28. Zharhary, D., Y. Segev, and H. E. Gershon. 1984. T-cell cytotoxicity and aging: Differing causes of reduced response in individual mice. *Mech. Ageing Dev.* 25:129.
29. Bruley-Rosset, M., I. Florentin, N. Kiger, M. Davigny, and G. Mathé. 1978. Effects of *Bacillus Calmette-Querin* and levamisole on immune responses in young adult and age-immunodepressed mice. *Cancer Treat. Rep.* 62:1641.

30. Bruley-Rosset, M., I. Florentin, N. Kiger, J. Schulz, and G. Mathé. 1979. Restoration of impaired immune functions of aged animals by chronic bestatin treatment. *Immunology*. 38:75.
31. Globerson, A., L. Abel, M. Barzilay, and I. Zan-Bar. 1982. Immunoregulatory cells in aging mice. I. Concanavalin A-induced and naturally occurring suppressor cells. *Mech. Ageing Dev.* 19:293.
32. Globerson, A., L. Abel, and T. Umiel. 1981. Immune reactivity during aging. III. Removal of peanut-agglutinin (PNA)-binding cells from aging mouse spleen cells leads to increased reactivity to mitogens. *Mech. Ageing Dev.* 16:275.
33. Globerson, A. 1986. Immunoregulatory cells in aging. *In* International Symposium on New Trends in Aging Research. In press.
34. Ellis, J. A., and J. C. Demartini. 1985. Ovine concanavalin A-induced suppressor cells: Generation, assay, age-related effects and re-evaluation of mechanism of suppression. *Immunology*. 54:353.
35. Gutowski, J. K., and M. E. Weksler. 1982. Studies on the syngeneic mixed lymphocyte reaction. Decline in the syngeneic mixed lymphocyte reaction with age. *Immunology*. 46:801.
36. Doria, G., C. Mancini, and L. Adorini. 1982. Immunoregulation in senescence: Increased inducibility of antigen-specific suppressor T cells and loss of cell sensitivity to immunosuppression in aging mice. *Proc. Natl. Acad. Sci. USA*. 79:3803.
37. Pike, B. L., T. W. Kay, and G.J.V. Nossal. 1980. Relative sensitivity of fetal and newborn mice to induction of hapten-specific B cell tolerance. *J. Exp. Med.* 152:1407.
38. Amagai, T., K. Nakano, and B. Cinader. 1982. Mechanisms involved in age-dependent decline of immune responsiveness and apparent resistance against tolerance induction in C57BL/6 mice. *Scand. J. Immunol.* 16:217.
39. Habicht, G. S. 1982. Acquired immunological tolerance in aged mice. I. The dose–response relationship. *Mech. Ageing Dev.* 19:53.
40. Habicht, G. S. 1985. Acquired immunological tolerance in aged mice. III. The contribution of lymphoid cells and their environments to the age-related resistance to tolerance induction. *Mech. Ageing Dev.* 30:37.
41. Hausman, P. B., E. A. Goidl, G. W. Siskind, and M. E. Weksler. 1985. Immunological studies of aging. XI. Age-related changes in idiotype repertoire of suppressor T cells stimulated during tolerance induction. *J. Immunol.* 134:3802.
42. Goidl, E. A., G. J. Thorbecke, M. E. Weksler, and G. W. Siskind. 1980. Production of auto-anti-idiotypic antibody during the normal immune response: Changes in the auto-anti-idiotypic antibody response and the idiotype repertoire associated with aging. *Proc. Natl. Acad. Sci. USA*. 77:6788.
43. Flood, P. M., J. L. Urban, M. L. Kripke, and H. Schreiber. 1981. Loss of tumor-specific and idiotype-specific immunity with age. *J. Exp. Med.* 154:275.

44. Gottesman, S.R.S., J. A. Kristie, and R. L. Walford. 1981. Proliferative and cytotoxic immune functions in aging mice. I. Sequence of decline of reactivities measured under optimal and suboptimal sensitization conditions. *Immunology.* 44:607.
45. Gottesman, S.R.S., R. L. Walford, and G. J. Thorbecke. 1984. Proliferative and cytotoxic immune functions in aging mice. II. Decreased generation of specific suppressor cells in alloreactive cultures. *J. Immunol.* 133:1782.
46. Gottesman, S.R.S., R. L. Walford, and G. J. Thorbecke. 1985. Proliferative and cytotoxic immune functions in aging mice. III. Exogenous interleukin-2 rich supernatant only partially restores alloreactivity in vitro. *Mech. Ageing Dev.* 31:103.
47. Chang, M. P., T. Makinodan, W. J. Peterson, and B. L. Strechler. 1982. Role of T cells and adherent cells in age-related decline in murine interleukin-2 production. *J. Immunol.* 129:2426.
48. Thoman, M. L., and W. D. Weigle. 1981. Lymphokines and aging: Interleukin-2 production and activity in aged animals. *J. Immunol.* 127:2102.
49. Miller, R. A., and O. Stutman. 1981. Decline in aging mice, of the anti-2,4,6-trinitrophenyl (TNP) cytotoxic T cell response attributable to loss of Lyt-2^-, interleukin 2-producing helper cell function. *Eur. J. Immunol.* 11:751.
50. Gillis, S., R. Kozak, M. Durante, and M. E. Weksler. 1981. Immunological studies of aging. Decreased production of and response to T cell growth factor by lymphocytes from aged humans. *J. Clin. Invest.* 67:937.
51. Joncourt, F., Y. Wang, F. Kristensen, and A. L. de Weck. 1982. Aging and immunity: Decrease in interleukin-2 production and interleukin-2-dependent RNA synthesis in lectin-stimulated murine spleen cells. *Immunobiology.* 163:521.
52. Gorczynski, R. M., M. Kennedy, and S. MacRae. 1984. Altered lymphoid recognition repertoire during ageing. III. Changes in MHC restriction patterns in parental T lymphocytes and diminution in T suppressor function. *Immunology.* 52:611.
53. Zharhary, D., and N. R. Klinman. 1983. Antigen responsiveness of the mature and generative B cell populations of aged mice. *J. Exp. Med.* 157:1300.
54. Harrison, D., C. Astle, and J. Doubleday. 1977. Stem cell lines from old immunodeficient donors give normal responses in young recipients. *J. Immunol.* 118:1223.
55. Goidl, E. A., J. W. Choy, J. J. Gibbons, M. E. Weksler, G. J. Thorbecke, and G. W. Siskind. 1983. Production of auto-antiidiotypic antibody during the normal immune response. VII. Analysis of the cellular basis for the increased auto-antiidiotype antibody production by aged mice. *J. Exp. Med.* 157:1635.
56. Kim, Y. T., E. A. Goidl, C. Samarut, M. E. Weksler, G. J. Thorbecke, and G. W. Siskind. 1985. Bone marrow function. I. Peripheral T cells are responsible for the increased auto-antiidiotype response of older mice. *J. Exp. Med.* 161:1237.

57. Naeim, F., and R. L. Walford. 1985. Aging and cell membrane complexes: The lipid bilayer, integral proteins and cytoskeleton. *In* Handbook of the Biology of Aging. C. E. Finch and E. L. Schneider, editors. Van Nostrand Reinhold Co., New York. 272.

13

Suppressor Cells in Aging

Diego Segre and Mariangela Segre

University of Illinois
Urbana, Illinois

I. INTRODUCTION

The mammalian immune system undergoes a number of changes during aging. The results of these changes are well known. The magnitude of the immune response to exogenous antigens decreases (1-3), as does the response of lymphocytes to mitogens (3). Thus, the efficiency of the immune system declines with advancing age. Paradoxically, these changes are accompanied by an increase in the incidence of autoantibodies in aged populations of humans and mice (1,4,5). Thus, the aging immune system is also poorly regulated.

While the end results of the age-related changes that occur in the immune system are well established, the cellular changes that are at the basis of the decreased efficiency and deregulation of the aging immune system are less well understood. It has long been known that the thymus involutes, beginning at sexual maturity (6-8); indeed, it has been suggested that the thymus acts as a clock that controls the aging of the immune system (9). In view of the age-related morphological changes in the thymus, the activity of T cells would be expected to be especially affected by aging. This is indeed the case; although the number of T cells remains relatively constant in aging humans (10,11) and mice (12), T-cell-dependent primary and secondary humoral responses (13,14), mixed lymphocyte culture reactivity (15), cytotoxic T-cell responses to allogeneic and hapten-modified syngeneic cells (16,17), and the response to T-cell mitogens (11,18) all decline with advancing age.

The immune response may be regarded as a manifestation of the individual's adaptation to its environment. A well-adapted, well-regulated immune system is responsive to exogenous antigens (pathogens) and tolerant to autoantigens (self components). The senescent immune system displays the opposite behavior; it responds poorly to exogenous antigens and produces autoantibodies with abnormally high frequency. This aberrant behavior, together with the morphological changes in the thymus that accompany aging, suggests that T suppressor cells, the major regulatory elements of the immune system (19,20), should be prominently affected by the aging process. This chapter reviews the evidence for age-related changes in suppressor cells and describes recent attempts to prevent these changes from occurring.

II. STUDIES IN HUMANS

A. Limitations

The major limitation to the study of suppressor activity in humans is that peripheral blood lymphocytes (PBL) are the only possible source of cells. However, the results obtained with PBL may not be representative of the behavior of the entire immune system. Furthermore, only certain types of immune response can be investigated with PBL which, for example, are not generally suitable for the in vitro antibody response. Finally, the health state of the elderly population studied may well affect the results, especially if the subjects are taking medications that might impinge on the immune system.

B. Numbers of T Suppressor Cells

Early attempts to enumerate T suppressor (T_s) cells in the peripheral blood relied on the presence of markers that were believed to be associated with the T_s subpopulation. Kishimoto et al. (21) found a statistically significant increase in the mean percentage of T_γ cells (T cells with receptors for IgG) in a group of aged individuals (60–89 years of age), as compared to a group of adults 14–59 years old. There was also a significant negative correlation between the magnitude of the phytohemagglutinin (PHA) response of PBL and the percentage of T_γ cells, suggesting that the latter cells were actively suppressing the PHA response. Similarly, Gupta and Good (22) reported an age-related increase in both the proportion and the absolute numbers of T_γ cells. This study utilized PBL of healthy, noninstitutionalized subjects who were not taking medication.

With the availability of monoclonal antibodies directed against surface markers characteristic of lymphocyte subpopulations, it became possible to enumerate lymphocyte subsets based on specific binding of monoclonal antibodies. Nagel et al. (23) used indirect immunofluorescence to analyze by flow cytometry the PBL reacting with antibodies OKT 3 (T cells), OKT 4 (helper/

inducer), and OKT 8 (cytotoxic/suppressor). Their sample consisted of 19 young subjects (age < 40 years; mean age 35 years) and 31 elderly individuals (age > 60 years; mean age 73 years). The subjects were not institutionalized. None of the subjects had a history of cancer, renal, hepatic, or hematologic disease, and none was taking medication. These authors found a decline in the relative proportion, but not in the absolute numbers, of T cells in the aged population. The decline was attributable to a decrease in both proportion and absolute numbers of the suppressor/cytotoxic subset, while there were no changes in the helper/inducer subset. The observed changes were statistically significant in male subjects, but not in the females, which, however, were represented in smaller numbers in the sample. In contrast with these results, Mascart-Lemone et al. (24) found that both the proportion and the absolute numbers of $T3^+$ and $T4^+$ cells were lower in aged than in young subjects. The proportion, but not the absolute number, of $T8^+$ cells was elevated in the elderly. Again, these changes were confined to male subjects, while no major age-related changes were observed in women. The sample was comprised of 32 people older than 70 years of age and 47 adults less than 40 years old. The elderly subjects were institutionalized but were judged healthy by the attending physician.

While these data are useful, they can give only a very approximate idea of the age-related changes that occur in circulating T_s cells. Neither of the markers used is present on suppressor cells only; T_γ cells contain effector cells for some immunological functions (22), and OKT 8 identifies cytotoxic as well as suppressor cells. Functional assays should, therefore, be considered to be more informative than quantitative measurements of cell populations of a given phenotype.

C. Suppressor Function

Suppression of the Response to Mitogens and to Allogeneic Cells

Hallgren and Yunis (25) tested the activity of concanavalin A (Con A)-induced suppressor cells derived from the PBL of 10 healthy individuals aged 79-98 years and 10 young donors aged 21-27 years. Lymphocytes from individuals of both age groups suppressed the uptake of tritiated thymidine by cultures of Con-A-stimulated allogeneic young human lymphocytes. The degree of suppression was highly variable, but the mean suppression was significantly lower in the aged group than in the young group. Age-related decreases in suppressor activity were also reported by Schulof et al. (26) and by Birnbaum and Swick (27). Schulof and collaborators measured the suppressor activity of Con-A-stimulated cells for the proliferative response to Con A of both autologous and allogeneic lymphocytes. While Con-A-induced suppressor cells from elderly subjects were less active than those from young individuals in suppressing the proliferation of allogeneic cells, no differences were observed between the two age groups in the suppression of proliferation of autologous lymphocytes. The authors concluded that two distinct populations of suppressor cells were involved, and that only cells capable of suppressing allogeneic proliferation were lost with age. Birnbaum and Swick (27) studied the suppression of the development of cytotoxic cells in mixed lymphocyte cultures (MLC). The suppressor cells were induced by Con A and were autologous to the responding cells in the MLC. They found that larger numbers of Con-A-inducible suppressor cells derived from the PBL of older individuals were necessary to obtain a 50% suppression of alloantigen-stimulated cytotoxicity than when Con-A-activated cells from younger individuals were used. Since these authors also found that the generation of cytotoxic cells induced by allogeneic stimulation was increased in older subjects, they advanced the hypothesis that the decrease in suppressor cells in aged individuals allows for greater expression of allogeneically induced cytotoxic cells.

Others who have investigated Con-A-induced suppression of the proliferative response to Con A of autologous cells, however, have concluded that this suppressor activity increases with advancing age. Thus, Antel et al. (28) found increased Con-A-induced suppression of the Con-A-proliferative response of autologous lymphocytes in old, as compared to young, PBL donors. Miller et al. (29) reported that Con-A-stimulated PBL from normal elderly people suppressed Con-A-induced proliferation of autologous PBL to a greater extent than did PBL from young subjects. Lymphocytes from a group of elderly Alzheimer's disease patients were even more suppressive than those from old, neurologically normal subjects. PBL from Alzheimer's patients had a lesser proliferative response to Con A than did PBL from old control subjects.

Suppression of Immunoglobulin Synthesis and of the Antibody Response in Vitro

While the antibody response of PBL in vitro requires special conditions and is not routinely performed in clinical or research laboratories, it is possible to induce immunoglobulin (Ig) production by cultures of B cells derived from PBL upon polyclonal activation with pokeweed mitogen (PWM) in the presence of T helper cells. The immunosuppressive effect of cells derived from young or old individuals can then be measured in this system.

Using this procedure, Kishimoto et al. (30) found that irradiation of the T cells added to allogeneic, PWM-stimulated B cells caused a significant enhancement of Ig production. This enhancement was attributed to inactivation of T_s cells by irradiation. The irradiation-induced enhancement of IgG production was greater when the T cells were derived from young adults (20–30 years old) or from newborns (cord blood) than it was with T cells from aged persons (70–90 years old). For IgM production, the enhancement was greater with neonatal T cells than with T cells from the old subjects, while no significant differences were found among the three age groups for IgA production. Similar results were obtained when T_s cells were inactivated by treatment with mitomycin C rather than by irradiation. On the basis of these results, it was concluded that there was an age-related impairment of the function of naturally occurring suppressor cells. The activity of Con-A-induced suppressor cells, measured by the decrease in IgG and IgM production upon addition to the cultures of T cells cultured with Con A, was also less when the Con-A-activated T cells were derived from aged subjects than when they were obtained from young adults. Thus, the function of Con-A-induced suppressor cells was also decreased in aging.

Ceuppens and Goodwin (31) also studied the PWM-stimulated Ig production by PBL and by combinations of T and B cells from young adult and old individuals. The cell donors comprised two groups of healthy, noninstitutionalized individuals who were not taking medication of any kind. These authors found that PBL from young (20–40 years old) and old (66–94 years old) subjects produced similar amounts of IgG and IgM. It was found, however, that old T cells consistently provided more help for both old and young B cells than did young T cells. The T cells were further fractionated according to their reactivity with monoclonal antibody OKT 4 (helper/inducer subset) or OKT 8 (suppressor/cytotoxic subset). It was found that $T4^+$ cells from old donors provided more help from either young or old B cells than did $T4^+$ cells from young people. Moreover, $T8^+$ cells from old individuals were less suppressive for cocultures of young B cells plus T helper cells from either young or old donors than were $T8^+$ cells from young subjects. Finally, it was found that T helper cells, which are the direct target of suppression, were more sensitive to suppression when they were derived from old donors than when they originated from young individuals. Appropriate controls showed that allogeneic helper effects or genetic restriction of cell interactions did not contribute to the observed differences in helper and suppressor activities. Cell marker analysis revealed a slight decrease in the proportion of $T4^+$ cells and an increase in $T8^+$ cells in the old subjects. These changes may compensate, in part, for the changes in activity reported above.

Barrett et al. (32) studied PWM-stimulated IgG production by PBL from healthy members of a retirement home, ranging in age from 65 to 103 years, and from a group of younger controls (22–41 years old). PBL from pairs of young and old subjects were cultured alone or in mixed cultures, and the quantity of IgG produced by cocultures was compared to the amount of IgG synthesized by each PBL population cultured alone. There was no significant difference between the mean quantity of IgG produced by young PBL and that produced by old PBL. No significant suppression or enhancement was noted in cocultures of allogeneic PBL from pairs of young controls or in cocultures of young and old PBL. Preincubation of PBL from either young or old individuals with Con-A-induced cells was capable of suppressing IgG secretion by young PBL, but similar degrees of suppression were observed with suppressor PBL from young or aged subjects. Thus, in this investigation, no age-related alterations of suppressor function were noticed.

Antel et al. (33) also measured the in vitro production of IgG by PBL, or by combinations of enriched T cells and B cells from PBL, upon stimulation with the T-cell-dependent mitogen PWM. They found that individual subjects could be classified as responders (R) or nonresponders (NR) according to the amount of IgG secreted by their PBL, and that the classification held true on repeated testing. These authors then measured the IgG production by mixed cultures, using various combinations of T cells and B cells from young (20–25 years of age) or old (65–84 years) R and NR individuals. The main results of this analysis were as follows:

1. T cells from old nonresponders (ONR) adequately supported IgG production by young responder (YR) B cells.
2. T cells from all sources (YR, YNR, OR, ONR) failed to increase IgG synthesis by B cells from ONR. Thus, it was concluded that nonresponsiveness in old individuals cannot be ascribed solely to changes in regulatory T cells, but must involve B cell defects.
3. YR T cells suppressed the response of OR B cells, but did not suppress the response of autologous or allogeneic YR B cells. This finding suggests that OR B cells are especially sensitive to suppressive signals.
4. The OR-T:YNR-B combination resulted in greater IgG production than did the combination of YNR-T:YNR-B, suggesting that YNR T cells had greater suppressor activity than did OR T cells.

The major conclusion that emerges from this analysis is that multiple changes in the immune function occur during aging. The interpretation of the changes is complicated by the observation that low responsiveness to PWM is not a characteristic of the elderly, but is an individual trait. Nevertheless, it appears that suppressor T cells are the major factor contributing to low responsiveness in young subjects, while in the elderly low responsiveness seems to be due mainly to a B-cell defect that may include heightened sensitivity to suppressor signals. There was some evidence suggesting loss of suppressor cell activity in the aged.

As mentioned earlier, PBL are not well suited for antibody production in vitro. Nevertheless, antibody production by PBL has been demonstrated under special conditions, and the ability of cells from young and old individuals to suppress the antibody response has been investigated.

Kishimoto et al. (34) obtained PBL from young adults (24–32 years old) and aged subjects (72–83 years of age) who had been primed and boosted with tetanus toxoid. Cell suspensions enriched for B cells and T cells were obtained from the PBL. B cells from individual donors were cultured in the presence of T cells from a single subject and of PWM, and the specific antitetanus toxoid antibodies produced by the cultures were measured by radioimmunoassay. These authors found that B cells from aged donors produced significantly fewer antibodies than B cells from young donors. The authors attributed the decreased antibody production by aged B cells to a decrease in numbers of precursors of B cells of the relevant clones. They also found a reduction in the frequency of radiation-resistant T helper cells in the aged subjects. Elimination of suppressor cells by irradiation of the T cells resulted in an enhancement of antibody production by cocultures of B cells and T cells. The irradiation-induced enhancement, however, was of the same magnitude whether the T cells originated from young or aged donors, leading to the conclusion that there was no age-related change in suppressor T-cell activity.

Delfraissy et al. (35) described a primary IgM response of PBL obtained entirely in vitro. The immunogen was the hapten trinitrophenyl conjugated to polyacrylamide beads (TNP-PAA). PBL from donors 70–90 years old had very poor responses, while PBL from young donors (18–35 years old) responded well. The lack of response with old PBL was attributed to lack of T-cell help, since addition of young T cells to old PBL or to old B cells restored the antibody response. PBL from young donors that were stimulated with Con A suppressed the response of allogeneic PBL in mixed cultures, while Con-A-stimulated PBL from old donors were unable to do so. Thus, the authors concluded that suppressor cells were not generated by Con A in PBL of old individuals. In a later paper (36), however, the same authors found that nylon wool-nonadherent old PBL responded as well as young PBL to TNP-PAA. The nonadherent cells were depleted of monocytes but contained substantial numbers of B cells. Further analysis revealed that adherent cells produced prostaglandin (PGE2) in culture and that PGE2 in turn induced T suppressor cells. Indeed, irradiated T cells from old individuals provided adequate T-cell help for both young and old T-depleted cells, resulting in antibody responses comparable to those obtained with irradiated or nonirradiated young T cells in conjunction with T-depleted cells from either young or old donors. Thus, the nonresponsiveness of old PBL was ultimately due to an exaggerated T-suppressor cell activity.

D. Conclusions

Table 1 summarizes the results obtained by various investigators. In most cases, changes in suppressor activity were observed by comparing PBL from aged and young donors. There is no consensus, however, as to the direction of the changes. The disparity of results cannot be attributed to the diversity of methodologies used or to the type of immune function assayed. Perhaps the only conclusion that can be made is that suppressor cell activity of PBL differs in elderly and in younger individuals, in agreement with the concept that aging results in deregulation of the immune system. Given the great individual variability that is characteristic of aged populations, it may be futile to expect a resolution of this question from cross-sectional studies. Longitudinal studies may prove more informative.

Table 1 Suppressor Cell Activity in Peripheral Blood Lymphocytes (PBL) of Aged Humans

Methodology	Immune function assayed	Suppressor activity	Ref.
Enumeration of T_γ cells	–	Increased	21
	–	Increased	22
Enumeration of OKT 8^+ cells	–	Decreased	23
	–	Increased	24
	–	Increased	31
Con-A induction	Con-A response	Decreased	25
		Decreased[a]	26
		Unchanged[b]	26
		Increased	28
		Increased	29
	MLC-generated CTL	Decreased	27
Inactivation of T_s	Ig production in vitro	Decreased	30
Con-A induction		Decreased	30
Addition of OKT 8^+ cells		Decreased	31
Mixed culture of PBL		Unchanged	32
Addition of Con-A-stimulated PBL		Unchanged	32
Mixed cultures of T and B cells		Decreased	33
Inactivation of T_s cells	Secondary antibody response in vitro	Unchanged	34
Addition of Con-A-stimulated PBL	Primary antibody response in vitro	Decreased	35
Inactivation of T_s cells	Primary antibody response in vitro	Increased	36

[a] Suppressor and responding cells were allogeneic.
[b] Suppressor and responding cells were autologous.

III. STUDIES IN ANIMALS

A. Advantages and Limitations

Most of the information on the age-related behavior of suppressor cells comes from studies in mice. Although the limitations mentioned above for human studies do not apply to experimental animals, other restrictions come into play. The spleen is the source of suppressor cells most commonly studied because, in the mouse, suppressor cells are spleen-seeking (19). Since the spleen can be sampled only once, longitudinal studies are precluded. However, much useful information has been gained from cross-sectional studies. The availability of inbred mouse strains is an obvious advantage in that genetic variation is largely eliminated. On the other hand, the results obtained with a given strain cannot necessarily be generalized to other strains. A distinction should be made between long-lived and short-lived strains of mice; the latter often exhibit pathological signs, and in many cases the pathology affects the immune system. Thus, results obtained with short-lived mouse strains may not reflect changes due to the aging process and must be interpreted with caution.

Another potential source of error derives from the finding of Jaroslow et al. (37) that spleen cells from mice with lymphoma suppress the antibody response to sheep red blood cells (SRBC) of cultures of syngeneic spleen cells from young, tumor-free mice. A transplantable lymphoma also proved to be highly immunosuppressive. Cells from the spleen of old mice that were tumor-free by visual inspection were immunosuppressive in some experiments, but not in others. Jaroslow and collaborators suggested that when apparently normal spleens of aged mice were immunosuppressive, the suppression was due to the presence of small numbers of tumor cells. It is equally plausible, however, that there was an age-related increase in suppressor activity in the absence of malignancy. At any rate, the possibility of malignant transformation of cells of the T suppressor lineage in old mice complicates the interpretation of assays for suppressor activity as a function of age.

B. T Suppressor Cells

Increased Suppressor Activity in Aged Animals

A number of reports have appeared in the literature indicating an increase in suppressor cell activity in the spleen of old mice. Gerbase-DeLima et al. (38) tested the proliferative response to allogeneic stimulator cells of spleen cells from 7- and 34-month-old $(129 \times LP)F_1$ mice in a one-way MLC reaction. Responder cells from the spleen of young and old mice were cultured, alone or mixed in various ratios, in the presence of stimulator cells. The response of mixtures of young and old spleen cells was lower than expected from the sum of individual responses of young and old spleen cells. The authors concluded that the MLC response was suppressed by spleen cells from old mice. Similar results were obtained with cells from old (BALB/c × C57BL/6)F_1 mice and from old outbred ICR mice, but not with cells from old C57BL/10 mice.

An age-related increase in suppressor cell activity in BC3F1 mice was reported by Makinodan et al. (39). They measured the plaque-forming cell (PFC) response to SRBC of cocultures of spleen cells from old and young mice and compared it to the sum of the responses of old cells and of young cells cultured alone. In 65% of the cases, they found that the response of mixed cultures was lower than that expected from the sum of the responses of young cells and old cells. This was attributed to the presence of suppressor cells in the spleen of old mice. Additive responses and responses higher than expected were also observed in mixed cultures, albeit with lower frequency than the suppressed responses. When the response of the mixed cultures was greater than the sum of the responses of young and old cells cultured separately, it was assumed that there was a decrease in number or activity of one type of immunocompetent cell in the spleen of old mice, and that the same cell type was present in excess in the young spleen. Makinodan and co-workers emphasized that the variability of the results obtained with spleen cells from individual old mice required that pooling of cells from different animals be avoided in experiments of this type.

Increased suppressor cell activity in the spleen of old BALB/c mice was described by Goidl et al. (40). They found that irradiated recipient mice given mixtures of spleen cells from young and old syngeneic donors had a lower PFC response to dinitrophenyl-bovine γ-globulin (DNP–BGG) than recipients of young spleen cells. The decreased response was attributed to the presence of suppressor cells in the spleen of old mice. It was already evident with 12-month-old donors, but it became more pronounced with 24- and 34-month-old mice. The nature of the suppressor cells was not investigated in this case. In a later paper from the same laboratory (41), however, immunosuppression was eliminated by treatment of the suppressive spleen cells with rabbit anti-mouse brain serum and complement, showing that the suppressor cells were T cells. In the later work, suppressor activity was assayed in mixed cultures of spleen cells responding to the T-dependent antigen, SRBC, or to the T-independent antigen, DNP-PAA. The PFC response of BALB/c spleen cells to both antigens was suppressed by spleen cells from 1- to 2-week-old and from 18- and 24-month-old syngeneic mice, but not by spleen cells from donors that were 3 weeks to 12 months of age.

Segre and Segre (14,42) studied the secondary PFC response of spleen cells from young adult and old BC3F1 mice to DNP–keyhole limpet hemocyanin (KLH). They utilized a cell transfer procedure in which the responding cells were propagated in Millipore diffusion chambers implanted into the peritoneal cavity of irradiated recipient mice. Age-related impairment of immune responsiveness was easily detected in this system. The mean response of 2-year-old mice was 25% of that of young mice, and the mean response of 2.5-year-old mice was only

2% of that of young mice. When spleen cells from primed young and old mice were cultured together in diffusion chambers, the response of the mixed cultures was less than the sum of the responses of cells from the two individual donors, indicating that the spleen of the old mice contained suppressor cells. Depletion of T cells by treatment of old spleen cells with rabbit anti-mouse brain serum and complement abolished the suppression. In fact, the response of cultures containing reference primed cells from young mice and T-depleted primed cells from old mice was often greater than the sum of the responses obtained with untreated primed young and old cells individually. It appears that removal of T suppressor cells allowed the B cells of old mice to respond to antigen, utilizing T-cell help present in the primed reference cells from young mice. Thus, excessive T suppressor cell activity seemed to be the major factor responsible for the low secondary response of spleen cells from old mice. Consistent with this conclusion was the finding of a significant negative correlation between the level of response of old cells alone and their ability to suppress the response of young cells.

The same authors (43) attempted to reconstitute the immunological activity of spleen cells from old mice. Spleen cells from aged mice primed with DNP-KLH were depleted of T cells and supplemented with T helper cells from KLH-primed young mice. The secondary response of these cell mixtures was generally much greater than the secondary response of untreated, unsupplemented cells from the same individual old mice. This indicated that suppressor cells were present in the old mice's spleen and that the B-cell function was intact. To obtain an indication of the activity of T helper cells, untreated spleen cells from the old mice were also supplemented with young, carrier-primed T helper cells. An increase in the secondary response in this case indicated that there was a decrease in T helper activity in the spleen of the old mice. This type of analysis revealed that increased T suppressor activity was by far the most frequent change detected in the aged mice. Decreased T helper cell activity was the next most frequent change, while loss of B-cell activity was relatively rare.

While the findings of Segre and Segre (42,43) were concerned with antigen-induced suppressor cells, those of Makinodan et al. (39), Goidl et al. (40), and Dekruyff et al. (41) reported above dealt with spontaneously occurring suppressor cells in mice that were not deliberately immunized. It must be pointed out, however, that exposure of the cells to antigen that is inherent in the assay for suppression may itself induce suppressor cells from spontaneously occurring precursors. Thus, in spite of methodological differences, similar suppressor cell populations may have been assayed by different workers.

Callard and Basten (44) also reported that spleen cells of old CBA mice were highly suppressive of the primary response to DNP-KLH, DNP-human γ-globulin (HGG), and horse red blood cells in adoptive transfer experiments. Suppression was obtained with nylon wool-nonadherent cells and was removed by treatment of the old spleen cells with anti-Thy-1.2 serum and complement, indicating that the suppressor cells were of the T lineage. In a later paper, Callard et al. (45) extended this observation to a T-independent antigen (DNP-Ficoll) and to the secondary response to DNP-HGG and investigated the phenotype of the suppressor cells. Suppression was abrogated by treatment of the old spleen cells with anti-Thy-1.2, anti-Lyt-1.1, anti-Lyt-2.1, or anti-Ia^k serum and complement. However, a mixture of two populations of old spleen cells, one of which was treated with anti-Lyt-1.1 and the other with anti-Lyt-2.1 in the presence of complement, was suppressive, leading to the conclusion that suppression was mediated by a T–T interaction between Lyt-1$^+$ and Lyt-2$^+$ cells, rather than by a single effector T cell with phenotype Lyt-1,2$^+$. Because of the wide range of antigen responses that were suppressed by old spleen cells, the suppressor cells were considered not to be antigen specific. In contrast, old mice primed with immunogenic HGG and challenged 4 weeks later with tolerogenic deaggregated HGG developed antigen-specific suppressor cells to about the same extent as did young mice. It was, therefore, concluded that the ability to generate antigen-specific suppressor cells did not change with age, while nonspecific suppressor cells increased in old age. These results are in conflict with those of Segre and Segre (42,43), who found an age-related increase in antigen-induced suppressor activity. The differences may be accounted for by the use of different mouse strains and by the different methodology employed for antigen induction of suppressor cells.

Evidence for an age-related increase in antigen-specific T suppressor cells was presented by Doria et al. (46). Azobenzene arsonate (ABA)-specific suppressor T cells were induced in 4- or 20-month-old DBF1 mice by injection of ABA conjugated to syngeneic spleen cells. Spleen cells from mice so treated, when added to cultures of spleen cells from mice primed with ABA-KLH, suppressed the TNP-specific PFC response to TNP-ABA-KLH, but not the response to TNP-KLH or to SRBC. Suppression was abrogated by treatment with anti-Thy-1.2 and complement. Thus, suppression was attributed to antigen (carrier)-induced, antigen-specific T cells. Titration of suppressor activity revealed that to obtain comparable degrees of suppression, 20 times more spleen cells from young mice were required than were cells from old mice. When the responding cells were derived from old mice, however, suppression was no longer demonstrable, regardless of whether the suppressor cells were generated in young or old mice. The authors concluded that there was an age-related increase in the inducibility of antigen-specific T suppressor cells, accompanied by an increased resistance to immunosuppression. There was no evidence of nonspecific suppression in either young or old mouse spleen cells, since the in vitro response to TNP-KLH or to SRBC was similar when spleen cells from young or old mice, primed or not primed with ABA-conjugated spleen cells, were added to the responding cells. It must be pointed out, however, that the "old" mice were only 20 months of age and may not yet have developed spontaneous suppressor cells.

Immunological functions other than the humoral response have also been found to be suppressed by cells from senescent animals. Globerson et al. (47) reported that the low responsiveness to the mitogens Con A and PHA exhibited by spleen cells from 24- to 30-month-old C3BF1 mice was due to the presence of suppressor cells that reacted with the lectin peanut agglutinin (PNA^+). Removal of PNA^+ cells from the spleen of old mice resulted in increased mitogen response by the PNA^- cells. PNA^+ cells also suppressed the mitogen response of young mouse spleen cells. The suppression was not abrogated by treatment of the PNA^+ cells with anti-Thy-1.2 and complement, suggesting that the suppressor cells were not mature T cells. Another report from the same laboratory (48) indicates that spleen cells from old mice, upon stimulation with Con A, develop less suppressor activity than do spleen cells from young mice for the proliferative response induced by mitogens (Con A and PHA), by mixed lymphocyte reactions, and by specific antigen. However, spleen cells from old mice exhibited a high degree of naturally occurring suppressor activity; treatment of old spleen cells with anti-Thy-1.2 serum and complement did not substantially reduce the suppressor activity, indicating that the suppressor cells were not mature T cells.

Bruley-Rosset et al. (49,50) reported that nylon wool-nonadherent spleen cells from 22-month-old $(C57BL \times BALB/c)F_1$ mice are capable of suppressing the proliferative response of spleen cells from young syngeneic mice to the T-cell mitogens PHA and Con A. The old mice were also deficient in delayed-type hypersensitivity, humoral response to T-cell-dependent antigens, and response to T-cell mitogens. Long-term treatment of the mice with levamisole led to a restoration of the impaired immune responses and, concomitantly, to absence of suppressor cells in the spleen of the treated mice. In contrast, long-term administration of the antibiotic bestatin restored the humoral response to SRBC and delayed-type hypersensitivity to oxazolone of 22-month-old mice, but failed to affect the response to T-cell mitogens and to prevent the appearance of suppressor cells. Thus, the responsiveness to T-cell mitogens of spleen cells from aged mice was correlated with the ability of the spleen cells to suppress the mitogen response.

Elevated suppressor cell activity was also found to occur in the spleen of hamsters 14 months of age or older (51). Suppressor activity was measured by the ability of old cells to decrease the proliferative response of young cells to the mitogen PHA. The age-related increase in suppressor activity was accompanied by decreases in responsiveness to PHA, natural killer cell activity, and monocyte chemotaxis. Interestingly, long-term administration of isoprinosine, beginning when the hamsters were 18 months of age, reduced the suppressor activity to the levels characteristic of young animals and restored the other immunological functions as well. The mode of action of isoprinosine as an immunopotentiator is not known.

Another immunological function that was found to diminish with advancing age is the syngeneic mixed lymphocyte reaction (SMLR), that is, the proliferative response of T lymphocytes cultured with syngeneic non-T lymphocytes. Gutowski and Weksler (52) reported that the spleen of 24-month-old BALB/c mice exhibited no significant SMLR reactivity. Mixed culture experiments showed that the loss of activity was due to inadequacy of both the stimulator cells and the responding T cells. The impaired ability of spleen cells from aged mice to stimulate an SMLR was due, at least in part, to the presence of suppressor cells.

Specific T-cell cytotoxic responses to allogeneic and hapten-modified syngeneic cells were also found to decrease with age. Zharhary et al. (53) investigated the causes of this decrease by comparing the cytotoxic responses of spleen cells from young and old (13-28 months of age) C57BL/6 mice with the response of mixtures of young and old cells. It was found that a low percentage of the aged mice had decreased helper cell activity or increased suppressor cell activity, while the majority of the mice showed no synergy, positive or negative, with the cells from young donors.

While suppressor cells have been repeatedly demonstrated in the lymphoid system of senescent experimental animals, soluble suppressor factors have not received much attention. A report by Delpierre et al. (54), however, indicates that extracts prepared from the lymph nodes of old cows, but not from those of young calves, inhibit the primary and secondary in vitro responses of mouse spleen cells to SRBC. The active factor is a protein having a molecular weight of 10,000-15,000, which appears to interfere with the differentiation of lymphocytes to antibody-producing cells. A similar inhibitor had been found by the same authors in long-term cultures of bovine lymphoid cells. The nature of the cells producing this factor is unknown.

Unchanged or Decreased Suppressor Activity in Aged Animals

In spite of a preponderance of evidence for an age-related increase in suppressor activity, there have been cases in which such an increase was not found. Krogsrud and Perkins (55) studied the ability of carrier-primed T cells from BC3F1 mice of various ages to collaborate with hapten-primed B cells from young mice in an adoptive transfer system. T-cell populations from old mice provided less help than those of young mice in the secondary response to DNP-BGG. The curves obtained by plotting the PFC response against graded numbers of T cells had similar slopes for T cells from mice of different ages; hence, the authors argued that suppressor cells were not involved in the decreased help provided by old T cells. There was, however, no attempt to demonstrate suppression directly by adding old T cells to the responding cells. Fujiwara and Kishimoto (56) reported that both the magnitude of the IgE response to DNP conjugated to ascaris extract and the avidity of the antibodies decreased with age in C57BL/6 mice. They attributed these results to age-related changes in the T helper cells. They thought that suppressor cells were unlikely to be involved in these phenomena, since they found that spleen cells of aged mice were incapable of abrogating an ongoing IgE response and of suppressing the primary IgE response when transferred into young syngeneic mice. Fujiwara and Kariyone (57) found that the number of both spontaneous and lipopolysaccharide (LPS)-stimulated PFC reactive with bromelain-treated syngeneic RBC increased with age in C57BL/6 and DDD mice. This phenomenon was demonstrable both in vivo and in vitro. Depletion of T cells before culture did not substantially increase the number of PFC, suggesting that the age-dependent increase in autoantibody reactive with syngeneic RBC was not due to loss of T-suppressor cells. No evidence of change in suppressor activity with age was found by coculture of young and old cells, nor could greater suppression be generated in old than in young cells by treatment with Con A. It must be noted that in this work, "old" cells were derived from 14-month-old mice.

There are also a few reports of an age-related decrease in suppressor activity. The best-documented case of loss of suppressor activity with age is that of autoimmune-prone NZB and (NZB × NZW)F_1 mice. This phenomenon may not be related to the aging process, but is likely to be a special case pertaining to the pathogenesis of autoimmune disease. Loss of suppressor cells in aging nonautoimmune mice has been reported by Smith (58), who found that treatment of BALB/c and C3H mice with antilymphocyte serum increased their PFC response to pneumococcal polysaccharide type III, presumably by inactivating T suppressor cells. The increase in response was greater for young mice than it was for 2-year-old mice, suggesting that there was an age-related loss of suppressor cell activity. Thoman and Weigle (59) found that spleen cells from 30-month-old C57BL/6 mice were deficient in the spontaneous generation of Lyt-2^+ suppressor cells in vitro. The deficiency was partially corrected by addition of IL-2 to the cultures in which suppressor cells were generated. Gottesman et al. (60) found that the generation of H-2-specific T suppressor cells in mixed lymphocyte cultures was significantly decreased in a portion of aged C57BL/6 mice as compared to young controls.

It is clear from the foregoing that there is solid evidence for an age-related increase in suppressor cell activity in normal mice. Some of the conflicting data (59,60) deal with the generation of suppressor cells in vitro and may reflect age-related changes in the requirements for the development of suppressor cells in culture, rather than in suppressor activity per se.

Relative Rate of Change in Suppressor Activity and Effects of Immunotherapy

The increase in suppressor activity during aging does not exclude the possibility of age-related changes taking place in other immunologically relevant cells. There is, in fact, solid evidence for decreased activity of T helper and B cells during aging (3). An important question concerns the relative rate of change in the different cell types. Liu et al. (61) measured the suppressor, T helper, and B-cell functions in BC3F1 mice of various ages. Spleen cells from individual mice were assayed for all three activities. Suppressor activity was measured by the ability of unfractionated spleen cells to suppress the secondary antihapten PFC response of young adult syngeneic spleen cells in mixed diffusion chamber cultures. Helper cell activity was assessed by measuring the ability of enriched T cells activated with carrier–anticarrier immune complexes to restore the response of hapten-primed, T-depleted syngeneic cells. Priming with immune complexes at the appropriate antigen-antibody ratio generates helper cells, but not suppressor cells (62). B-cell activity was assessed by measuring the response of B-enriched spleen cells to the T-independent antigen, DNP-Ficoll. It was found that suppressor cell activity increased rapidly from 4 to 15 months of age and remained elevated thereafter. In contrast, T helper and B-cell activity decreased at a constant, exponential rate from 4 to 30 months of age. Thus, middle-aged mice exhibited a high degree of suppressor activity but had still relatively vigorous T helper and B-cell activity.

This finding suggested that if it were possible to correct the suppressor cell defect at the appropriate time, further deterioration of the immune system might be delayed or arrested. This was attempted in subsequent work by the same group (63). BC3F1 mice were injected weekly with monoclonal anti-I-J antibody or with saline from 18 months of age until natural death. Since the I-J determinant is expressed on T cells of the suppressor circuit (64), it was thought that the anti-I-J antibody would principally affect the suppressor cells. The mice were primed and boosted with a protein antigen at 27 and 29 months of age, respectively, and were bled one week after each immunization, but otherwise they were left undisturbed. It was found that the secondary IgG response of anti-I-J-treated mice was significantly greater than that of saline-treated controls, and in fact was equal to the response of untreated young mice.

Additional findings of interest were a correlation between the magnitude of the secondary response of the old mice and their longevity and the apparently greater longevity of the anti-I-J-treated mice compared to the saline-treated controls. These results have important implications which, however, must be considered to be tentative at this time. The preservation of the immune potential in old age by immunological intervention on suppressor cells suggests that these cells play a central role in the age-related deterioration of the immune system. Changes in other cell types may be triggered by changes in suppressor cells. The correlation between immune responsiveness and longevity, and the effect of anti-I-J immunotherapy on life span, suggest that the immune system may be a pace setter for the aging process itself, as proposed by Walford's immunologic theory of aging (1).

The age-related changes in suppressor activity discussed above relate to T-suppressor cells. In many instances, the suppressor activity was abolished by treatment of the cells with anti-Thy-1 and complement, or it was shown to reside with the nylon wool-nonadherent fraction of the spleen cells. In other cases, the nature of the suppressor cells was not specifically investigated, but no effort was made to exclude T cells from the suppressive cell population. However, immunosuppression by non-T cells has also been reported, and there are a few papers describing the age-related behavior of non-T suppressor cells.

C. Non-T Suppressor Cells

Macrophages can suppress the immune response (19,65). Callard (66) found that macrophages from old mice functioned normally in a number of immunological roles. Removal of adherent cells increased the response of both young and old cells to allogeneic stimulation in MLC to the same extent, suggesting that there was no age-related increase in macrophage-mediated suppression. Furthermore, no evidence of suppression was obtained in cocultures of old and young cells responding to PHA, LPS, or allogeneic cells. Thus, it appears that the activity of suppressor macrophages does not change with advancing age.

Age-related changes have been described in another type of non-T suppressor cells. Since these cells lack characteristic markers, they are classified as null cells. They can be identified only by their biological properties and by the absence of markers associated with other cell types. Suppressor null cells were generated at the University of Illinois by injecting mice with cyclophosphamide at a dose of 200 mg per kilogram of body weight (67). Cells capable of nonspecifically suppressing the humoral response to T-dependent antigens were found in the spleen of the mice 5–14 days after administration of the drug. These cells, designated cyclophosphamide-induced suppressor (Cy-S) cells, were nonadherent to nylon wool and plastic, had no surface immunoglobulin, and were negative for the membrane markers Thy-1, Lyt-1, Lyt-2, I-J, Ia, Qa-5, and MAC-1. The Cy-S cells were generated with equal ease in normal mice, in athymic mice, and in adult thymectomized, irradiated, bone-marrow-reconstituted mice (67–69). On the basis of these characteristics, the Cy-S cells are probably identical to suppressor cells found in the spleen of mice subjected to total lymphoid irradiation (70,71) or injected with radioactive strontium (72). Similar or identical suppressor cells appear spontaneously in the spleen of neonatal mice (70,73), in the bone marrow of mice of several strains (74), and in the genital tract of pregnant and pseudopregnant mice (75).

Because of their presence in newborn mice and in the regenerating spleen of adult mice that have been subjected to lymphocytotoxic treatments such as administration of cyclophosphamide or total lymphoid irradiation, it was suspected that suppressor null cells are involved in the establishment and maintenance of self tolerance (67,71,73). This hypothesis was confirmed by experiments in which transfer of Cy-S cells to young NZB mice prevented their conversion to Coombs' reactivity and the development of thymocytotoxic antibodies (76). Since the incidence of autoimmunity increases in old age (1,4,5), it would be expected that suppressor null cell activity would decrease with advancing age. The experimental findings, however, indicate that the activity of suppressor null cells increases in old age. Segre et al. (77) found increased Cy-S cell activity in the spleen of 31-month-old C57BL/6 mice as compared to young adult mice of the same strain. Roder et al. (78) found a gradual, age-related increase in spontaneous suppressor null cells in the spleen and bone marrow of mice of several strains. The suppressor cells were assayed by their ability to suppress the in vitro response of young syngeneic spleen cells to SRBC. The increase in suppressor activity was correlated with the age-related decrease in the in vitro response to SRBC.

The same authors (78,79) found that suppressor null cells appeared spontaneously in the spleen of NZB and (NZB × NZW)F_1 autoimmune mice. The proportion of mice with suppressor null cells increased gradually and reached 100% at about 8 months of age. Similar findings were reported by Greeley et al. (80). While suppressor null cells were induced by cyclophosphamide administration in both young and old NZB mice, spontaneous suppressor null cells were detected in the spleen of 28- to 52-week-old, but not in the spleen of 3- to 8-week-old NZB mice. Spontaneous suppressor null cells were also found in the spleen of BXSB mice, but there was no difference between the more autoimmune males and the less autoimmune females.

Michalski et al. (81) demonstrated that spleen cells from (NZB × NZW)F_1 mice (15–20 months of age) have severely impaired reactivity to the T-cell mitogen PHA and contain suppressor null cells that inhibit the PHA response of spleen cells from young syngeneic mice. There was an inverse correlation between the response to PHA of individual spleens and their suppressor activity. Suppressor activity was not detected in the spleen of middle-aged (10–19 months old) mice of four nonautoimmune strains. The same authors (83) reported that androgen therapy increased the longevity of male (NZB × NZW)F_1 mice. Spleen cells of the treated mice had increased responsiveness to PHA and decreased suppressor activity.

D. Conclusions

In contrast to the findings in humans, the preponderance of evidence in experimental animals points to an age-related increase in suppressor cell activity. The age-related behavior of suppressor cells of the T lineage has been thoroughly studied. There is solid evidence for an increase in nonspecific T suppressor cells in aging individuals. Whether all the T-cell subsets that constitute the suppressor circuit (64) are equally affected by age is unknown. At any rate, since suppressor cells are the major regulatory element of the immune response, any change in the suppressor cell compartment, in either direction, can be viewed as an indication of deregulation of the immune system. In this connection, it is interesting that treatments that preserved the immune responsiveness in aged animals also resulted in a decrease in suppressor activity (49,51), and a treatment that should affect only T suppressor cells also resulted in a vigorous immune response in old mice (63). These results suggest a major role for T suppressor cells in the aging of the immune system.

The age-related behavior of non-T, or null, suppressor cells is just beginning to be investigated. The results obtained suggest that there is an association between autoimmunity and the spontaneous development of suppressor null cells. Experimentally, however, it has been shown that suppressor null cells prevent the development of autoantibodies in NZB mice (76). To resolve this apparent paradox, it has been suggested (77) that the suppressor cells represent an indicator of an ongoing autoimmune process that has stimulated their generation, but which they have failed to prevent or reverse. Indeed, one may argue that when the suppressor cells do succeed in preventing autoimmunity, they would soon be inhibited or lost and would not be detectable.

ACKNOWLEDGMENTS

The authors' work cited in this chapter was supported by grant AG-00451 from the National Institutes of Health.

REFERENCES

1. Walford, R. L. 1969. The Immunologic Theory of Aging. Munksgaard, Copenhagen.
2. Makinodan, T., E. H. Perkins, and M. G. Chen. 1971. Immunologic activity of the aged. *Adv. Gerontol. Res.* 3:171.
3. Makinodan, T., and M.M.B. Kay. 1980. Age influence on the immune system. *Adv. Immunol.* 29:287.
4. Hallgren, H., C. Buckley, V. Gilbertsen, and E. Yunis. 1973. Lymphocyte phytohemagglutinin responsiveness, immunoglobulins and autoantibodies in aging humans. *J. Immunol.* 111:1101.
5. Stutman, O. 1974. Cell-mediated immunity and aging. *Fed. Proc.* 33:2028.
6. Boyd, E. 1932. The weight of the thymus gland in health and disease. *Am. J. Dis. Child.* 43:1162.
7. Santisteban, G. A. 1960. The growth and involution of lymphatic tissue and

its interrelationships to aging and to the growth of the adrenal glands and sex organs in CBA mice. *Anat. Rec.* 136:117.
8. Makinodan, T. 1978. The thymus in aging. *Aging.* 5:217.
9. Burnet, F. 1970. An immunological approach to aging. *Lancet.* 1:358.
10. Portaro, J. K., G. I. Glick, and J. Zighelboim. 1978. Population immunology: Age and immune cell parameters. *Clin. Immunol. Immunopathol.* 11:339.
11. Adler, W. H., and J. E. Nagel. 1981. Studies of the immune function in a human population. *In* Immunological Aspects of Aging. D. Segre and L. Smith, editors. Marcel Dekker, New York. 295–311.
12. Kay, M.M.B., T. Denton, N. Union, J. Mendoza, J. Diven, and M. Lajiness. 1979. Age-related changes in the immune system of 8 medium and long-lived strains and hybrids. I. Weight, cellular and activity changes. *Mech. Ageing Dev.* 11:295.
13. Makinodan, T., and W. J. Peterson. 1964. Growth and senescence of the primary antibody-forming potential of the spleen. *J. Immunol.* 93:886.
14. Segre, M., and D. Segre. 1976. Humoral immunity in aged mice. I. Age-related decline in the secondary response to DNP of spleen cells propagated in diffusion chambers. *J. Immunol.* 116:731.
15. Meredith, P., W. Titter, M. Gerbase-DeLima, and R. Walford. 1975. Age-related changes in the cellular immune response of lymph node and thymus cells in long-lived mice. *Cell. Immunol.* 18:324.
16. Gottesman, S.R.S., J. A. Kristie, and R. L. Walford. 1981. Proliferative and cytotoxic immune functions in aging mice. I. Sequence of decline of reactivities measured under optimal and suboptimal sensitization conditions. *Immunology.* 44:607.
17. Gershon, H., E. C. Lattime, and O. Stutman. 1980. Host age and H-2 tolerance in chimeric mice. Mixed lymphocyte reactivity, cell-mediated lympholysis and responses to hapten-modified self. *Mech. Ageing Dev.* 13:253.
18. Callard, R. E., and A. Basten. 1977. Immune function in aged mice. I. T-cell responsiveness using phytohemagglutinin as a functional probe. *Cell. Immunol.* 31:13.
19. Gershon, R. K. 1974. T cell control of antibody production. *Contemp. Top. Immunobiol.* 3:1.
20. Cantor, H., and E. Boyse. 1977. Regulation of the immune response by T-cell subclasses. *Contemp. Top. Immunobiol.* 7:47.
21. Kishimoto, S., S. Tomino, K. Inomata, S. Kotegawa, T. Saito, M. Kuroki, H. Mitsuya, and S. Hisamitsu. 1978. Age-related changes in the subsets and functions of human T lymphocytes. *J. Immunol.* 121:1773.
22. Gupta, S., and R. A. Good. 1979. Subpopulations of human T lymphocytes. X. Alterations in T, B, third population cells, and T cells with receptors for immunoglobulin M (T_{μ}) or G (T_{γ}) in aging humans. *J. Immunol.* 122:1214.
23. Nagel, J. E., F. J. Chrest, and W. H. Adler. 1981. Enumeration of T lymphocyte subsets by monoclonal antibodies in young and aged humans. *J. Immunol.* 127:2086.

24. Mascart-Lemone, F., G. Delespesse, G. Servais, and M. Kunstler. 1982. Characterization of immunoregulatory T lymphocytes during aging by monoclonal antibodies. *Clin. Exp. Immunol.* 48:148.
25. Hallgren, H. M., and E. J. Yunis. 1977. Suppressor lymphocytes in young and aged humans. *J. Immunol.* 118:2004.
26. Schulof, R. S., J. A. Garofalo, R. A. Good, and S. Gupta. 1980. Concanavalin A-induced suppressor cell activity for T-cell proliferative responses: Autologous and allogeneic suppression in aging humans. *Cell. Immunol.* 56:80.
27. Birnbaum, G., and L. Swick. 1981. Human suppressor lymphocytes. II. Changes in concanavalin A inducible suppressor cells with age. *J. Gerontol.* 36:410.
28. Antel, J. P., M. Weinrich, and B.G.W. Arnason. 1978. Circulating suppressor cells in man as a function of age. *Clin. Immunol. Immunopathol.* 9:134.
29. Miller, A. E., P. A. Neighbour, R. Katzman, M. Aronson, and R. Lipkowitz. 1981. Immunological studies in senile dementia of the Alzheimer type: Evidence for enhanced suppressor cell activity. *Ann. Neurol.* 10:506.
30. Kishimoto, S., S. Tomino, H. Mitsuya, and H. Fujiwara. 1979. Age-related changes in suppressor functions of human T cells. *J. Immunol.* 123:1586.
31. Ceuppens, J. L., and J. S. Goodwin. 1982. Regulation of immunoglobulin production in pokeweed mitogen-stimulated cultures of lymphocytes from young and old adults. *J. Immunol.* 128:2429.
32. Barrett, D. J., S. Stenmark, D. W. Wara, and A. J. Ammann. 1980. Immunoregulation in aged humans. *Clin. Immunol. Immunopathol.* 17:203.
33. Antel, J. P., J.J.-F. Oger, L. G. Wrabetz, B.G.W. Arnason, and J. E. Hopper. 1983. Mechanisms responsible for reduced in vitro immunoglobulin secretion in aged humans. *Mech. Ageing Dev.* 23:11.
34. Kishimoto, S., S. Tomino, H. Mitsuya, and H. Nishimura. 1982. Age-related decrease in frequencies of B-cell precursors and specific helper T cells involved in the IgG anti-tetanus toxoid antibody production in humans. *Clin. Immunol. Immunopathol.* 25:1.
35. Delfraissy, J. F., P. Galanaud, J. Dormont, and C. Wallon. 1980. Age-related impairment of the in vitro antibody response in the human. *Clin. Exp. Immunol.* 39:208.
36. Delfraissy, J. F., P. Galanaud, C. Wallon, J. F. Balavoine, and J. Dormont. 1982. Abolished in vitro antibody response in elderly: Exclusive involvement of prostaglandin-induced T suppressor cells. *Clin. Immunol. Immunopathol.* 24:377.
37. Jaroslow, B. N., K. M. Suhrbier, R.J.M. Fry, and S. A. Tyler. 1975. In vitro suppression of immunocompetent cells by lymphomas from aging mice. *J. Natl. Cancer Inst.* 54:1427.
38. Gerbase-DeLima, M., P. Meredith, and R. L. Walford. 1975. Age-related changes, including synergy and suppression, in the mixed lymphocyte reaction in long-lived mice. *Fed. Proc.* 34:159.
39. Makinodan, T., J. W. Albright, C. P. Peter, and M. L. Heidrick. 1976. Reduced humoral immune activity in long-lived old mice: An approach to elucidating its mechanisms. *Immunology.* 31:903.

40. Goidl, E. A., J. B. Innes, and M. E. Weksler. 1976. Immunological studies of aging. II. Loss of IgG and high avidity plaque forming cells and increased suppressor cell activity in aging mice. *J. Exp. Med.* 144:1037.
41. DeKruyff, R. H., Y. T. Kim, G. W. Siskind, and M. E. Weksler. 1980. Age-related changes in the in vitro immune response: Increased suppressor activity in immature and aged mice. *J. Immunol.* 125:142.
42. Segre, D., and M. Segre. 1976. Humoral immunity in aged mice. II. Increased suppressor T cell activity in immunologically deficient old mice. *J. Immunol.* 116:735.
43. Segre, D., and M. Segre. 1977. Age-related changes in B and T lymphocytes and decline of humoral immune responsiveness in aged mice. *Mech. Ageing Dev.* 6:115.
44. Callard, R. E., and A. Basten. 1978. Immune function in aged mice. IV. Loss of T cell and B cell function in thymus-dependent antibody responses. *Eur. J. Immunol.* 8:552.
45. Callard, R. E., B. Fazekas de St. Groth, A. Basten, and I.F.C. McKenzie. 1980. Immune function in aged mice. V. Role of suppressor cells. *J. Immunol.* 124:52.
46. Doria, G., C. Mancini, and L. Adorini. 1982. Immunoregulation in senescence: Increased inducibility of antigen-specific suppressor T cells and loss of cell sensitivity to immunosuppression in aging mice. *Proc. Natl. Acad. Sci. USA.* 79:3803.
47. Globerson, A., L. Abel, and T. Umiel. 1981. Immune reactivity during aging. III. Removal of peanut-agglutinin binding cells from aging mouse spleen cells leads to increased reactivity to mitogens. *Mech. Ageing Dev.* 16:275.
48. Globerson, A., L. Abel, M. Barzilay, and I. Zen-Bar. 1982. Immunoregulatory cells in aging mice. I. Concanavalin A-induced and naturally occurring suppressor cells. *Mech. Ageing Dev.* 19:293.
49. Bruley-Rosset, M., I. Florentin, N. Kiger, J. Schulz, M. Davigny, and G. Mathe. 1979. Age-related changes in the immune response and immunorestoration by stimulating agents. *In* The Immune System: Functions and Therapy of Dysfunction. G. Doria and A. Eshkol, editors. Academic Press, Orlando, Fla. 171–187.
50. Bruley-Rosset, M., I. Florentin, N. Kiger, J. Schultz, and G. Mathe. 1979. Restoration of impaired immune functions of aged animals by chronic bestatin treatment. *Immunology.* 38:75.
51. Tsang, K. Y., H. H. Fudenberg, and M. J. Gnagy. 1983. Restoration of immune responses of aging hamsters by treatment with isoprinosine. *J. Clin. Invest.* 71:1750.
52. Gutowski, J. K., and M. E. Weksler. 1982. Studies on the syngeneic mixed lymphocyte reaction. II. Decline in the syngeneic mixed lymphocyte reaction with age. *Immunology.* 46:801.
53. Zharhary, D., Y. Segev, and H. E. Gershon. 1984. T-cell cytotoxicity and aging: Differing causes of reduced response in individual mice. *Mech. Ageing Dev.* 25:129.

54. Delpierre, M.-A., J. Panijel, and M. Terquem. 1980. Lymphoid cells from senescent animals contain specific inhibitors of immune response. *Cell. Immunol.* 52:204.
55. Krogsrud, R. L., and E. H. Perkins. 1977. Age-related changes in T cell function. *J. Immunol.* 118:1607.
56. Fujiwara, M., and S. Kishimoto. 1979. IgE antibody formation in aging. I. Age-related changes in IgE antibody formation and avidity for the DNP-determinant in mice. *J. Immunol.* 123:263.
57. Fujiwara, M., and A. Kariyone. 1981. Lipopolysaccharide-induced auto-antibody response. II. Age-related change in plaque-forming cell response to bromelain-treated syngeneic erythrocytes. *Int. Arch. Allergy Appl. Immunol.* 66:161.
58. Smith, A. M. 1976. The effects of age on the immune response to type III pneumococcal polysaccharide (SIII) and bacterial lipopolysaccharide (LPS) in BALB/c, SJL/J, and C3H mice. *J. Immunol.* 116:469.
59. Thoman, M. L., and W. O. Weigle. 1983. Deficiency in suppressor T cell activity in aged animals. *J. Exp. Med.* 157:2184.
60. Gottesman, S.R.S., R. L. Walford, and G. J. Thorbecke. 1984. Proliferation and cytotoxic immune functions in aging mice. II. Decreased generation of specific suppressor cells in alloreactive cultures. *J. Immunol.* 133:1782.
61. Liu, J. J., M. Segre, and D. Segre. 1982. Changes in suppressor, helper, and B-cell functions in aging mice. *Cell. Immunol.* 66:372.
62. Ding, D.-H., M. Segre, and D. Segre. 1979. Activation of helper T cells by immune complexes. *Cell. Immunol.* 46:281.
63. Liu, J. J., D. Segre, H. B. Gelberg, H. H. Fudenberg, K. Y. Tsang, N. Khansari, C. R. Waltenbaugh, and M. Segre. 1984. Effects of long-term treatment of mice with anti-I-J monoclonal antibody and dialyzable leukocyte extract on immune function and lifespan. *Mech. Ageing Dev.* 27:359.
64. Green, D. R., P. M. Flood, and R. K. Gershon. 1983. Immunoregulatory T-cell pathways. *Annu. Rev. Immunol.* 1:429.
65. Ptak, W., and R. K. Gershon. 1975. Immunosuppression effected by macrophage surfaces. *J. Immunol.* 115:1346.
66. Callard, R. E. 1978. Immune function in aged mice. III. Role of macrophages and effect of 2-mercaptoethanol in the response of spleen cells from old mice to phytohemagglutinin, lipopolysaccharide, and allogeneic cells. *Eur. J. Immunol.* 8:697.
67. McIntosh, K. R., M. Segre, and D. Segre. 1979. Inhibition of the humoral response by spleen cells from cyclophosphamide-treated mice. *Immunopharmacology.* 1:165.
68. McIntosh, K. R., M. Segre, and D. Segre. 1982. Characterization of cyclophosphamide-induced suppressor cells. *Immunopharmacology.* 4:279.
69. Segre, M., E. Tomei, and D. Segre. 1985. Cyclophosphamide-induced suppressor cells in mice: Suppression of the antibody response in vitro and characterization of the effector cells. *Cell. Immunol.* 91:443.
70. Oseroff, A., S. Okada, and S. Strober. 1984. Natural suppressor (NS) cells

found in the spleen of neonatal mice and adult mice given total lymphoid irradiation (TLI) express the null surface phenotype. *J. Immunol.* 132:101.

71. Strober, S. 1984. Natural suppressor (NS) cells, neonatal tolerance, and total lymphoid irradiation. *Annu. Rev. Immunol.* 2:219.
72. Merluzzi, V. J., E. M. Levy, V. Kumar, M. Bennet, and S. R. Cooperband. 1978. In vitro activation of suppressor cells from spleens of mice treated with radioactive strontium. *J. Immunol.* 121:505.
73. Calkins, C. E., and O. Stutman. 1978. Changes in suppressor mechanisms during postnatal development in mice. *J. Exp. Med.* 147:87.
74. McGarry, R. C., and S. K. Singhal. 1982. The immunoregulatory role of bone marrow. III. Further characterization of the suppressor cell and its mode of action. *Immunology.* 46:387.
75. Slapsys, R., and D. A. Clark. 1982. Active suppression of host-vs.-graft reaction in pregnant mice. IV. Local suppressor cells in decidua and uterine blood. *J. Reproductive Immunol.* 4:355.
76. Greeley, E. H., M. Segre, and D. Segre. 1985. Modulation of autoimmunity in NZB mice by cyclophosphamide-induced, nonspecific suppressor cells. *J. Immunol.* 134:847.
77. Segre, D., E. H. Greeley, and M. Segre. 1981. Cyclophosphamide induction of non-T suppressor cells and their possible role in self-tolerance. *In* Immunological Aspects of Aging. D. Segre and L. Smith, editors. Marcel Dekker, New York. 151-164.
78. Roder, J. C., A. K. Duwe, D. A. Bell, and S. K. Singhal. 1978. Immunological senescence. I. The role of suppressor cells. *Immunology.* 35:837.
79. Roder, J. C., D. A. Bell, and S. K. Singhal. 1977. Regulation of the immune response in autoimmune NZB/NZW F_1 mice. I. The spontaneous generation of splenic suppressor cells. *Cell. Immunol.* 29:272.
80. Greeley, E. H., M. Segre, and D. Segre. 1981. Suppressor cells in cyclophosphamide-treated mice. *Immunopharmacology.* 4:355.
81. Michalski, J. P., C. C. McCombs, and N. Talal. 1979. Suppressor cells and immunodeficiency in (NZB $\times$ NZW)F_1 hybrid mice. *Eur. J. Immunol.* 9:440.
82. Michalski, J. P., C. C. McCombs, J. R. Roubinian, and N. Talal. 1983. Effect of androgen therapy on survival and suppressor cell activity in aged NZB/NZW F_1 hybrid mice. *Clin. Exp. Immunol.* 52:229.

14

Zinc Metabolism and Immune Aging

Richard A. Winchurch

Baltimore Regional Burn Center
Johns Hopkins University
School of Medicine
and Francis Scott Key Medical Center
Baltimore, Maryland

I. INTRODUCTION

A variety of definitions have been applied to the aging process. By and large one's perspective and consequently one's working definition often depend on one's expertise and the area of investigation that is being pursued. However, a holistic approach to the study of the aging process demands that any physiological event that is being examined be considered in the light of all the other age-dependent changes that are occurring at the level of the whole organism. Ultimately the changes that occur in one system can be expected to affect other organs and systems. Thus aging may be viewed as a progressive degeneration of homeostatic control mechanisms at the organism level, and any analyses of age-related alterations in a single system must be considered from the perspective of what is occurring or has already occurred elsewhere in the body.

The study of immune aging and the attendant decline of the host's immune defense network has been the subject of intense effort in many laboratories in recent years. Much progress has been made in defining the parameters of immunity that are influenced by age but, as yet, the causes of immunosenescence are unknown. Ultimately it will be shown that immune aging is not the result of a single physiological failure but is the net result of decreased or altered function at the level of the whole organism and that a number of genetic, environmental, and metabolic factors are all responsible to some degree. Insights into the interrelationships among endocrine processes, neurological functions, and the immune system are only recently becoming more clearly understood, and it is growing more apparent that optimal immune function is regulated by many processes outside the lymphoreticular system.

The relationship between metabolic and nutritional processes and immunity has been a subject of intense study over the past two decades or so, and a large number of studies have shown that deficiencies in nutrition and even a marginal deficiency in a single essential nutrient can produce profound effects on immunity. One such nutrient that has received an extraordinary amount of attention and has been shown to play a critical role in immune function is the element zinc.

II. EFFECTS OF ZINC DEFICIENCY ON IMMUNITY

The essential role played by zinc in human physiology came to prominence more than two decades ago following the initial reports by Prasad and his colleagues concerning patients in the Middle East (1). Among the clinical features observed by this group were growth retardation, impaired sexual development, and skin disorders. Dietary habits of these patients suggested that the syndrome might have been related to some nutritional insufficiency, and subsequent studies revealed that zinc insufficiency was responsible for both growth retardation and gonadal hypofunction (2). Subsequent studies showed that supplemental dietary zinc reversed the symptoms and restored normal development (3). About a decade later it became apparent that apart from dietary insufficiency, other conditions could result in disorders related to zinc deficiency. In 1973 Barnes and Moynahan (4) showed that acrodernatitis enteropathica, a disease characterized by impaired growth, skin lesions, and gastrointestinal disorders was in fact due to a congenital defect resulting in malabsorption of dietary zinc. The course of the disease could be completely reversed by supplemental dietary zinc (5). Similarly, studies of the A 46 mutants in Danish Fresian cattle also revealed that an inherited disorder resulting in zinc malabsorption was responsible for the disease (6). It was significant that these animals also showed evidence of deficient T-cell-mediated immunity, hypoplastic thymuses, and increased susceptibility to infection in addition to stunted growth and skin lesions. Finally, clinical studies showed that some of patients suffering from common variable immunodeficiency disease also suffered from zinc deficiency and that T-cell functions improved after treatment with dietary supplements (7).

These clinical studies and experiments of nature revealed a strict physiological requirement for zinc and provided some clues for a possible role of zinc in host immune resistance. However, a clear understanding of the requirement for zinc in immunity and the scope of the role played by zinc in host resistance was not fully appreciated until the late 1970s, when the first reports appeared concerning the effects of experimentally induced zinc deficiency on specific immune responses. At that time Pamela Fraker and her colleagues showed that zinc deficiency impaired the ability of mice to generate specific antibody in response to immunization with a T-dependent antigen (8). This finding was confirmed and extended shortly thereafter by the studies of Gabriel Fernandes, Philip Frost, and their colleagues (9,10). Fernandes et al. also showed that zinc insufficiency was associated with thymic involution, depressed cell-mediated cytotoxicity, and decreased natural killer cell activity, as well as with a general decrease in the numbers of Thy-1.2-bearing lymphocytes (9). Further investigations showed that zinc deficiency appears to affect both primary and secondary antibody responses, and a deficiency induced after primary immunization seems to decrease the responses of memory cells even if these cells are transferred to zinc-adequate recipients (11). Delayed-type hypersensitive responses are reduced in zinc-deficient mice (12), as are mitogen responses (13). While the sum total of these data indicates a clear dependence of T-cell activity on adequate zinc levels, other data suggest that both B cells and macrophage activities are altered by changes in zinc status. Wirth et al. have demonstrated changes in the systemic distribution and activity of macrophages from deficient animals (14), and Fraker and her colleagues have shown diminished phagocytosis and killing of *Trypanosoma cruzi* in zinc-deficient macrophages (15). An arrest in B-cell development has also been inferred from the differential responses to T-cell-independent antigens and mitogens (16,17).

While it is clear that zinc is essential for the optimal functioning of the immune system, and particularly for T-cell-mediated functions, the mechanism(s) underlying the impaired responsiveness of immunocytes from zinc-deficient animals are unknown. Indeed it is questionable whether a single mechanism is involved, since more than 200 enzymes are known to depend on or to require zinc for their catalytic activity or structural integrity. Many of these enzymes are involved in protein synthesis, while others are essential to nucleic acid metabolism, e.g., RNA polymerases, thymidine kinase, or purine catabolic enzymes (18). The list of the various enzymes and enzymatic activities that are affected by zinc is too long for even a passing comment on each in this chapter. Suffice it to say that zinc inadequacy could influence lymphocyte functions by affecting the activity of any of a large number of specific enzymes. Whether any specific activity among these is solely responsible for the effects of zinc deprivation on immune responsiveness is problematic at this point. Clearly a diminution of activity of the enzymes involved in lymphocyte proliferation or a reduction in the activity of specificities essential for the synthesis of regulatory lymphokines is certain to impair immune responsiveness.

The question of whether lymphokine production is regulated by zinc-dependent enzymes has already been approached by some investigators. It has been reported that the thymic hormone, facteur thymique serique (FTS), described and studied by Bach and his associates, is dependent on zinc for its activity (19). Moreover, Bendtzen and his colleagues have recently published data suggesting that macrophage-derived leukocyte migration inhibitory factor (LIF) production by specifically stimulated cells is regulated by a carboxypeptidaselike, zinc-dependent enzyme (20,21). Similarly, Dessaint et al. have speculated that "lymphocyte-activating factor" (interleukin-1) activity is dependent on carboxypeptidase B, an enzyme whose catalytic activity is zinc dependent (22). It is tempting to speculate further that one of the chief effects of zinc deficiency is a reduced production of regulatory cytokines, but thus far the evidence is inconclusive.

Regardless of the mechanism(s) by which zinc deficiency affects immune responses, it is nonetheless clear that zinc does play a critical if not essential role in immunity. In the context of this discussion the question is whether either changes in zinc levels or alterations of zinc metabolism contribute in any way to the demise of immune function in the aged. A clear, unequivocal demonstration that immunosenescence is related to changes in zinc status requires that two conditions be satisfied. First, some change in zinc metabolism in aged subjects should be demonstrable at either the cellular or the systemic level. Second, if the age-associated decrease in immune potential is due to an inadequate level of zinc, the restoration of zinc levels by supplementation regimes should enhance immunity in an age-dependent manner.

III. AGING AND ZINC STATUS

The question of whether zinc metabolism is affected by age has received scant attention in the literature. In general, the results of most studies indicate no dramatic differences in circulating zinc levels in older subjects. Certainly no gross deficiencies have been documented in normal subjects, provided they enjoy an adequate and balanced diet (23). However, some studies have shown that plasma zinc levels do indeed decrease slightly with age, and these changes are statistically significant (24). Recently Turnlund et al. (25), in a carefully controlled study, have demonstrated that the intestinal absorption of dietary zinc in a group of normal, aged male humans is about half that of a young adult population sample. Moreover, these investigators confirmed the earlier findings that plasma levels are indeed decreased slightly with age (Turnlund, personal communication). Confirmation of these clinical findings in experimental animals was also recently reported by Woodward et al. (26), who showed that the serum levels of CBA/J mice maintained on a zinc-adequate diet decreased with age. In all these studies the age-related changes in zinc levels were not dramatic and did not by any means result in a deficiency or in any apparent zinc-related abnormality. The main import of these findings is that zinc status is altered with age. Whether the changes truly reflect alterations of systemic regulation is a matter for continued study and debate. Our own data suggest that hepatic regulation of zinc uptake and the intracellular zinc levels in subpopulations of lymphocytes are altered with age, but these results await further confirmation.

IV. EFFECTS OF ZINC ON AGED IMMUNE RESPONSES

While the analytic data suggested that there may indeed be some changes in zinc metabolism with age, there is, as yet, no direct support for the hypothesis that the changes in immune status in the aged are a consequence of these metabolic perturbations. However, our own studies have provided information suggesting that zinc supplementation can correct some of the immune defects in aged mice. In considering the problem, we reasoned that if the changes in immune potential in aged subjects were due to changes in the levels or distribution of zinc within immunocytes, then the addition of zinc itself to the cells might restore the normal zinc status and at the same time allow for the expression of normal immune potential. We elected to examine the effects of zinc supplementation on antibody formation in vitro, since this T-cell-dependent system required all the cellular components of the immune system. By employing an in vitro milieu, we could be assured that any effects we might observe were due to direct effects of zinc on the activities of the cells themselves rather than indirect effects related to changes in systemic metabolism. Initially we compared the influence of zinc supplementation on the antibody-forming potential of young adult and 12-month-old mice (27). At 12 months of age mice of the C57Bl/6 (B6) strain already show a diminished capacity to form antibody (28). Zinc chloride was added at the initiation of antibody-forming cultures in concentrations ranging from 10^{-6} to 10^{-3}M. The results (Figure 1) showed that concentrations between 10^{-5} and 10^{-4}M did indeed enhance antibody formation. Doses below 10^{-5} were ineffective, while doses above 10^{-4} were inhibitory. The data showed further that while zinc enhanced the responses of both age groups, responses in the older animals showed much greater increases, on the order of 300%, compared to the young adults (approximately 60%). This disproportionate increase in the older group, of course, occurred because the baseline response of the older mice was about half that of the young adults. Ultimately, the responses achieved in both groups were virtually identical (Figure 2). These data suggested that despite an apparent decrease in plaque responses, the potential for antibody formation in 12-month-old mice was equal to that of the younger, more robust animals. This potential could be achieved in the presence of supplemental zinc.

While 12-month-old mice show clear evidence of age-related immune decline, these animals are not by any means immunosenescent. Hence we next examined the effects of zinc supplementation on the responses of 24-month-old animals. Other investigators have shown that the immune responses of 2-year-old mice, while clearly depressed, vary considerably (29). Moreover, in aged

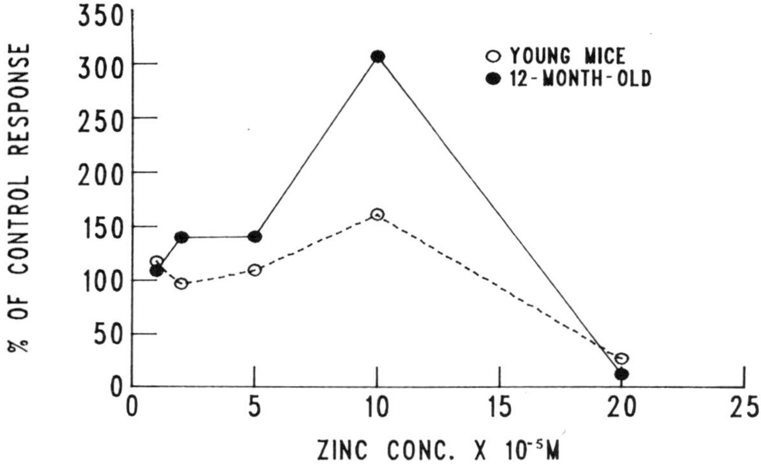

Figure 1 Comparison of the effects of varying concentrations of supplemental zinc on in vitro plaque-forming cell (PFC) responses of young adult (open points) and 12-month-old (solid points) C57Bl/6 mice expressed in terms of percentage increases of baseline (no zinc added) responses. (From Ref. 27.)

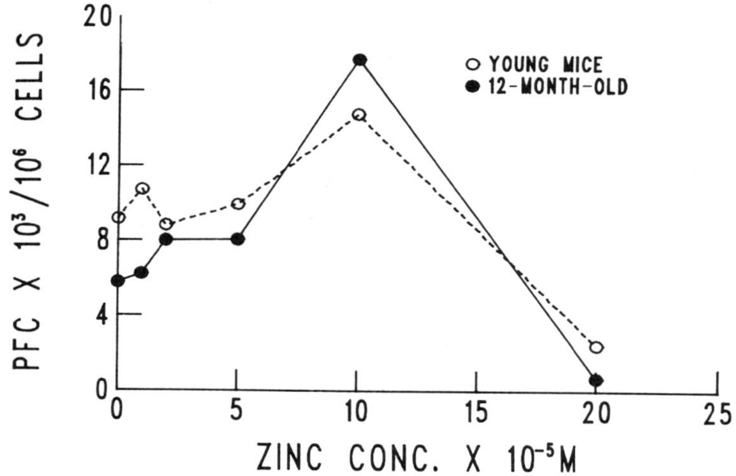

Figure 2 The data presented in Figure 1 expressed in terms of actual plaque-forming cells per million cultured cells.

populations the responses of pooled suspensions is usually equivalent to or less than the lowest individual response of cells making up the pool. For this reason it was imperative to examine the effects of zinc supplementation on individual mice rather than on pools of cells. Figure 3 and Table 1 illustrate the results of these experiments. As expected, antibody formation in the absence of zinc varied widely—from virtually no response in some cases (mouse 4) to approximately 600 plaque-forming cells (PFC) per million cultured cells. Zinc enhanced the response in every individual, although the magnitude of the increase was again variable. For example, mouse 3 (Figure 3) achieved a response nearly equal to young adults. In contrast, mouse 12 (Table 1), which produced about 1000 PFC per million in the absence of zinc, showed little more than a twofold increase when zinc was added to the cultures. Other animals demonstrated intermediate increases that were independent of the baseline (no zinc added) response. Cultures of pooled young adult cells were also enhanced, but the increase amounted to only 20% of the unsupplemented response. Moreover, intermediate concentrations of zinc that also enhanced the aged responses actually depressed the young adult response to some extent. These data clearly showed that the enhancement of antibody formation by zinc supplementation is an age-dependent phenomenon.

The in vitro results obtained at Johns Hopkins University have been confirmed and extended in other in vivo studies. Goidl et al. (unpublished data)

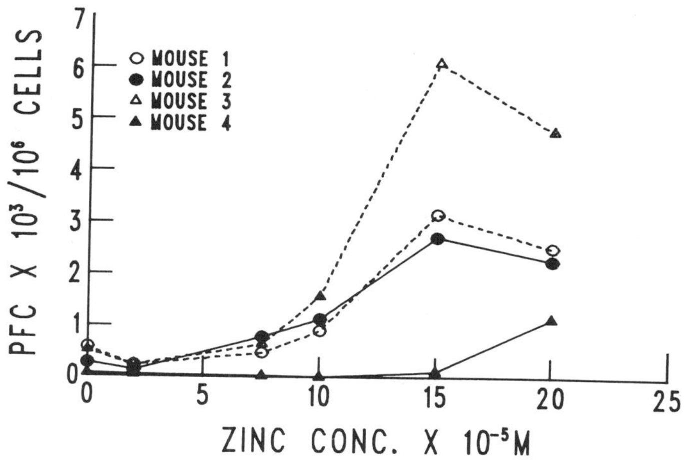

Figure 3 The effects of various concentrations of supplemental zinc on plaque-forming responses of four individual 24-month-old C57Bl/6 mice. The data are expressed as plaque-forming cells (PFC) per million cultured spleen cells. (From Ref. 27.)

Table 1 The Effects of Supplemental Zinc on Antibody Response in Young Adult and 24-month-old Mice[a]

Zinc concentration ($\times 10^{-5}$ M)	PFC/10^6 cultured cells				
	Young adult mice	24-month-old mice			
		Mouse 9	Mouse 10	Mouse 11	Mouse 12
0	5265	791	346	343	1111
1.0	4193	2038	1180	1165	1927
1.5	6299	3428	3959	1947	2313

[a]Exposure to supplemental zinc in vitro, as described in Figure 3.

have demonstrated that antibody formation in response to TNP-Ficoll in 10 to 12-month-old C57Bl/6 mice could be increased substantially if the animals were subjected to a regimen of zinc supplementation by injection over a 2 week period just before immunization. In these experiments, zinc chloride was administered at a dose rate of 2.5 mg/kg thrice weekly. Analyses of both direct (IgM) and indirect (IgG) plaque-forming responses indicated that the capacity to produce both isotypes was increased considerably. Of greater interest was the finding that the zinc-treated animals displayed changes in auto-anti-idiotype antibody production and manifested an anti-idiotype response that was characteristic of a young adult response. Previous studies by this group had shown that aging results both in increased anti-idiotype production and in changes in the antibody repitoire (30). Thus their recent observations on the effects of zinc supplementation further supported the concept that zinc was somehow effecting age-related changes in immune status.

While it was clear from the aforementioned studies that zinc could enhance immune processes in aged mice both in vivo and in vitro, the mechanism(s) responsible for this effect were unknown. For example, it was not known whether zinc was simply facilitating the production of antibody by B cells or whether an early activation step at the level of either the macrophage or T cell was involved. The question of B-cell involvement was particularly relevant because it had been reported that zinc can sometimes act as a B-cell mitogen (31). Our own experimental data did not suggest that the increases we observed were due to polyclonal B-cell activation, since zinc alone never produced any increases in plaque formation unless specific antigen was also included in the cultures. When we examined the time course of the zinc effect, we observed that the maximum effect was produced when the metal was added to the cultures at 24 h. Additions at 48 h were less effective, and if the addition was delayed until 96 h, one day before harvest, no effect whatever was produced (Figure 4). The

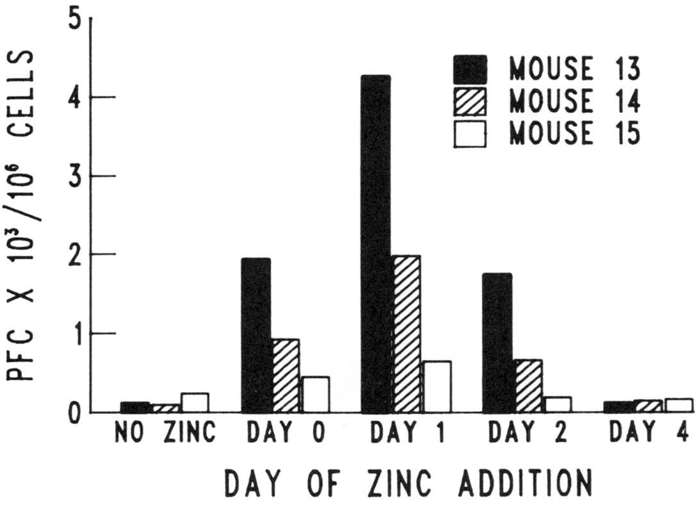

Figure 4 The effects of delayed addition of zinc on plaque-forming responses of individual 24-month-old C57Bl/6 mice. Zinc, at a concentration of 1.5×10^{-4} M was added on the days indicated and was maintained for the 5-day incubation period. (From Ref. 27.)

failure of delayed additions to produce a strong response also argued against a polyclonal effect, since polyclonal activation is usually manifested within 2-3 days after culture initiation. These results also suggested that zinc was acting at some early, activation step in the response. In further studies in which cultures were pulsed for discrete intervals, washed to remove excess zinc, and recultured, we showed again that the early addition of zinc produced optimal effects, provided the cultures were left undisturbed for at least 48 h after the metal was added (Figure 5). Shorter intervals of zinc exposure were apparently ineffective, and a 48-h exposure beginning at time zero also produced no enhancement. Curiously, a short 4-h exposure beginning at time zero consistently produced some enhancement. We reasoned that exposures of 0–48 h and 24–48 h were ineffective either because the duration of exposure was too short or because the washing procedure removed soluble mediators generated in response to the presence of zinc. The shorter pulse of 4 h at the onset of the culture period was sufficient to load the cells with enough zinc to facilitate subsequent activation of mediator-producing cells. Maximum production of mediator occurred around 25 h, and maximum uptake of these soluble immune activators by the appropriate target cells occurred within 72 h.

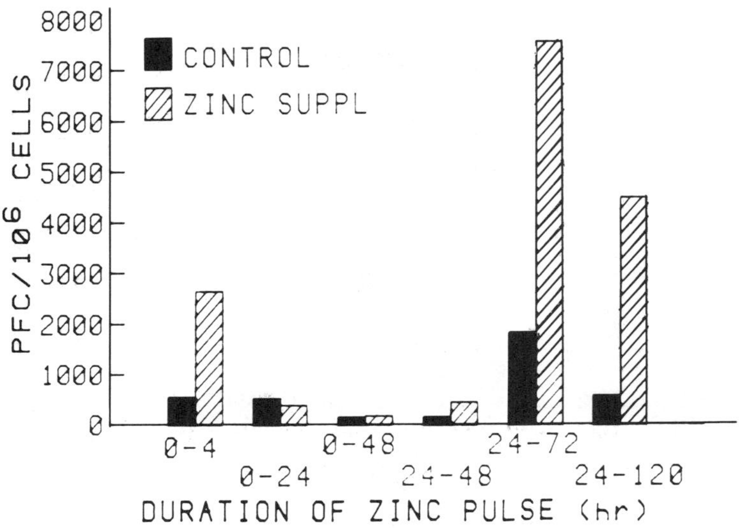

Figure 5 In vitro antibody responses of spleen cells from 24-month-old C57Bl/6 mice to sheep red blood cells. Zinc, at a final concentration of 1.5×10^{-5} M, was added to the cultures for the periods indicated. At the termination of zinc exposure, the cells were washed and reseeded in culture with fresh culture medium. Plaque responses were determined at day 5.

We next attempted to demonstrate directly that the zinc-supplemented cultures did indeed generate increases in soluble mediators capable of supporting the responses of aged immunocytes. A series of zinc-pulsed cultures were set up as described above and, at the termination of each pulse, the culture supernatants were collected. These supernatants were dialyzed exhaustively, first against phosphate-buffered saline to eliminate the excess zinc, then against culture medium, and subsequently against fully supplemented culture medium containing fetal calf serum and 2-mercaptoethanol, to reconstitute the composition of the medium. All supernatants were then analyzed for zinc levels. To determine whether these supernatants contained soluble factors capable of supporting antibody formation half-milliliter aliquots were added to half-milliliter volumes of aged spleen cell, antigen was added, and the cultures were incubated for 5 days.

As expected, the spleen cells cultured in media alone responded poorly in comparison to those from young adults. Similarly, cells cultured in supernatants obtained from aged cells preincubated without added zinc did not respond well. In contrast, culture supernatants obtained from cells exposed to zinc between 0 and 24 h produced a good response (Figure 6). All other supernatants were inactive. The ability of 0–24 h zinc-conditioned medium to support antibody formation was not due to the presence of residual zinc. While all the zinc-conditioned media did contain elevated levels of the metal that could not be completely removed by dialysis, this residual zinc concentration was only about 10^{-5} M, a concentration that does not support a response in aged spleen cells. Moreover, all the zinc-conditioned supernatants, including those that were inactive, contained equivalent levels of the metal. Thus our results showed that zinc affected an early phase of antibody formation, and our data suggest that zinc acts by facilitating the production of some soluble mediator. The identification of the mediator(s) remains uncertain. Thoman and Weigle had reported earlier that supplementation of aged spleen cell cultures with interleukin 2 (IL-2) restored antibody formation to about the same degree as our regimen of zinc supplementation (32). When we analyzed zinc-conditioned supernatants for IL-2 levels, we could detect no increases of a magnitude sufficient to support the responses of aged cells. Thus the identity of the factor or factors generated in response to zinc supplementation remains unknown.

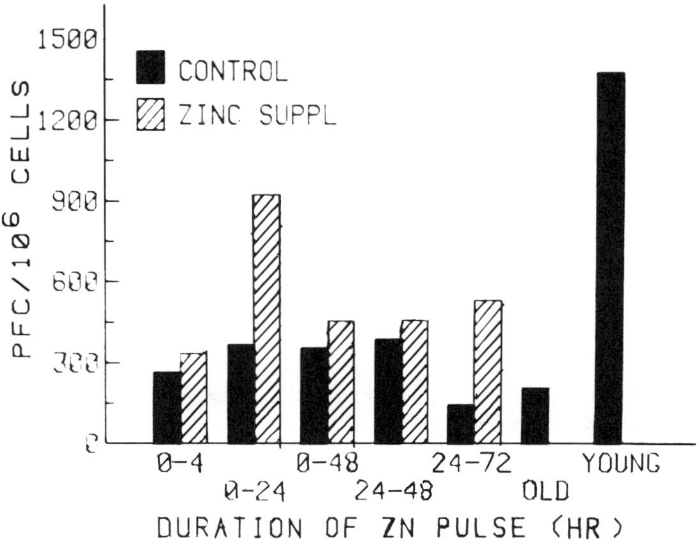

Figure 6 In vitro antibody responses of fresh spleen cells from 24-month-old mice cultured in the presence of dialyzed, conditioned medium from aged cells exposed to supplemental zinc. The conditioned media were obtained from cells maintained as described in Figure 5.

V. CONCLUSIONS

The analytic and metabolic studies that have been carried out thus far indicate that zinc metabolism may be affected by the aging process. Clearly all the data are not in yet, and much work remains to be done to establish the relationships between aging and zinc status. This point is critical, but beyond this we need to learn more about the relationships between immune aging and zinc metabolism. The evidence obtained thus far clearly indicates a relation between zinc status and the ability of the aged immune system to produce antibody. However, it is highly unlikely that alterations of zinc metabolism are solely responsible for the demise of immune function in the aged.

The important questions at this point are to determine the extent to which the putative age-related changes in zinc metabolism influence immunity and to establish what other physiological changes affect the dependence on or requirement for zinc in the aging immune system. The body is an integrated whole, and each system is ultimately dependent on the functions of other organs and systems. It is not at all surprising that immunity depends on an adequate zinc nutriture, and it is entirely reasonable to speculate that the demise of immune function that accompanies advanced age may be related to age-dependent changes in zinc metabolism.

"The immune system belongs to the body" is the title of a recent new article in the journal *Science* (33). This statement, expressed by Karen Bulloch of the State University of New York at Stony Brook, very appropriately underscores the significance of some recent findings dealing with the relationships between nervous function and immunity. All the more, these words might be the catchphrase for studies of immune aging, and they might help us bear in mind that all the other physiological events that accompany aging will eventually affect host immune resistance.

REFERENCES

1. Prasad, A. S., J. A. Halsted, and M. Nadimi. 1961. Syndrome of iron deficiency anemia, hepatosplenomegaly, hypogonadism, dwarfism and geophagia. *Am. J. Med.* 31:522.
2. Prasad, A. S., A. Miale, Z. Farid, A. Schulert, and H. H. Sandstead. 1963. Zinc metabolism in patients with the syndrome of iron deficiency anemia, hypogonadism and dwarfism. *J. Lab. Clin. Med.* 61:537.
3. Halsted, J. A., H. A. Ronagy, P. Abadi, M. Haghshenass, G. H. Amirkakimi, R. M. Barakat, and J. G. Reinhold. 1972. Zinc deficiency in man: The Shiraz experiment. *Am. J. Med.* 53:277.
4. Barnes, P. M., and E. J. Moynahan. 1973. Zinc deficiency in acrodermatitis enteropathica: Multiple dietary intolerance treated with synthetic diet. *Proc. R. Soc. Med.* 66:327.
5. Oleske, J. M., M. L. Westphal, S. Shore, D. Gordon, J. Bodgen, and A.

Nahmias. 1979. Correction with zinc therapy of depressed cellular immunity in acrodermatitis enteropathica. *Am. J. Dis. Child.* 133:915.

6. Brummerstedt, E., T. Flagstad, A. Basse, and E. Andresen. 1971. The effect of zinc on calves with hereditary thymus hypoplasia (lethal trait A 46). *Acta Pathol. Microbiol. Scand.* 79:686.
7. Cunningham-Rundles, C., S. Cunningham-Rundles, J. Garofaio, T. Iwata, G. Incefy, J. Twomey, and R. A. Good. 1979. Increased T lymphocyte function and thymopoietin following zinc repletion in man. *Fed. Proc.* 38:1222.
8. Fraker, P. J., S. M. Haas, and R. W. Lueke. 1977. Effect of zinc deficiency on the immune response of the young adult A/J mouse. *J. Nutr.* 107:1889.
9. Fernandes, G., M. Nair, K. Onoe, T. Tanaka, and R. A. Good. 1979. Impairment of cell-mediated immunity function by dietary zinc deficiency in mice. *Proc. Natl. Acad. Sci. USA.* 79:452.
10. Frost, P., P. Rabbani, J. Smith, and A. Prasad. 1981. Cell-mediated cytotoxicity and tumor growth in zinc deficient mice. *Proc. Soc. Exp. Biol. Med.* 167:333.
11. DePasquale-Jardieu, P., and P. J. Fraker. 1984. Interference in the development of a secondary immune response in mice by zinc deprivation; persistence of effects. *J. Nutr.* 114:1762.
12. Fraker, P. J., C. M. Zwickl, and R. W. Luecke. 1982. Delayed type hypersensitivity in zinc deficient mice: Impairment and restoration of responsivity to dinitrofluorobenzene. *J. Nutr.* 111:309.
13. Gross, R. L., N. Osdin, L. L. Fong, and P. M. Newberne. 1979. Depressed immunologic function in zinc-deprived rats as measured by mitogen responses of spleen, thymus and peripheral blood. *Am. J. Clin. Nutr.* 32: 1260.
14. Wirth, J. J., P. J. Fraker, and F. Kierszenbaum. 1984. Changes in the levels of marker expression by mononuclear phagocytes in zinc-deficient mice. *J. Nutr.* 114:1826.
15. Fraker, P. J., R. Caruso, and F. Kierszenbaum. 1982. Alteration of the immune and nutritional status of mice by synergy between zinc deficiency and infection with *Trypanosoma cruzi*. *J. Nutr.* 112:1224.
16. Hildebrandt, K., R. Luecke, and P. J. Fraker. 1982. Effect of maternal dietary zinc on growth and mitogenic responses in suckling mice. *J. Nutr.* 112:1921.
17. Beach, R. S., M. E. Gershwin, and L. S. Hurley. 1979. Altered structure and mitogen responsiveness in postnatally zinc-deprived mice. *Dev. Comp. Immunol.* 3:725.
18. Chesters, J. K. 1982. Metabolism and biochemistry of zinc. *In* Clinical, Biochemical and Nutritional Aspects of Trace Elements. A. Prasad, editor. Alan R. Liss, New York. 221–238.
19. Dardenne, M., J.-M. Pleau, P. Lefrancier, and J.-F. Bach. 1981. Role du zinc et d'autres métaux dans l'activité biologique du FTS (thymuline). *C.R. Acad. Sci. Paris.* 292:793.
20. Bendtzen, K. 1982. Induction of antigen-specific lymphocyte unresponsive-

ness in vitro: Possible role of divalent cations and defective function of human T-cell-activating factor (TAF). *Cell. Immunol.* 66:152.
21. Bendtzen, K., and L. Mayland. 1982. Role of zinc and other divalent metal ions in human lymphokine production in vitro. *Scand. J. Immunol.* 15:81.
22. Dessaint, J.-P., S. P. Katz, and B. H. Waksman. 1979. Catheptic carboxypeptidase B as major component in "lymphocyte activating factor" of macrophages. *J. Immunopharmacol.* 1:399.
23. Solomons, N. W. 1982. Biological availability of zinc in humans. *Am. J. Clin. Nutr.* 35:1048.
24. Lindeman, R. D., M. L. Clark, and J. P. Colmore. 1971. Influence of age and sex in plasma and red cell zinc concentration. *J. Gerontol.* 26:358.
25. Turnlund, J. R., N. Durkin, and S. Margen. 1984. Zinc absorption in young and elderly men. *Fed. Proc.* 43:850.
26. Woodward, W. D., S. M. Filleau, and O. B. Allen. 1984. Decline in serum zinc level throughout adult life in the laboratory mouse. *J. Gerontol.* 39:521.
27. Winchurch, R. A., D. J. Thomas, W. H. Adler, and T. J. Lindsay. 1984. Supplemental zinc restores antibody formation in cultures of aged spleen cells. *J. Immunol.* 133:569.
28. Winchurch, R. A., W. Birmingham, C. Hilberg, and A. Munster. 1982. Effects of endotoxin on immunity in aging mice. *Cell. Immunol.* 67:384.
29. Nordin, A. A., and W. H. Adler. 1979. The effects of aging on in vitro cellular interactions. *In* Developmental Immunobiology. G. W. Siskind, S. D. Litwin, and M. E. Weksler, editors. Grune & Stratton, New York. 215.
30. Goidl, E. A., G. T. Thorbecke, M. E. Weksler, and G. W. Siskind. 1980. Production of auto-anti-idiotypic antibodies during the normal immune response: Changes in the auto-anti-idiotype antibody response and the idiotype repertoire associated with aging. *Proc. Natl. Acad. Sci. USA.* 77:6788.
31. Cunningham-Rundles, S., C. Cunningham-Rundles, B. Dupont, and R. A. Good. 1980. Zinc-induced activity of human B lymphocytes. *Clin. Immunol. Immunopharmacol.* 16:115.
32. Thoman, M. L., and W. O. Weigle. 1981. Lymphokines and aging: Interleukin-2 production and activity in aged animals. *J. Immunol.* 127:2102.
33. Bulloch, K. 1984. The immune system belongs in the body. *Science.* 227:1190.

15

Idiotype Shifts

Aging or Maturation

Sybille Müller, Hui-chen Chang, Mary M. Ward, Jyh-Hsiung Huang, Ronald E. Ward, and Heinz Köhler

Roswell Park Memorial Institute
Buffalo, New York

I. INTRODUCTION

One of the most intriguing features of the immune system is the homeostasis of the network. As described by Niels Jerne (1), the immune system consists of an interacting web of idiotypes and anti-idiotypes. The terminology of idiotypes and anti-idiotypes is operational only as derived from experiments in which certain antibodies (idiotypes) were selected to make anti-idiotypic antibodies. Within the network concept, the idiotype–anti-idiotype nomenclature denotes the complementarity of binding sites (paratopes) and idiotypic determinants (idiotopes). Paratopes and idiotopes are present on B-cell receptors, antibodies, and on the antigen-specific receptors of T cells. Thus, the entire immune system with its B- and T-cell arms is tied together by complementarity fits of paratopes and idiotopes.

Network immunologists have been doing idiotype suppression experiments for more than 10 years (for review, see Ref. 2) and more recently, protocols have been devised to stimulate a given idiotype or to raise its level through idiotypic manipulations (for review, see Ref. 3). Because it is relatively easy to disturb idiotype expression experimentally, it has been speculated that the cause for certain immunological diseases may be an altered idiotype network balance. Since diseases like autoimmune disorders occur more frequently in older people, the idiotype network may lose stability with age and abnormal idiotype shifts may become causatively involved. Similar explanations for the increased incidence of cancer in older persons have been given. Finally, the increased susceptibility with age to infections has also been linked to a failing immune system.

In the following discussion we summarize literature on age-associated changes in humoral and cellular immune responses, related and not related to autoimmune diseases. Furthermore, we present data from the Roswell Park Memorial Institute on evidence for changes of a dominant idiotype expressed in an experimental animal system. We ask whether the observed changes are signs of an aging and failing immune system, or whether these idiotype shifts occur as part of a normal maturation process. We also address the question of the stability of T helper cell idiotype loops and discuss manipulations to reverse idiotype shifts.

II. INCREASE OF AUTOIMMUNE DISEASES WITH AGE

The question here is, which changes in the immune system should be considered pathological and which should be considered normal?

Physiological factors of the aging process imply turnover of the immune system, which is subject to the breakdown of immunoregulation and to a disturbance of homeostatic control. None of the autoimmune diseases occur in young individuals with well-maintained immune systems; most of the disorders occur in individuals in which age-related malfunction of the immune system is ongoing. In animal models and patients with apparent clinical autoimmune diseases, acceleration of immunological aging is observed. Probably these two phenomena—acceleration of immunological aging and clinical manifestations of autoimmune disease—mutually affect each other, leading to a vicious cycle of disease.

A. Classification of Autoimmune Diseases

Autoantibodies that are directly related to the cause of the disease, such as antibodies against thyroid-stimulating hormone (TSH) in Graves' disease, produce one type of autoimmune disease. Another type of autoimmune disease is caused by the accumulation of immune complexes, such as antinuclear antibody in systemic lupus erythematosus (SLE) and rheumatoid factor in rheumatoid arthritis (RA). The third type consists of those that are not yet proven in terms of causality, such as antiparietal cell antibody and anti–smooth muscle antibody (4,5). These autoantibodies can be classified into three categories: autoantibodies against a cellular constituent or product, those against the cell wall as a whole, and those against hormone receptors. The latter play a major role in the induction of so-called organ-specific autoimmune diseases such as myasthenia gravis and insulin-resistant diabetes.

It is important to note that there is an age-related increase in the incidence of routinely measured autoantibodies in humans and laboratory animals in association with an age-related decline in many normal immune functions (6-8). Such antibodies as antinucleus, antiparietal cell, and antithyroglobulin were reported in healthy individuals without apparent clinical manifestations, as well as in long-lived, non-autoimmune-prone mice, which showed an increasing incidence of autoantibodies with advancing age. Both phenomena, increasing autoimmune functions and decreasing normal immune functions, could be due to the age-related inefficiency of T-cell functional capacity, especially regulatory T-cell functions (9). Although a causal relationship between autoantibody and vascular lesions is not known, several studies suggest that accumulating nonspecific autoantibodies appear to play a major role in the occurrence of vascular diseases, such as coronary heart disease and artherosclerosis of the aorta through the immune complex pathway (10-12).

B. Age-Related Alteration of Humoral and Cellular Immune Functions

Age-related alterations in normal immune functions have been well documented in humans and rodents at the level of lymphoid tissues and cellular and humoral immune functions (4). A major contribution to the decline of the response to T-dependent antigens is due to reduced T-cell help (13) or increased T-cell suppression (14,15), as well as depression of suppressor cell function with age (16).

When the response at the clonal level of B cells of aged mice to a T-dependent antigen, dinitrophenylated hemocyanin (DNP–Hy), was investigated, to determine the origin of the impaired humoral response in aged mice, a lower number of clones producing anti-DNP-antibody were found in aged mice. The isotype distribution was slightly different in young and old mice. The frequency of DNP-responsive cells in the bone marrow cell suspensions and the surface-immunoglobulin-negative (sIg^-) subpopulation was not significantly different when such cells were isolated from aged versus young mice. Therefore the authors suggested that this defect is associated with the maturation of B-cell clones in the aged environment and occurs during the migration of cells from the bone marrow to the spleen (17).

In a study (18) of the responsiveness to the influenza virus and its HA moiety, it was found that the frequency of mature B cells responsive to the intact virion and the HA moiety is not reduced in BALB/c mice 24-26 months old, as compared with the frequency of responsive B cells in young mice (3-4 months). Consequently, for this response, there is no evidence of the preexistence of regulatory or suppressive mechanisms in aged mice. This coincides with the absence of any apparent deficit in the capacity of bone marrow cell populations of aged animals to generate both B-cell precursors and B cells.

Therefore, limitations or changes in repertoire expression observed in response to various antigens in aged animals are likely to be due to regulatory mechanisms that affect the particular responses than to a central defect in the generation of the normally diverse repertoire.

On the other hand, recent findings from Averill and Wolf (19) indicate that an intrinsic mechanism could be responsible for the decline of polyclonally induced proliferation of B and T lymphocytes; bone marrow cells (BMC) derived from old or young donor $AB6F_1$ mice were transplanted into the neutral environment of young, lethally irradiated recipients. The response levels of phytohemagglutinin (PHA) and lipopolysaccharides (LPS) exhibited by old donors as well as their recipients were 30 and 70% of those of young donors and their recipients, respectively. Thus, even under the influence of a young recipient environment, old BMC were incapable of giving rise to mitogen-responding cells that function the same as their younger counterparts.

It has been reported that spleen cells enriched for T lymphocytes derived from old Coombs' positive NZB mice were not capable of producing suppression of the in vitro antisyngeneic mouse erythrocyte (MRBC) autoimmune response, whereas enriched splenic T lymphocytes from young NZB mice suppressed this antiresponse (16). It was of interest to investigate whether CBA/N mice, which have a sex-linked defect in antibody formation, were also defective in their autoantibody response and how age would affect this autoimmune response (20). Bromelain-modified syngeneic mouse erythrocytes (Br-MRBC) were injected and plaque-forming cells (PFC) were determined. The results showed that the B-cell response to modified self erythrocytes was also under sex-linked control in both homozygous and heterozygous mice. Only a low number of PFC was found when Br-MRBC injection was enhanced with LPS or 17XL *Plasmodium yoelii* in young homozygous mice and male F_1 offspring of CBA/N-mothered crosses, e.g., $(CBA/N \times NZB)F_1$ males. This defect, however, is largely overcome with age; in mice older than 5-7 weeks, PFC response to Br-MRBC gradually increased with age, becoming comparable to the level in normal mice. Probably this is a result of environmental stimulation, indicating the presence of low frequencies of the specific precursors, which can be triggered and expanded with age.

Various laboratories have demonstrated that immunodefective CBA/N mice are able to overcome their X-linked genetic inability to respond to TI-2 antigens with increasing age (21-23). In the CBA/N mice, the inability to respond to such antigens as type III pneumococcal polysaccharide and dinitrophenyl conjugates of Ficoll has been generally ascribed to the absence of a mature subpopulation of $Lyb5^+$ B cells. Over time, it appears that this $Lyb5^-$ population proceeds through various activation steps so that, after induction by TI-2 antigens, the CBA/N mice can respond to such antigens (24-26).

To study the stability of the profile of idiotypic antibodies to phosphorylcholine-keyhole limpet hemocyanin (PC-KLH), the ontogeny of BALB/c and anti-PC idiotypes in lethally irradiated BALB/c hosts was studied (27). The T15-positive ($T15^+$) idiotype initially 100% of the anti-PC response at day 16 after the reconstitution with neonatal liver cells of irradiated BALB/c mice, declined to less than 50% at day 96, to be replaced by non-T15-positive ($T15^-$) idiotypes. The authors concluded that the transition from an initial $T15^+$ expression to a later non-T15 dominance is due to an ontogenic preference of $T15^+$ clones in BALB/c mice. This loss of dominance would occur when the normal generative environment of intact BALB/c mice is disrupted by events as irradiation tolerance, induction, or adoptive transfer (28). It remains to be seen whether aging may have an impact, too, on clonal shifts within the idiotype profile to PC-KLH.

C. Age and Auto-Anti-Idiotypic Antibody

It has been shown that in mice there is an age-related increase of auto-anti-idiotypic antibody, which is believed to play a suppressive role in the immune response network of idiotype–anti-idiotype (29).

C57Bl/6 and BALB/c mice were immunized intravenously with trinitrophenyl (TNP), and their spleens removed and B cells assayed for auto-anti-idiotypic antibody activity by hapten augmentation of plaque formation according to Schrater et al. (30). The increased auto-anti-idiotype (Id) response can be transferred to young recipient mice with splenic T cells from aged donor mice (31). Lethally irradiated mice reconstituted with BM from aged donors manifest a low auto-anti-Id response comparable to young mice, suggesting that the BM of old and young animals is similar. When mice were exposed to a normally lethal dose of irradiation while their BM was partly shielded, they survived and regained immune function, including a modest occurrence of auto-anti-Id antibodies as observed in normal young mice. This is seen as a result of repopulation of the peripheral lymphoid system in the irradiated mice by the cells that originated from the shielded BM. High levels of auto-anti-idiotypic antibodies were found, as determined by hapten-augmentable PFC response, when splenic T cells from old donor mice were transferred into recipient mice, irradiated with BM shielded previously. Thus, the production of enhanced levels of auto-anti-idiotypic antibodies is dependent on changes in the T-cell repertoire with increasing age. Changes in Id expression and anti-auto-Id responses in old animals are connected with shifts in clonal distribution of long-lived T cells, as a consequence of life-long interactions with internal and external antigens. Specifically, the repertoire of hapten-specific suppressor cells, elicited by TNP-conjugated syngeneic spleen cells, which make mice tolerant to hapten response, undergoes an age-related shift (32): suppressor T cells induced in young mice depressed the PFC response of young, but not old, mice to TNP-Ficoll or TNP-bovine γ-globulin. Similarly, suppressor T cells induced in old mice depressed the response in old mice, but not young mice, to both antigens. Changes in idiotype repertoire may consequently influence the specificity of suppressor T cells present in tolerant mice.

D. Autoimmune Diseases and Auto-Anti-Idiotypic Antibody

Auto-anti-idiotypic antibodies can be considered to be regulatory molecules in the physiological process of aging, as well as in the occurrence of autoimmune diseases. For the latter, some experimental evidence emphasizes the role of auto-anti-Id. According to the network theory, one idiotype generates a complementary anti-idiotypic antibody, which in turn generates an anti-idiotypic antibody (33). Anti-idiotypic antibodies share structural similarities with the inducing antigenic isotype (34-38) and thus can trigger B and T cells as if those anti-idiotypic antibodies were antigen. This would be an example of a positive abnormality in which auto-antibody-specific B-cell proliferation and auto-antibody production result via network stimulation without antigen becoming involved. It has been found that idiotypes on immunoglobulin V regions are serologically cross-reactive with an idiotope or idiotopes on T lymphocytes (34-39). This finding raises the possibility of idiotypic intervention in the ongoing immune response. It was demonstrated several years ago that immune responses may be suppressed or enhanced by the administration of appropriate anti-Id antibodies (40-43). Since then, experimental evidence for regulatory functions of the internal antigen-Ab2β has grown (44).

For example, it has been shown that rabbit anti-idiotypic antibody to human rheumatoid factor autoantibodies bears the "internal image" of the antigen, human IgG (45). Furthermore, auto-anti-idiotypic antibodies may modulate autoantibody production in myasthenia gravis (46) and SLE (47,48). Studies have been done on idiotype expression in experimental allergic encephalomyelitis and multiple sclerosis (49). It has been demonstrated that C_8-substituted guanine ribonuclosides could restore PFC response to sheep red blood cells (SRBC) in senescent mice (50).

Therapy in autoimmune diseases is often approached by restoring immune functions of middle-aged mice to the level of young mice. Double-stranded polynucleotides, certain free-radical inhibitors (antioxidant), and sulfhydryl compounds have been shown to mitigate the aging process. Thymic products and grafting of cells and tissues also restored age-related immune deficiencies (4). Nutritional factors have been shown to influence the life span and susceptibility autoimmune disease development in mouse strains of differing genetic backgrounds (51).

Also, anti-idiotypic antibodies directed against monoclonal antibodies to autoantibodies have been used for immunomodulation of autoimmune responses in murine models (52). For example, anti-idiotypic antiserum to monoclonal antiribonucleoprotein (SM)-antibody inhibited the SM-autoantigen-induced proliferation response. This antibody was able to suppress the T-cell (Lyt $1^+,2^-$) proliferative in normal and autoimmune [lpr/lpr] MRL/MPJ or C3H/HeJ mice. This suggests that normal mouse strains also have T lymphocytes bearing determinants that are structurally similar to the Id determinants of autoantibodies, supporting the concept that autoreactive lymphocytes are present in normal mice but remain silent unless activated in some way. Thus, spontaneous production of anti-SM antibodies in normal mice can be manipulated through Id signals that have potential therapeutic value in vivo.

The question arises whether suppression of autoimmune diseases such as autoimmune tubolointerstitial nephritis, myasthenia gravis, and spontaneous autoimmune thyrotditis can be effected by the addition of exogeneous anti-idiotypic antibodies from the Abβ-type. Teitelbaum et al. (53) studied the influence of the production of autoantibodies with the high-frequency idiotype of MRL-lpr/lpr (H130) mice by administration of corresponding anti-idiotypic antibodies. They found that these anti-idiotypic antibodies induced antibodies with the H130 idiotype. When $(Fab')_2$ fragments of anti-idiotypic antibodies were administered, a rise of antibodies could be observed. Therefore, it appears that the treatment of autoimmune diseases with anti-Id antibodies may have the undesired effect of augmenting the production of autoantibodies.

Nevertheless, experiments were performed to determine whether anti-Id to autoantibodies from patients with SLE or RA can be used in the differential diagnosis of these diseases (54). To improve assays for the measurement of fluctuating anti-DNA antibodies in patients with SLE in different stages of the disease, rabbit anti-idiotypic antisera raised against hybridoma anti-DNA autoantibodies were obtained. The hybridoma anti-DNA autoantibodies were produced from the fusion of peripheral blood lymphocytes (PBL) from SLE and RA patients. These studies indicate that some anti-idiotypic antisera may detect specific idiotypes found only on SLE-derived anti-DNA autoantibodies, whereas other antisera detect shared idiotypes found on both RA and SLE DNA-binding and non-DNA-binding antibodies. The latter may be an Ab2 directed against an idiotype located outside the antigen combining site and therefore termed "α-type anti-idiotype antibody" according to the nomenclature discussed by Kohler (2). Specific idiotypes found only in SLE-derived anti-DNA autoantibodies may belong to either Abβ or Abγ, since these anti-idiotypes can be directed against an idiotype in or near the antigen combining site (γ) or can bear an internal image of the antigen to which anti-DNA antibody (Abl) binds by virtue of this similarity with antigen.

E. Cancer Increase with Age

The different forms of cancer are influenced by multiple factors such as life styles (e.g., diet or smoking habits) and endemic environmental and occupational factors. Against a background of drastic environmental modification and rapid technological change, cancer appears to be an "epidemic" threat to civilization.

However, since more people are living longer and cancer rates are higher among older people, adjustment for age corrects the impression that cancer rates are being driven upward dramatically by an increasing environmental threat. On the other hand, one could argue that older people are exposed longer to external factors favoring cancer development and therefore these factors still pose a threat. Despite the large body of phenomenalistic observations regarding changes of the immune system with age and their correlation to the increase of cancer incidence with age, we will not review here findings that may explain incidence of cancer within the context of functional changes of the immune system in age.

F. Idiotype Shifts in BALB/c Mice Hyperimmunized with Alloantigen and Normal BALB/c Mice Within 12 Months

Recent data from our laboratory demonstrate changes in the frequency of the major, dominant TEPC 15 idiotype in aging BALB/c mice injected with alloantigens.

It was shown before that an autoimmunization with allogeneically induced T-cell blasts against one haplotype generates strong suppression-affecting responses against the respective, corresponding major histocompatibility complex (MHC) specificity (55). Because of the known T-cell cross-reactivity between self and external antigens, the idiotype network stability might be impaired by multiple exposure to allogeneically different autoblasts. Therefore, we attempted to induce the network perturbation by multiple alloimmunization with different H-2 haplotypes. Since mice must be kept for more than one year in this experimental protocol, a parallel study of the network stability under normal aging conditions was required. In Section II.G we describe network stability of T helper cell function in normal aging mice. Furthermore, we show data on the number of T helper/T suppressor cells as well as shifts in T15 idiotype, after PC-Hy-1 immunization in normal and allogeneically immunized aged BALB/c mice.

G. Network Stability of T helper Cell Function in Aging Mice

We first determined the network stability of the T helper cell function in aging mice. The previously established idiotype-specific helper T-cell system (56,57) was used to compare the immune network specificity in young and old mice

(58). T helper cells recognize a shared idiotope on the T15 and M167 idiotypes as a carrier determinant and thereby deliver help to B cells responding to a hapten–idiotype antigen. Such helper cells are induced by priming with PC-Hy. T cells from PC-Hy-primed donors are transferred to nu/nu BALB/c recipients. Fragment cultures from these recipients respond to immunization with both TNP-T15 and TNP-M167.

The number of T helper cells for the T15 and M167 shared determinant can be determined under limiting dilution conditions in the adoptive transfer to nude BALB/c mice. The frequency is then calculated according to the Poisson distribution. The numbers of T helper cells for T15 and M167 of young and old mice are identical within the experimental error of the method (58): there is approximately one T15/M167-specific T helper cell for every 16,000 T cells in both young and 15-month-old mice. The number of T15- and M167-specific T helper cells does not change in older mice (15 months old). Thus, it appears that the T-cell helper activity for network recognition remains stable with age under normal response situations. Network stability therefore could be provided for by a relatively invariant T-cell population restricted in its recognition of antigen or idiotope repertoires over time.

H. Accelerated T15 Idiotype Shifts in Alloimmunized BALB/c Mice

The rationale for using hyperalloimmunization to create a network imbalance has been reviewed recently by us (59). Briefly, multiple exposures to alloantigens induce suppression, which accumulates and affects the network regulation. Changes in network homeostasis can be detected by analyzing the expression of dominant idiotypes. For this study we used the T15 idiotype, which is the major protective antibody against a bacterial pneumococal infection in BALB/c mice (60). Groups of BALB/c mice were given 10 different non-H-2^d haplotype immunizations at 10-day intervals. Group I mice were immunized with autolymphoblasts generated in vitro against one particular H-2 haplotype. Group II mice were immunized with spleen cells from alloimmunized BALB/c mice, which were immunized with one particular H-2 haplotype. Normal age-matched controls served as group III. These mice were then rested for 2 months before being challenged with PC-KLH. The resultant anti-PC response and T15 expression were analyzed by enzyme-linked immunoadsorbent assay (ELISA). The anti-PC antibody level and the percentage of T15 in the sera of immunized mice are shown in Table 1. There is a significant reduction of T15 expression in all sera from groups I and II. In contrast, group III mice demonstrate T15 dominance in preimmune sera and in sera tested 16 days after immunization. However, group III mice also show a relative reduction of T15 expression in sera tested 22 days after immunization. In addition, sera samples from groups I and II tested 16 days after immunization show a significant reduction in the

Table 1 Anti-PC Antibody Levels and Percentages of TEPC-15 Idiotype in BALB/c Mice Immunized with PC-Hy After Allogeneic Hyperimmunization

	Preimmune level (SEM)[c]		Day 16 level (SEM)[d]		Day 22 level (SEM)[d]	
Animal group[a,b]	anti-PC	% T15	anti-PC	% T15	anti-PC	% T15
I. T-cell autoblasts	29.7 (8.2)	54.3 (8.9)	1250 (306)	69.1 (9.2)	1727 (493)	37.9 (4.8)
II. Primed spleen	29.7 (6.2)	54.5 (8.2)	1613 (231)	61.0 (11.9)	1728 (631)	38.9 (4.8)
III. Normal	21.9 (3.2)	95.6 (6.3)	2656 (387)	102 (11.0)	3000 (758)	64.9 (10.1)

[a]Each group consisted of 10 mice. The antibody titer against PC was determined by enzyme-linked immunoadsorbent assay (ELISA) using T15 as standard. The T15 idiotype was measured by ELISA using enzyme-linked anti-T15 (F6-3) monoclonal antibody for color development.

[b]The three groups were as follows: Group I: BALB/c mice were injected subcutaneously (S.C.) 10 times with 5×10^6 T-cell autoblasts suspended in incomplete Freund's adjuvant (IFA). T-cell autoblasts were prepared from MLC cultures derived from BALB/c lymph node cells (responder cells) stimulated with irradiated spleen cells of one of 10 different non-H-2^d haplotypes. BALB/c mice donating lymph node cells as responder cells had been sensitized 6 days previously with the respective haplotypes, used later for MLC culture, i.e., irradiated spleen cells of one non-H-2^d type were injected intraperitoneally (I.P.) into responder BALB/c mice. Group II: BALB/c mice were injected S.C. 10 times with 5×10^6 non-H-2^d-primed BALB/c spleen cells suspended in IF Adjuvant. The primed spleen cells were obtained from BALB/c mice that had been sensitized 6 days previously with the respective haplotype. Group III: Normal, age-matched BALB/c mice were kept under identical conditions for the same time period, injected with IFA but not with allogeneic cells.

[c]The three groups of mice rested for 2 months and were injected I.P. with 100 μg of PC-Hy in IFA. Four days before immunization, the preimmune sera of mice were collected to determine the background anti-PC-antibody level and the percentage of TEPC 15 idiotype.

[d]Anti-PC antibody levels and percentage of TEPC 15 idiotype profile was determined 16 and 22 days after immunization, respectively.

anti-PC response, (where $p < .05$ in the Student t test) compared to controls (group III). The results shown here suggest that multiple alloimmunization can accelerate the immunological shifts that occur during the course of the immune response, i.e., that hyperalloimmunization induced an earlier decline of the PC response and a loss of the T15 dominance in BALB/c mice.

I. Changes in the Ratio of T Helper to T Suppressor Cells in Alloimmunized BALB/c Mice

Since allogenic hyperimmunization is considered to be an enhancing cofactor to viral agents in the development of clinical acquired immunodeficiency syndrome (AIDS) in humans (61-63), we determined the T helper and T suppressor cells in the allogeneically hyperimmunized mice. The relative reduction of the helper cells in comparison to the number of T suppressor cells is an important symptom indicating AIDS.

Lane et al. (64) showed by cell-mixing experiments with purified subpopulations from AIDS patients that the hyporesponsiveness of the unfractionated lymphocytes was not due to active suppression. They concluded that the relative intactness of T8 suppressor function with a selective defect in T4 function with respect to inducer signals, in the form of either lymphokines or helper/inducer T cells, fits well with the hypothesis that T4 lymphocytes are selectively attacked by the human retrovirus (HTLV-III or LAV), leading to clinical symptoms of AIDS.

We have analyzed the peripheral blood leukocytes and lymph node cells from mice derived from the three groups described above for their numbers of T helper (T_h) and T suppressor (T_s) cells using monoclonal anti-Lyt antibodies (Table 2). As seen in Table 3, the T_h/T_s ratio is significantly changed, due to a decline of the number of T_h cells and to a relative increase of T_s cells (Table 2). This indicates also that allogeneic hyperimmunization without viral agents can lead to a profound alteration of immune homeostasis, as expressed as the number of T helper and suppressor cells. Aged BALB/c mice (15 months old) showed no differences in T helper and suppressor cells from young BALB/c mice (6-8 weeks old; see Tables 2 and 3) and therefore display stability in these T-cell subpopulations in age.

J. Induced Phosphorylcholine-Specificity Loss in Alloimmunized BALB/c Mice

Epitope specificity of the response to PC was determined by inhibition assays using as inhibitors *p*-nitrophenylphosphorylcholine (NPPC). Rittenberg and colleagues (65) have shown that the specificity of the secondary antibody response of normal BALB/c mice to PC coupled to hemocyanin shifts from T15 dominant and PC specificity to T15 nondominance and NPPC specificity. Using an

Table 2 Percentage of T-Helper (T_h) and T Suppressor (T_s) Cells in Peripheral Blood Lymphocytes (PBL) in Young and Old BALB/c Mice Injected with Multiple Alloantigens[a–c]

Cells taken from:	Number of animals	T_h/PBL (%, mean ±SEM)	T_s/PBL (%, mean ±SEM)
Normal BALB/c mice (6–8 weeks old)	3	35.0 ±2.0	9.2 ±0.1
Normal BALB/c mice (15 months old)	3	35.0 ±4.0	9.4 ±0.5
Set a: 16-month old BALB/c mice treated with IFA only	10	33.0 ±2.0	11.5 ±1.1
Set b: 16-month old BALB/c mice treated with autolymphoblast in IFA	10	23.0 ±2.0	27.8 ±2.8
Set c: 16-month-old BALB/c mice treated with primed spleen cells in IFA	10	26.0 ±3.0	22.5 ±2.8

[a]Peripheral blood T-helper and T-suppressor cell phenotypes were determined by fluorescent staining: 0.5 ml peripheral blood was suspended in 1% of BSA-PBS containing 100 heparin. The lymphocyte cells were isolated by Ficoll-Hypaque medium. Then, the isolated lymphocyte cells were centrifuged into a pellet and the supernatant discarded. T_h and T_s cells were detected by adding fluorescine isothiocyanate-conjugated rat anti-mouse anti-Lyt-1 monoclonal antibody and FITC-conjugated rat anti-mouse anti-Lyt-2 monoclonal antibody, respectively. The suspensions were incubated for 30 min at room temperature and then washed two times with BSA-PBS. After the treatment, the cells were resuspended in 0.02 ml of BSA-PBS, mounted on a slide, and fluorescent cells were enumerated. The numbers shown here are the percentage of Th and Ts in peripheral blood cells. For details of the different mouse groups, see note b, Table 1.
[b]Significant difference between sets a and b determined by Student t test ($p < .05$).
[c]Significant difference between sets a and c determined by Student t test ($p < .05$).

PC/NPPC assay, they classify these anti-PC antibodies into three groups. Group I antibodies can be inhibited by both PC and NPPC and can also bind to the pneumococcal antigen R36A. Group II antibodies can be inhibited appreciably only by NPPC and cannot bind to pneumococcal R36A. Group III antibodies cannot be inhibited by PC or NPPC. We found that there is an idiotype shift from T15 idiotype-specific anti-PC antibodies to non-T15 idiotype and NPPC-specific anti-PC antibodies in late primary immune response to PC-ovalbumin. Preliminary results show that in sera of allogeneically hyperimmunized mice a general shift from PC specificity to NPPC specificity could be observed in comparison to age-matched control mice (Chang, Muller, and Kohler, unpublished).

Recently we compared the response to nominal and idiotope antigens (Huang, Ward, and Kohler, submitted for publication). The hapten, idiotype,

Table 3 Ratio of T Helper (T_h) to T Suppressor (T_s) Cells in Peripheral Blood of BALB/c Mice[a–c]

Cells taken from:	Number of animals	T_h/T_s (Mean ±SEM)
Normal BALB/c mice (6–8 weeks old)	3	3.80 ±0.30
Normal BALB/c mice (15 months old)	3	3.69 ±0.22
Set a: 16-month-old BALB/c mice treated with IFA only	10	2.81 ±0.17
Set b: 16-month-old BALB/c mice treated with autolymphoblast in IFA	10	0.91 ±0.05
Set c: 16-month-old BALB/c mice treated with primed spleen cells in IFA	10	1.30 ±0.22

[a]For further details of different mouse groups, see notes to Tables 1 and 2.
[b]Significant difference between sets a and b determined by Student t test ($p < .001$).
[c]Significant difference between sets a and c determined by Student t test ($p < .001$).

and isotype specificities of the antibody responses to PC-ovalbumin (nominal antigen) and the anti-idiotope antigens, 4C11-Hy (Ab2β) and F6-Hy (Ab2α), were compared. The results show that differential antibody responses are induced in mice by these three antigens. Early during the course of the immune response to all three antigens, the response is dominated by PC-specific, T15-Id$^+$ antibody. But, for the PC-ovalbumin immunization, there is a shift, late in the response, to non-T15, non-PC-specific antibody. In contrast, there is no such shift in the late response to 4C11-Hy and F6-Hy immunization. The late anti-PC response to both F6-Hy and 4C11-Hy remains T15 dominant. The later IgG_1 populations induced by F6-Hy are more heterogeneous with respect to idiotype and antigen specificity and probably consist of both T15-Id$^+$ non-PC-binding Ab3β and F6-binding Ab3α populations. In contrast to PC-ovalbumin, both the idiotope antigens preferentially stimulate IgG_1 antibodies. The results support the concept of differential stimulation using nominal or idiotope antigen.

By injecting 4C11-Hy (Ab2β) and F6-Hy (Ab2α) into the different groups (I, II, III, see Table 1) of aged mice, we hoped to reverse the experimentally induced T15/PC antibody level changes. Therefore, in these experiments, we examined the response of the groups of alloimmunized BALB/c mice to 4C11-Hy and F6-Hy. As a control, groups of alloimmunized mice were immunized with PC-KLH, and the total amount of anti-PC antibodies, as well as the idiotope and epitope specificity of the response, were examined. It is postulated that anti-idiotype vaccines may be able to reverse the T15 idiotype shift observed in allogeneically sensitized groups I and II (Table 1). It will be interesting to find out if age-related shifts in T15 can be reversed also. A positive result would emphasize the hypothesis that shifts in the immune network with age should be considered basically as a maturation process rather than as a malfunctioning of normal immune responses maintained through growth and adulthood.

III. CONCLUSION

In this chapter we discussed data that show changes in the immune system with respect to the expressed idiotype repertoire and the generation of somatic variants. Some of these changes appear to be involved in the causation of autoimmune disease; other are without obvious pathological consequences. We also discussed results from our laboratory on the stability of the T15 idiotype network and the involvement of T cells. Experiments to induce idiotype shifts were presented, and a protocol was proposed to correct these idiotype changes in the anti-PC response.

These discussions led to the key question of whether these observed or experimentally induced changes are pathological or are part of an ongoing maturation process. While asking this question, it is important to remember that aging per se is not a pathological process but is part of normal physiology. On the other hand, certain chronic diseases occur more frequently in older than in younger individuals. The causal connection between disease and immunological changes cannot be made convincingly, in particular with the finding of variant clones that produce autoantibodies.

It is important to distinguish between age-related changes that appear to be normal and those that cause or aggravate diseases. For example, the loss of the T15-dominant idiotype in the response to the bacterial PC antigen might make the mouse more susceptible to pneumococcal infection because the T15 anti-PC antibody is by far the best protective antibody. On the other hand, the increase of auto-anti-idiotypic antibodies in aging mice does not need to produce disease but could be merely the result of repertoire maturation and more efficient regulation of the immune response. There is also a clear indication of the central role of regulatory T cells that are germ-line encoded and do not show changes in their frequency or repertoire during aging. Such T cells exist to provide stability in the B-cell repertoire and to maintain a functional immune network.

In the final analysis the controversy of maturation versus aging in the immune response is artificial, but it is necessary to dissect clearly the observed changes into those that cause disease and other that are normal.

ACKNOWLEDGMENT

We thank Mrs. Cheryl Zuber for preparation of the manuscript. The studies were supported in part by grant C000533 from the New York State Department of Health, AIDS Institute, by grant IM-405 from the American Cancer Society, by grant AG-04180 from the National Institute on Aging, U.S. Department of Health and Human Services, and by grant CTR1565 from the Council for Tobacco Research–U.S.A., Inc.

REFERENCES

1. Jerne, N. K. 1974. Towards the network theory of the immune system. *Ann. Immunol. (Paris)*. 125C:373.
2. Kohler, H. 1984. The immune network revisited. *In* Idiotypy in Biology and Medicine. H. Kohler, J. Urbain, and P. A. Cazenave, editors. Academic Press, Orlando, Fl. 3.
3. Bona, C., C. Victor-Korbin, C. Manheimer, A. J. Belloni, and C. J. Rubinstein. 1984. Regulatory arms of the immune network. *Immunol. Rev.* 79: 25.
4. Hirokawa, K. 1985. Autoimmunity and aging. *In* Concepts of Immunopathology, Vol. 1. M. Cruse and R. E. Lewis, Jr., editors. Karger, Basel. 251.
5. Aho, K. 1980. Autoantibodies and the risk of death. *Med. Biol.* 58:8.
6. Rowley, M. J., H. Buchman, and I. R. Mackay. 1968. Reciprocal change with age in antibody to extrinsic and intrinsic antigens. *Lancet.* 2:24.
7. Makinodan, T. 1979. Immunity and aging. *In* Handbook of the Biology of Aging. C. Finch and L. Hayflick, editors. Van Nostrand and Reinhold, London. 379.
8. Bullock, J. Y., R. J. Booth, and J. D. Wilson. 1979. Tissue antibodies in a healthy New Zealand population. *N. Z. Med. J.* 89:11.
9. Hirokawa, K., M. Utsuyama, and K. Kuramoto. 1984. Differential rate of age-related decline in immune functions in genetically defined mice with different tumor incidence and life span. *Gerontology.* 30:223.
10. Mikkelsen, W. M., H. J. Dodge, I. F. Duff, and H. Kato. 1967. Estimates of the prevalence of rheumatic diseases in the population of Tecumseh, Michigan. *J. Chron. Dis.* 20:351.
11. Bastenie, P. A., L. Vanhaelst, J. Goldstein, P. H. Smets, A. Keys, M. J. Karmonen, and S. Punsar. 1977. Asymptomatic autoimmune thyroiditis and coronary heart disease. Cross-sectional and prospective studies. *Lancet* 1:155.
12. Mackay, I. R., S. F. Whittingham, and J. D. Matthews. 1978. The immunoepidemiology of aging. *In* Immunology and Aging. T. Makinodan and E. J. Yunis, editors. Plenum Publishing, New York. 35.
13. Krogsrud, R. L., and E. H. Perkins. 1977. Age-related changes in T cell function. *J. Immunol.* 118:1607.
14. Segre, D., and M. Segre. 1976. Humoral immunity in aged mice. II. Increased suppressor T cell activity in immunologically deficient old mice. *J. Immunol.* 116:735.
15. Goidl, E. A., J. B. Innes, and M. E. Weksler. 1976. Immunological studies of aging. II. Loss of IgG and high avidity plaque-forming cells and increased suppressor cell activity in aging mice. *J. Exp. Med.* 144:1037.

16. Moore, J. S., and C. E. Calkins. 1985. In vitro regulation of the pathogenic auto-antibody response of New Zealand Black Mice. I. Loss with age of suppressive activity in T cell population. *J. Immunol.* 134:3838.
17. Zharhary, D. and N. R. Klinman. 1983. Antigen responsiveness of the mature and generative B cell populations of aged mice. *J. Exp. Med.* 157: 1300.
18. Zharhary, D., and N. R. Klinman. 1984. B cell repertoire diversity to PR8 influenza virus does not decrease with age. *J. Immunol.* 133:2285.
19. Averill, L. A., and N. S. Wolf. 1985. The decline in murine splenic PHA and LPS responsiveness with age is primarily due to an intrinsic mechanism. *J. Immunol.* 134:3859.
20. Rosenberg, Y. T. 1979. Influence of the sex-linked defect in CBA/N mice on autoimmune responses to isologous erythrocytes. Ability to overcome the defect with age. *J. Exp. Med.* 150:1561.
21. Schroer, K. R., K. J. Kim, B. Prescott, and P. J. Baker. 1979. Generation of anti-type III pneumococcal polysaccharide hydridomas from mice with a x-linked B lymphocyte defect. *J. Exp. Med.* 150:698.
22. Fidler, J. M., E. L. Morgan, and W. O. Weigle. 1980. B lymphocyte differentiation in the CBA/N mouse: A delay in maturation rather than a total arrest. *J. Immunol.* 124:13.
23. Scher, I., A. K. Berning, S. Kessler, and F. D. Finkelman. 1980. Development of B lymphocytes in the mouse: studies of the frequency and distribution of surface IgM and IgD in normal and immune defective CBA/N F_1 mice. *J. Immunol.* 125:1686.
24. Scher, I., S. O. Sharrows, and W. E. Paul. 1976. X-Linked B lymphocyte defect in CBA/N mice. III. Abnormal development of B-lymphocyte populations defined by their density of surface immunoglobulins. *J. Exp. Med.* 144:507.
25. Ahmed, A., and I. Scher. 1976. Studies on non-H-2-linked lymphocyte activating determinants. III. Nonexpression of MlS determinants in a mouse strain with a x-linked B lymphocyte immune defect. *J. Immunol.* 117: 1922.
26. Scher, I. 1982. CBA/N immune defective mice: evidence for the failure of a B cell subpopulation to be expressed. *Immunol. Rev.* 64:117.
27. Quan, Z. S., and J. Quintans. 1981. Alteration of clonal profile. III. T15 ontogenetic advantages are not sufficient for establishing idiotype dominance in adoptive transfer. *J. Exp. Med.* 154:1475.
28. Kaplan, D. R., J. Quintans, and H. Kohler. 1978. Clonal dominance: loss and restoration in adoptive transfer. *Proc. Natl. Acad. Sci. USA.* 75:1967.
29. Goidl, E. A., Y. T. Kim, and M. E. Weksler. 1981. Studies on autoimmunity in aging. *In* Immunological aspects of aging. D. Segre and L. Smith, editors. Marcel Dekker, New York. 165.
30. Schrater, A. F., E. A. Goidl, G. J. Thorbecke, and G. W. Siskind. 1979. Production of auto-antiidiotypic antibody during the normal immune response to TNP-Ficoll. I. Occurrence in AKR/J and BALB/c mice of hapten-augmentable, anti-TNP plaque-forming cells and their accelerated appearance in recipients of immune spleen cells. *J. Exp. Med.* 150:138.

31. Kim, Y. T., E. A. Goidl, C. Samarut, M. E. Weksler, G. J. Thorbecke, and G. W. Siskind. 1985. Bone marrow function. I. Peripheral T cells are responsible for the increased auto-antiidiotypic response of older mice. *J. Exp. Med.* 161:1237.
32. Hausman, P. B., E. A. Goidl, G. W. Siskind, and M. E. Weksler. 1985. Immunological studies of aging. XI. Age-related changes in idiotype repertoire of suppressor T cells stimulated during tolerance induction. *J. Immunol.* 134:3802.
33. Kluskens, L., and H. Kohler. 1974. Regulation of the immune response by autologous antibody against receptor. *Proc. Natl. Acad. Sci. USA.* 71: 5083.
34. Nisonoff, A., S.-T. Ju, and F. L. Owen. 1977. Studies of structure and immunosuppression of a crossreactive idiotype in strain A mice. *Immunol. Rev.* 34:89.
35. Cazenave, P.-A. 1977. Idiotypic-anti-idiotypic regulation of antibody synthesis in rabbits. *Proc. Natl. Acad. Sci. USA.* 74:5122.
36. Urbain, J., M. Wikler, J. D. Fraussen, and C. Collignon. 1977. Idiotype regulation of the immune system by the induction of antibodies against anti-idiotype antibodies. *Proc. Natl. Acad. Sci. USA.* 74:5126.
37. Eichmann, K., and K. Rajewsky. 1975. Induction of T and B cell immunity by anti-idiotypic antibody. *Eur. J. Immunol.* 5:661.
38. Cosenza, H., M. H. Julius, and A. Augustin. 1977. Idiotypes as variable region markers: Analogies between receptors on phosphorylcholine-specific T and B lymphocytes. *Immunol. Rev.* 34:3.
39. Binz, H., and H. Wigzell. 1975. Shared idiotypic determinants on B and T lymphocytes reactive against the same antigenic determinants. I. Demonstration of similar or identical idiotypes on IgG molecules and T-cell receptors with specificity for the same alloantigens. *J. Exp. Med.* 142: 197.
40. Eichmann, K. 1978. Expression and function of idiotypes on lymphocytes. *Adv. Immunol.* 26:195.
41. Cosenza, H., and H. Kohler. 1972. Specific suppression of the antibody response by antibodies to receptors. *Proc. Natl. Acad. Sci. USA.* 69:2701.
42. Hart, D. A., A. L. Wang, L. L. Paulak, and A. Nisonoff. 1972. Suppression of idiotypic specificities in adult mice by administration of anti-idiotypic antibody. *J. Exp. Med.* 135:1283.
43. Eichmann, K., I. Falk, and K. Rajewsky. 1978. Recognition of idiotypes in lymphocyte interactions. II. Antigen-independent cooperation between T and B lymphocytes that possess similar and complementary idiotypes. *Eur. J. Immunol.* 8:853.
44. Kohler, H., S. Müller, and C. Bona. 1985. Internal antigen and immune network. *Proc. Soc. Exp. Biol. Med.* 178:189.
45. Fong, S., R. A. Gilbertson, P. P. Chen, J. H. Vaughan, and D. A. Carson. 1984. Modulation of human rheumatoid factor specific lymphocyte responses with a cross-reactive anti-idiotype bearing the internal image of antigen. *J. Immunol.* 132:1183.
46. Dwyer, D. S., R. J. Bradly, C. U. Urquhart, and J. F. Kearney. 1983.

Naturally occurring anti-idiotypic antibodies in myasthenia gravis patients. *Nature (Lond.)*. 301:611.
47. Abdou, N. I., H. Wall, H. B. Lindsly, J. F. Halsey, and T. Suzuki. 1981. Suppression of serum anti-DNA antibody binding to DNA by anti-idiotypic antibody in SLE. *J. Clin. Invest.* 67:1297.
48. Nasa, H., D. S. Chia, O. Taniguchi, and E. V. Barnett. 1982. Characterization of anti-F$(Ab')_2$ antibodies in SLE patients. Evidence for cross-reacting auto-anti-idiotypic antibodies. *Clin. Immunol. Immunopathol.* 25:5058.
49. Fritz, R. B. 1984. Idiotypy in autoimmune central nervous system demyelinating disease: Experimental allergic encephalomyelitis and multiple sclerosis. *In* Idiotypy in Biology and Medicine. H. Kohler, J. Urbain, and P. A. Cazenave, editors. Academic Press, Orlando, Fl. 329.
50. Goodman, M. G., and W. O. Weigle. 1985. Restoration of humoral immunity in vitro in immunodeficient aging mice by C8-derivatized guanine ribonucleosides. *J. Immunol.* 134:3808.
51. Fernandes, G., R. A. Good, and E. J. Yunis. 1981. Responses of autoimmune diseases of aging to dietary restriction. *In* Immunological Aspects of Aging. D. Segre, and L. Smith, editors. Marcel Dekker, New York. 207.
52. Dang, H., M. Fischbach, and N. Talal. 1985. Anti-idiotypic antiserum to monoclonal anti-sm inhibits the autoantigen-induced proliferative response. *J. Immunol.* 134:3825.
53. Teitelbaum, D., J. Rauch, B. D. Stollar, and R. S. Schwartz. 1984. In vivo effects of antibodies against a high frequency idiotype of anti-DNA antibodies in MRL mice. *J. Immunol.* 132:1282.
54. Rauch, J., H. Massicotte, and H. Tannenbaum. 1985. Specific and shared idiotypes found on hybridoma anti-DNA autoantibodies derived from Rheumatoid Arthritis and systemic lupus erythematosus patients. *J. Immunol.* 135:2385.
55. Anderson, L. C., M. Aguet, E. Wight, R. Andersson, H. Binz, and M. Wigzell. 1977. Induction of specific immune unresponsiveness using purified mixed leukocyte culture-activated T lymphoblasts as autoimmunogens. I. Demonstration of general validity as to species and histocompatibility barriers. *J. Exp. Med.* 146:1124.
56. Gleason, K., and H. Kohler. 1982. Regulatory idiotypes. T helper cells recognize a shared V_H idiotype on phosphorylcholine-specific antibodies. *J. Exp. Med.* 156:539.
57. McNamara, M., K. Gleason, and H. Kohler. 1983. Idiotype-specific T-helper cells. *Ann. N.Y. Acad. Sci.* 418:65.
58. McNamara, M., C-Y. Kang, and H. Kohler. 1985. Analysis of a $T_{H1} \rightarrow T_{H2}$ helper cell circuit. *J. Immunol.* 135:1603.
59. Suciu-Foca, N., D. W. King, K. Reemtsma, S. Müller, and H. Kohler. 1985. Autoimmunity and self-antigens. *Concepts Immunopathol.* 1:173.
60. Briles, D. E., C. Forman, S. Hudak, and J. L. Claflin. 1982. Antiphosphocholine antibodies found in normal mouse serum are protective against intravenous infection with type 3 *Streptococcus pneumoniae*. *J. Exp. Med.* 156:1177.

61. Shearer, G. M., and R. B. Levy. 1984. Noninfectious cofactors in susceptibility to AIDS. Possible contributions of semen, HLA alloantigens and lack of natural resistance. *Ann. N.Y. Acad. Sci.* 437:49.
62. Kim, B. S., and K. H. Mui. 1985. Induction of infectious immunodeficiency in BALB/c mice by serial transfer of lymphocytes immune to alloantigens. *J. Immunol.* 135:255.
63. Raghunathan, R., T. M. Mundy, J. Faust, and S. Misra. 1985. Allogeneic leukocyte and germ cell-induced murine immunodeficiency. *J. Immunol.* 135:2429.
64. Lane, C. H., J. M. Depper, W. C. Greene, G. Whalen, G. Waldman, and A. S. Fauci. 1985. Qualitative analysis of immune function in patients with the acquired immunodeficiency syndrome: Evidence for a selective defect in soluble antigen recognition. *New Engl. J. Med.* 313:79.
65. Chang, S. P., M. Brown, and M. B. Rittenberg. 1982. Immunologic memory to phosphorylcholine II. PC-KLH induces two antibody populations that dominate different isotypes. *J. Immunol.* 128:702.

16

Rheumatoid Factors and Aging
Functional and Molecular Aspects

Audrey J. Manheimer-Lory, Blanche Bellon,* and Constantin A. Bona

Mount Sinai School of Medicine
New York, New York

I. INTRODUCTION

Rheumatoid factors (RF) are autoantibodies specific for antigenic determinants of autologous immunoglobulin G (IgG) (1). These autoantibodies have been discovered in patients with rheumatoid arthritis and later were detected in other autoimmune diseases. Recently, RF were found in normal subjects subsequent to vaccination or during acute phases of infectious diseases (2,3).

The nature and origin of the autoimmune antibodies and their relationship to immune function during senescence have been the subject of in-depth analysis. However, little is known about the origin of RF in old subjects and animals, the mechanisms leading to their occurrence, or their beneficial or deleterious functions. RF are usually IgM but may be IgG or IgA and bind to the Fc fragment of autologous or homologous IgG. The affinity of these autoantibodies for antigenic determinants of Fc_{γ} is generally low 10^5 liters/mole) (4). However, it can be increased by subtle conformational alteration of Fc by heating at 63°C for 15 min or binding of IgG to antigen. The low affinity of RF for Fc_{γ} suggests there might well exist another antigen to which they would bind with high affinity and therefore the RF could be an example of multispecific antibodies. The discovery of epibodies strongly supports this concept.

**Current affiliation*: CNS ERA 48, INSERM U28, and Hôpital Broussais, Paris, France

Epibodies are a category of antibodies that react not only with the idiotype expressed on monoclonal human RF but also with the antigenic determinants of Fc fragment of human IgG. Indeed, we found that a set of antibodies produced in A/J mice after immunization with an IgM KIII paraprotein, which displayed RF activity and bore a cross-reactive idiotype (Wa IdX), bound not only to various Wa IdX^+ RF but also to human IgG (5).

The structural correlate of Wa IdX^+ probably corresponds to the complementarity-determining region I (CDRI) amino acid sequence of the V_KIII light chain, which is generally used by the majority of IgM paraproteins with rheumatoid activity. Chen et al. (6) synthesized a polypeptide corresponding to the amino acid sequence of CDRI of the V_KIII light chain of an IgM KIII paraprotein, including the cysteine residue from the first framework. A fraction of antibodies obtained in rabbits against this synthetic polypeptide bind to both IgM KIII RF, as well as to human IgG. Chen et al. (6) established that these antibodies/epibodies recognize a shared sequence Val-Ser-Ser-Ser (residue 28–31) on CDRI of V_KIII and Ser-Ser-Ser at position 195–197 on Fc_γ.

We also found that anti-idiotype antibodies against "a" or "b" series rabbit allotype bind to human Fc_γ and probably represent another example of epibodies (7). These results strongly support the concept indicating that RF are multispecific antibodies specific for idiotypes or nominal antigens that can secondarily bind to Fc_γ.

Recent experimental data support several mechanisms that may contribute to the activation of clones that produce rheumatoid factors: (a) stimulation by antigen–antibody complexes in a T-independent way, (b) stimulation of clones by antigens or idiotypes (these clones produce antibodies or anti-idiotype antibodies that secondarily bind to Fc_γ, (c) activation by polyclonal B-cell mitogens, and (d) alteration of the ratio of T helper to T suppressor cells, which leads to the expansion of antigen-specific or idiotype-specific helper T cells able to favor the proliferation of RF precursors.

II. HIGH INCIDENCE OF RHEUMATOID FACTORS DURING AGING

A high incidence of RF was found in the aged human population. Experimental studies were carried out to investigate the cellular mechanisms responsible for increased RF activity in the elderly. Thus, Rodriguez et al. (8) and Koopman and Schrohenloher (9) have investigated the functional aspects of B and T cells from older individuals in an in vitro system. That is, by coculturing B lymphocytes from either old or young people with T cells from older persons in the presence of pokeweed mitogen, the highest production of IgM RF in the supernatants of the cultures was observed. These results indicated that there is an altered functional state in the T-cell population in older individuals. Although in vitro human studies can provide interesting results, it is certainly more desirable to have at hand animal models for diseases to investigate the mechanisms responsible for the occurrence of RF. Indeed, this was reported in 129/Sv mice (10). This mouse strain has allowed investigators to extensively analyze the age-dependent occurrence of RF. The RF has been detected in a colony of apparently healthy 129/Sv mice. Their levels increase with age as in the human population. RF in this strain have been well characterized as immunoglobulins of the μ and α isotypes (9). Van Snick and Masson (10) noted that while in young animals the IgM RF predominate, IgA RF predominate in adults.

A study of the distribution of RF in various lymphoid organs by measuring the amount of anti-IgG autoantibodies demonstrated that before 20 weeks RF production was predominant in the mesenteric and caudal lymph nodes and only after 20 weeks does it extend to the spleen (11). This observation indicates that there is stimulation via environmental antigens of intestinal origin. No RF at this age was observed in the 129/J substrain, implying that an unknown alteration of intestinal permeability after 20 weeks occurs in 129/Sv mice. Van Snick and Coulie (12) have prepared monoclonal antibodies from 129/Sv mice injected with lipopolysaccharides (LPS). About 3% of the hybridomas obtained secreted RF. No IgA RF monoclonal antibody was obtained from 129/Sv mice not stimulated with LPS. The majority of IgM RF bound to a single mouse IgG subclass; i.e., 58 bound to IgG_1, 1 bound to IgG_{2a}; 8 were specific for IgG_1 but cross-reacted to some extent with IgG_{2a}, and 1 was multispecific for IgG subclasses.

Utilization of mutant IgG_1 that lacks either CH_1 or the CH_3 domain allowed Stassin et al. (13) to establish that the CH_3 domain is essential for the binding of RF to IgG_1. Deletion of CH_3 completely abolished the reactivity of 70/71 monoclonal RF. With IgG_{2a}-IgG_{2b} hybrids, it was also established that the determinants recognized by RF preferentially binding to IgG_{2a} span the C-terminal 8 residues of the CH_2 domain and the complete CH_3 domain.

Thus, 129/Sv mice, like old human populations, exhibit an age-dependent increase in the level of RF. The RF produced in this mouse strain are generally specific for IgG subclasses. Their fine specificity depends on isotype of RFs as well as the type of lymphoid organ housing the cells producing autoanti-IgG antibodies.

III. OCCURRENCE OF RHEUMATOID FACTORS DURING CONVENTIONAL IMMUNE RESPONSES

RF have been considered to have deleterious effects in the pathogenesis of such autoimmune diseases in humans as systemic lupus erythematosus (SLE), rheumatoid arthritis (RA), scleroderma, and subacute endocarditis. Similarly, in animals prone to develop SLE- or RA-like diseases, RF may be involved in the deposition of immune complexes in the kidney, which could lead to the appearance of nephritis. However, the occurrence of RF during acute infections or even subsequent to vaccination is generally not associated with immune complexes mediating pathological phenomena. It seems that this is also true in the case of old subjects with high titers of RF who do not present with any disease, as well as in 129/Sv mice in which no well-defined autoimmune disease has been described.

These data prompted us to investigate the synthesis of RF in 129/Sv mice after antigenic stimulation. The study was carried out on 129/Sv mice of various ages (1, 3, and 6 months), as well as on 129/J mice, a substrain not prone to develop RF during aging.

A. Antibody Response Induced by a TI_1 Antigen: TNP-BA

Both 129/J and 129/Sv mice immunized intraperitoneally with trinitrophenyl brucella abortus (TNP-BA) develop an anti-TNP plaque-forming cell (PFC) response varying from 8 to 40×10^3 PFC/spleen (Figure 1) (11). In 129/Sv mice, an age-dependent increase of the magnitude of the PFC response was observed (39,519 PFC/spleen in 129/J and 31,200 PFC/spleen in 129/Sv), which is in agreement with the observation made by Hooijkaas et al. (15) demonstrating that there is no decrease in the frequency of anti-TNP precursors during aging in various mouse strains. However, a significant increase of RF specific for $\gamma 2_a$ was observed not only in old 129/Sv mice but also in old 129/J animals.

B. Antibody Responses Induced by TI_2 Antigens: TNP-Ficoll, Bacterial Levan, and $\alpha_{1,3}$ Dextran

Immunization with TNP-Ficoll, a prototypic TI_2 antigen, also results in an age-dependent increase in the magnitude of the anti-TNP PFC response. This is expected, since there is a known ontogenic delay of the $Lyb\text{-}5^+$ subset, which is stimulated by TNP-Ficoll. Here too immunization with TNP-Ficoll induced the production of RF in all age groups of 129/Sv and 129/J mice tested (14).

Immunization with bacterial levan also led to the occurrence of RF with specificity for only γ2a in old (6 months) 129/J and 129/Sv mice (Figure 2). Dextran immunization induced the production of RF specific for γ2a in 6-month old 129/J and 129/Sv mice, while anti-γ1 antibodies were induced in 3- and 6-month-old 129/J mice (Figure 3) (16).

C. Antibody Responses Induced by T-Dependent Antigens: TNP-KLH

The induction of RF was also studied during the secondary response elicited by the T-dependent antigen TNP-KLH (trinitrophenylated keyhole limpet hemocyanin).

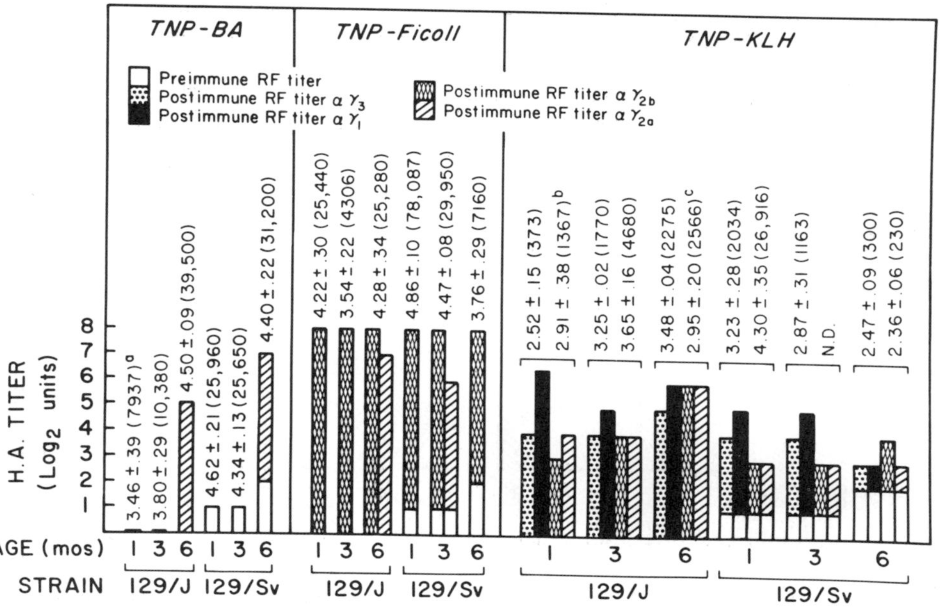

Figure 1 Anti-TNP-PFC response and titer of RF produced by 129/Sv mice after immunization with TI_1, TI_2, and TD antigens. Mice were immunized (*A*) intraperitoneally with 0.1 ml of 0.1% TNP-BA solution, (*B*) 20 μg of TNP-Ficoll, or (*C*) 100 μg of TNP-KLH in complete Freund's adjuvant (CFA). TNP-KLH-primed mice were boosted intraperitoneally with 10 μg of TNP-KLH in saline 1 month later. The PFC response was measured after 5 days in the case of TI_1 and TI_2 antigens and 7 days after challenge with the TD antigen. (Left) Direct TNP-PFC-log CM + SEM (arthmetic mean) of 3–5 mice for each group, (center) indirect PFC response (IgG), (right) only 4 out of 5 mice expressed a γ response. Titers of RF were determined in hemagglutination (HA) assays. Sera were absorbed with sheep red blood cells (SRBC) before testing. SRBC were coupled to p-azophenylarsonate. Subagglutinating amounts of isotype specific monoclonal anti-Ars antibodies were incubated with the Ars-coupled SRBC and sera from the mice (preimmune or postimmune) were then added and HA titers were determined ($1/\log_2$) of the highest dilution giving agglutination. (From Ref. 16.)

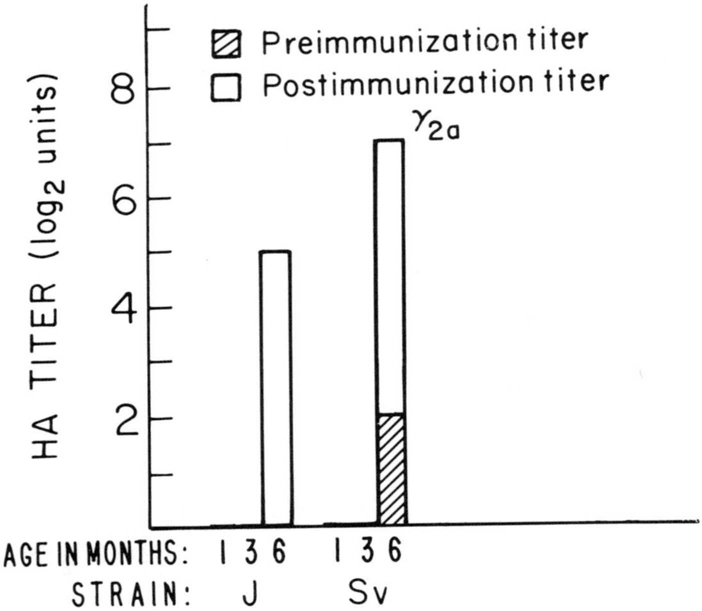

Figure 2 Titers of RF produced by 129/Sv mice after immunization with bacterial levan BL. (From Ref. 16.)

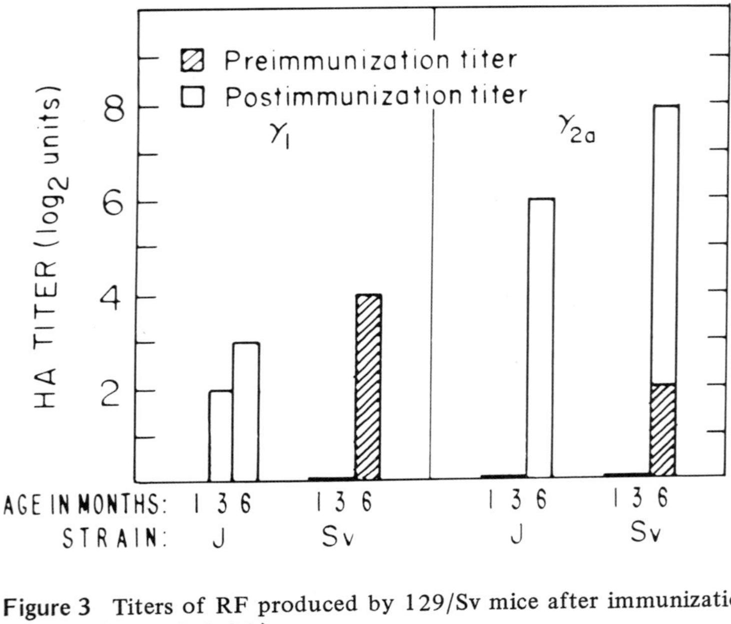

Figure 3 Titers of RF produced by 129/Sv mice after immunization with dextran. (From Ref. 16.)

The sera of mice immunized and boosted with the immunogen were collected at various timepoints and tested in hemagglutination assays to determine the titer of RF postimmunization. That is, subagglutinating amounts of monoclonal antiarsonate antibodies ($\gamma 3$, $\gamma 1$, $\gamma 2b$, $\gamma 2a$) were coupled to arsonate-coated sheep red blood cells and incubated with immune sera. Titers were determined $1/\log_2$ of the highest dilution giving agglutination. In all cases, anti-γ-globulin antibodies were produced and these were multispecific (Figure 1). In addition, our analysis of the kinetics of this response revealed that there was a long-lasting persistence of serum RF (17). Taken together, these results showed that the synthesis of RF is associated with conventional immune responses induced by TI_1, TI_2, or TD antigens. These RF occur in 129/Sv mice, a strain prone to make RF, as well as in 129/J, which is not prone. There is no simple explanation for the induction of Fc-isotype-specific RF after immunization with these antigens. The variation in specificity of RF induced by conventional immunization may be related to the nature of the immunogen, the route of immunization, or even the dose of the antigen.

IV. REGULATORY EFFECT OF RHEUMATOID FACTORS

Since we and others have shown that RF can occur after normal antigenic stimulation, it has been proposed that there may exist two categories of RF: one associated with various autoimmune diseases and having pathological implications, and another that includes RF but may be beneficial for the host. Consequently, one may ask whether in general, RF exhibit a regulatory role on lymphocytic function as has been shown for anti-isotypic, anti-allotypic, and anti-idiotype antibodies (18–20).

Therefore, the effect of monoclonal RF on in vitro immune responses was investigated and compared to the effect of the corresponding anti-idiotypic antibodies.

A. Anti-TNP PFC Response Elicited by the TI_1 Antigen TNP-NWSM

The effects of anti-idiotype and RF monoclonal antibodies was studied on spleen cells from BALB/c, 129/J, or 129/Sv mice cultured with the optimal dose of trinitrophenylated *Nocardia* water-soluble mitogen (TNP-NWSM) and increasing concentrations of monoclonal anti-460-Id antibodies (FD5-13) or monoclonal RF (LPS 10-1 or 129-48). The 460-Id is a minor component of anti-TNP response elicited by TI_1 (21) and dominates secondary response induced by a TNP-ovalbumin conjugate, a TD antigen (22). As expected, anti-Id antibody strongly decreased the primary anti-TNP responses of the three strains (Figure 4). High doses of LPS 10-1, an RF antibody originated from BALB/c mice with

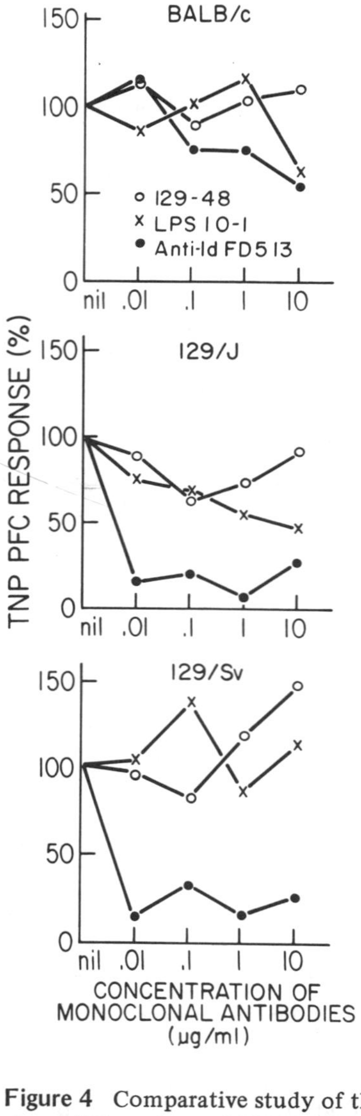

Figure 4 Comparative study of the effect of anti-idiotype antibody and monoclonal RF on the anti-TNP PFC response obtained from BALB/c or 129 mice. The anti-TNP-PFC response is expressed as percent versus PFC obtained from cultures stimulated with TNP-NWSM considered as 100%. LPS 10-1 129-48 FD-5-13.

a high affinity for IgD, decreased the primary anti-TNP response of BALB/c and 129/J mice, but did not affect the 129/Sv response. Conversely, high doses of 129-48, an RF originating from 129/Sv mice exhibiting a high affinity for IgG_1, increased the 129/Sv anti-TNP responses and did not alter the BALB/c and 129/J anti-TNP responses.

B. Anti-Bacterial Levan (BL) and Inulin (Inu) PFC Response Elicited by the TI_2 Antigen BL

Spleen cells from BALB/c mice were cultured with an optimal dose of BL and increasing amounts of monoclonal anti-Id antibodies (anti-E109 IdX) or monoclonal RF (LPS 5-7, 129-48, or MRL 5-51). Anti-Id antibodies strongly inhibit the primary anti-BL response and although to a lesser extent, the anti-inulin response (Figure 5). High concentrations of LPS 5-7 (same specificity as LPS 10-1) considerably enhance both the BL and Inu PFC responses, whereas high doses of 129-48 inhibit them, but lower doses of 129-48 exhibit an enhancing effect. MRL 5-51 generated from MRL/lpr mice, which bind $\gamma 3$, displayed a dose-dependent effect inhibition of both the anti-BL and anti-Inu responses.

As virgin, mature, IgD-IgM-bearing cells are involved in the primary response to TI_1 and TI_2 antigens, one may expect that RF specific for δ may bind to these IgD-IgM-bearing cells and then either expand mature lymphocytes or give a negative signal to the IgM response. Our results suggest that the former hypothesis could prove true when TI_2 antigens are involved and the latter when TI_1 antigens are involved. Furthermore, RF that bind $\gamma 1$ may not bind virgin, mature cells and then not affect the immune response. According to our data, RF display a regulatory effect on the in vitro primary response independent of their isotypic specificity. A simple explanation could be that RF are multi-specific antibodies and this situation required another antigenic specificity.

V. V_H REGION OF MONOCLONAL ANTIBODIES USED BY RHEUMATOID FACTORS OF VARIOUS ORIGINS

From earlier studies by Henry Kunkel, it appears that a restricted number of variable (V) genes encode autoantibodies (23). Monoclonal RF IgM paraproteins with RF activity that bear the major IdX (i.e., Wa IdX) were shown to belong to V_KIII. We have been interested in studying the V_H gene families that are utilized by one panel of monoclonal antibodies.

Monoclonal antibodies with RF activity were generated in our laboratory following four separate fusion events. That is, 6-month-old 129/Sv spleen cells, 5-month-old MRL/lpr spleen cells, and BALB/c spleen cells stimulated in vitro with LPS and BALB/c spleen cells postimmunization with *Yersinia enterocolitica* were fused with the nonsecretory tumor cell line sp2/0. The fine specificity of these antibodies was tested in an enzyme-linked immunoadsorbent

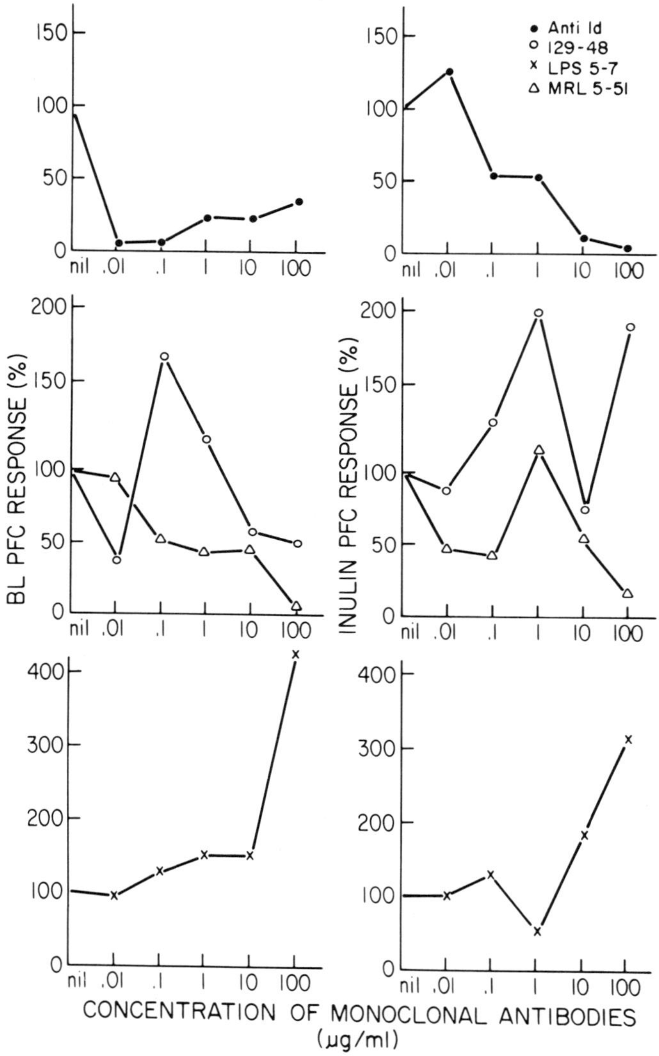

Figure 5 Comparative study of the effect of anti-idiotype antibody and monoclonal RF or the anti-BL and anti-Inu PFC response obtained from BALB/c mice. The anti-BL and anti-Inu PFC response is expressed as percent versus PFC obtained from cultures stimulated with BL considered as 100%. LPS 5-4 129-48 MRL 22-46 Anti-E-109 IdX.

Table 1 Specificity of Monoclonal Rheumatoid Factors

Monoclonal antibody	Origin of monoclonal antibody	Binding[a] of monoclonal antibodies to microtiter plates coated with:						
		IgD	IgG_3	IgG	IgG_{2b}	IgG_{2a}	IgE	IgA
129-48	6-month-old naive 129/Sv mice	0.09	0.35	0.80	0.33	0.62	0.08	0
129-78		0.02	0.11	0.90	0.08	0.08	0.01	0
MRL 50-8	5-month-old naive MRL/lpr mice	0.05	0.22	1.16	0.07	0.18	0.01	0.07
MRL 22-46		0.01	0.10	0.77	0.10	0.34	0.01	0.05
MRL 5-51		0	0.02	0.80	0.07	0.17	0	0.03
LPS 5-4	BALB/c spleen cells stimulated in vitro with LPS	0.17	0.02	0.10	0.15	0.48	0.82	0.10
LPS 7-3		0.55	0.20	0.20	0.05	0.36	0.16	0.30
LPS 10-1		0.53	0.24	0.55	0.23	0.60	0.15	0.51
Y19-10	BALB/c mice injected with 10 μg of *Y. enterocolitica*	0.11	0.33	0.27	0.60	0.12	0.12	0.20
Y19-16		0.15	0.29	0.38	0.40	0.17	0.17	0.26

[a]O.D. at 405 nm. The binding of monoclonal RF to various isotypes was measured with alkaline-phosphatase-labeled goat anti-μ antibodies (1:1500 dilution).

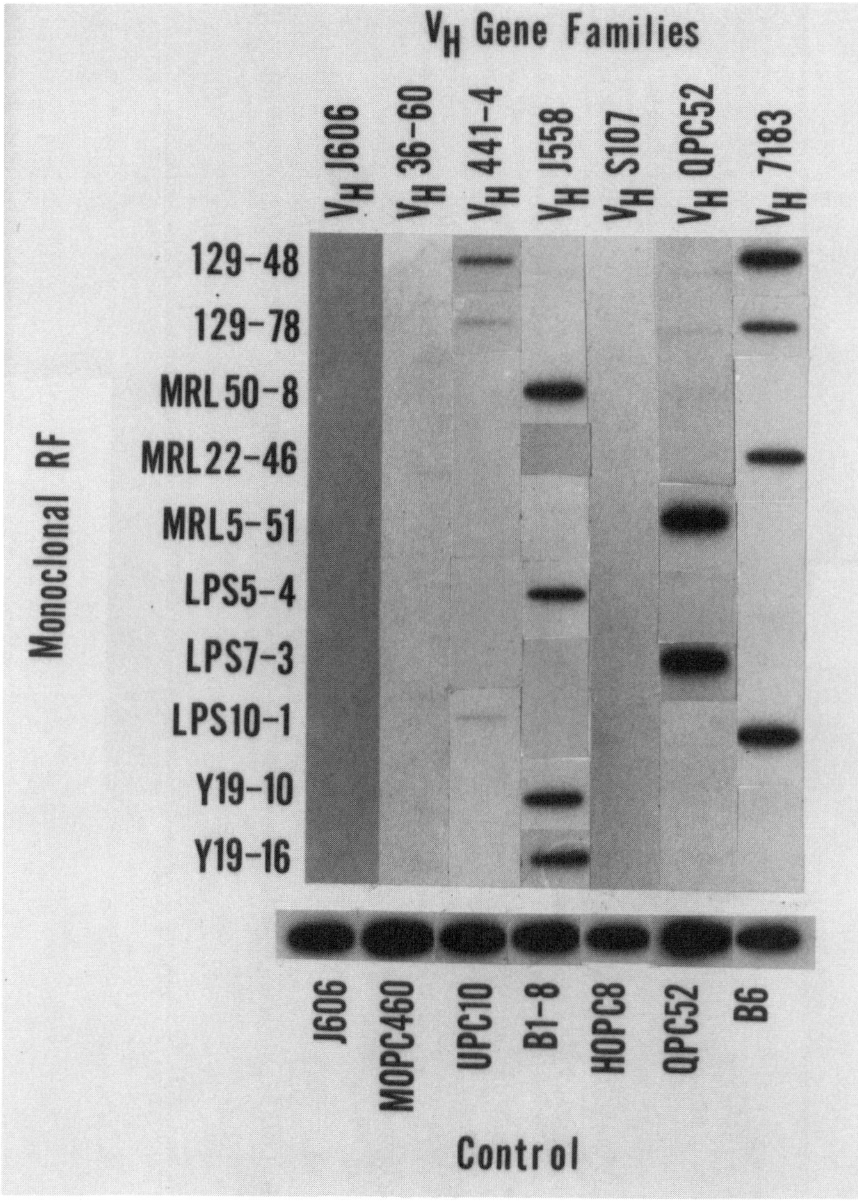

Figure 6 Slot-blot analysis of cytoplasmic RNA lysates obtained from hybridoma secreting RF from four sources (129/Sv and MRL/lpr mice, in vivo LPS-stimulated BALB/c mice, and BALB/c mice immunized with *Yersinia enterocolitica*). RNA was blotted on nitrocellulose and subsequently hybridized to the ^{32}P nick-translated V_H gene probes. Control lines for each V_H gene family are shown at the bottom of the figure.

assay (ELISA) (Table 1) in which microtiter wells were coated with heat-aggregated monoclonal antibodies of various isotypes. Since all monoclonal RF that were obtained were of the IgM isotype, we detected the binding of these antibodies via an alkaline-phosphatase-labeled goat anti-IgM antibody at a dilution of 1:1500. Subsequently, we prepared cytoplasmic RNA from hybridoma-secreting RF and hybridized nitrocellulose containing these lysates to various V_H-region gene probes in a Northern slot-blot analysis. Of the seven V_H gene families that have been well characterized (24), V_H 36-60, V_H 441-4, V_H J606, V_H J558, V_H S107, V_H QPC52, and V_H 7183, only three have been utilized by our monoclonal RF: V_H J558, V_H QPC52, and V_H 7183. Of greater interest and import may be that the V_H 7183 germ-line gene, the most 3′ of the V_H gene cluster, has been shown to be preferentially rearranged in only pre-B cells (25); yet four of the monoclonal RF appear to utilize a gene in this family. One may speculate that in autoimmune disease some disregulation might occur that allows a pre-B-cell V_H gene to be expressed by a mature B cell (Figure 6).

VI. CONCLUSION

The nature of the autoimmune response and its relation to aging and disease has not been well understood. However, recently investigators have begun to explore the mechanisms of the anti-self response by employing animal models that exhibit autoimmune pathology. Furthermore, the availability of congenic mouse strains in which one animal is prone to produce RF with aging versus another that is not, provides the researcher with a controlled system. These factors have allowed us and others to study conventional immune responses and the auto-anti-immunoglobulin responses in animals such as the 129 mouse strain. We have found that we could induce RF production in 129/Sv mice, the subline that spontaneously produces autoantibodies as they age, as well as in the 129/J congenic strain (which does not), after immunization with several T-independent antigens (16) and T-dependent antigens (26). These and other data have caused us to doubt the "dogma" that RF have only a deleterious function in the immune system, leading to pathological states. Instead, it has been hypothesized (26) that RF may act as enhancing antibodies and may participate in clearing antigen-antibody complexes, thereby facilitating the recovery phase of disease. In light of this, we have studied the regulatory effects of monoclonal RF on the in vitro immune response. Our results indicated that there is a differential effect on the in vitro anti-BL, anti-Inu (TI_2), and anti-TNP-NWSM (TI_1) responses when one incubates primed spleen cells with monoclonal RF of differing specificities, derived from different sources. One may speculate that the monoclonal RF that bind δ could bind IgM-IgD immature B cells and affect the response by transmitting either a negative signal (inhibition) or a positive signal (stimulation).

Taken together, these results prompted us to learn about the variable region gene(s) that encode RF. The study of our panel of hybridomas generated in completely different ways revealed that only three families of V_H genes—V_H J558, V_H QPC52, and V_H 7183—have been utilized by these autoantibodies.

The study of the structure of active V_H genes expressed in hybridomas secreting RF obtained from old 129/Sv mice or MRL/lpr with autoimmune disease as well as from BALB/c not prone to develop RF spontaneously will certainly provide new insights on the molecular basis of genes encoding autoantibodies.

ACKNOWLEDGMENT

This work was supported by grant AG/A10271601A from the U.S. Public Health Service.

REFERENCES

1. Waaler, E. 1940. On the occurrence of a factor in human serum activating the specific agglutination of sheep red blood corpuscles. *Acta Pathol. Microbiol. Scand.* 17:72.
2. Welch, M. J., S. Fong, J. H. Vaughan, and D. A. Carson. 1983. Increased frequency of rheumatoid factor precursor B lymphocytes after immunization of normal adults with tetanus toxoid. *Clin. Exp. Immunol.* 51:299.
3. Carson, D. A., J. L. Pasquali, C. D. Tsoukas, S. Fong, S. F. Slovin, S. K. Lawrance, L. Slaughter, and J. H. Vaughan. 1981. Physiology and pathology of rheumatoid factors. *Springer Semin. Immunopathol.* 4:161.
4. Mannick, M. 1979. *In* Rheumatoid Factors in Arthritis and Allied Conditions. J. C. Hollander and D. S. McCarthy, Jr., editors. Lea & Febiger, Philadelphia. 504.
5. Bona, C. A., S. Finley, S. Waters, and H. G. Kunkel. 1982. Anti-immunoglobulin antibodies. III. Properties of sequential anti-idiotypic antibodies to heterologous anti-γ-globulins. Detection and reactivity of anti-idiotype antibodies with epitopes of Fc fragments (homobodies) and with epitopes and idiotopes (epibodies). *J. Exp. Med.* 156:986.
6. Chen, P. P., S. Fong, R. A. Houghten, and D. A. Carson. 1985. Characterization of an epibody. An anti-idiotype that reacts with both idiotype of rheumatoid factors (RF) and the antigen recognized by RF. *J. Exp. Med.* 161:323.
7. Bona, C. A., B. Goldberg, D. Metzger, J. Urbain, and H. G. Kunkel. 1984. Anti-immunoglobulin antibodies. IV. Cross-reaction of anti-idiotypic antibodies specific for rabbit and murine anti-a-allotype antibodies with Fc fragment of human immunoglobulins. *Eur. J. Immunol.* 14:548.
8. Rodriguez, M. A., J. L. Ceuppens, and J. S. Goodwin. 1982. Regulation of IgM RF production in lymphocyte cultures from young and old subjects. *J. Immunol.* 128:2422.

9. Koopman, W. J., and R. E. Schrohenloher. 1980. In vitro synthesis of IgM RF by lymphocytes from healthy adults. *J. Immunol.* 125:934.
10. Van Snick, J. L., and P. L. Masson. 1979. Age dependent production of IgA and IgM autoantibodies against IgG_{2a} in a colony of 129/Sv mice. *J. Exp. Med.* 149:1519.
11. Van Snick, J. L. 1981. The production of anti-IgG_{2a}, autoantibody in the 129/Sv mouse: Onset in the lymph nodes draining the intestinal tract and prevention by neonatal thymectomy. *J. Immunol.* 126:815.
12. Van Snick, J. L., and P. Coulie. 1982. Monoclonal anti-IgG autoantibodies derived from lipopolysaccharide-activated spleen cells of 129/Sv mice. *J. Exp. Med.* 155:219–230.
13. Stassin, V., P. G. Coulie, B. K. Birshtein, D. S. Secher, and J. Van Snick. 1983. Determinants recognized by murine rheumatoid factors: Molecular localization using a panel of mouse myeloma variant immunoglobulins. *J. Exp. Med.* 158:1763.
14. Manheimer, A. J., and C. A. Bona. 1986. Are rheumatoid factors produced during conventional immune responses beneficial to the host? *In* Paradoxes in Immunology. G. W. Hoffmann, J. G. Levy, and G. T. Nepom, editors. CRC Press, Boca Raton, Fla. In press.
15. Hooijkaas, H., A. A. Pressman, A. Van Oudernaren, R. Benner, and J. J. Haaijman. 1983. Frequency analysis of functional immunoglobulin C and V gene expression in murine B cells at various ages. *J. Immunol.* 131:1629.
16. Manheimer, A. J., C. Victor-Kobrin, K. E. Stein, and C. A. Bona. 1984. Anti-immunoglobulin antibodies. V. Age-dependent variation of clones stimulated by polysaccharide TI-2 antigens in 129 and MRL mice spontaneously producing antigamma globulin antibodies. *J. Immunol.* 133:562.
17. Manheimer, A., and C. Bona. 1986. Anti-immunoglobulin antibodies. VII. Age-dependent isotype and autoanti-immunoglobulin variation during secondary immune response in 129 mice. *Mech. Ageing Dev.* 30:187.
18. Weiss, S., K. Lehmann, W. C. Raschke, and M. Cohn. 1984. Mice completely suppressed for the immunoglobulin κ light chain. *Proc. Natl. Acad. Sci. USA.* 81:211.
19. Eskinazi, D. P., A. Gilman-Sachs, A. Dray, and S. Knight. 1979. Suppression of the paternal IgA-f and IgA-g allotypes in heterogyzous rabbits suppressed for the paternal IgM allotype. *Mol. Immunol.* 16:1019.
20. Bona, C., K. Stein, R. Lieberman, and W. E. Paul. 1979. Direct and indirect suppression induced by anti-idiotype antibody in the insulin bacterial levan antigenic system. *Mol. Immunol.* 16:1093.
21. Bona, C., R. Hooghe, P. A. Cazenave, C. Leguern, and W. E. Paul. 1979. Cellular basis of regulation of expression of idiotype. II. Immunity to anti-MOPC460 idiotype antibodies increases the level of anti-trinitrophenyl antibodies bearing 460 idiotypes. *J. Exp. Med.* 149:815.
22. Dzierzak, E., R. W. Rosenstein, and C. A. Janeway. 1981. Expression of an idiotype (Id-460) during in vivo anti-dinitrophenyl antibody responses. II. Transient idiotype dominance. *J. Exp. Med.* 154, 1432.
23. Kunkel, H. G., R. J. Winchester, F. G. Joslin, and J. D. Capra. 1971. Simi-

larities in the light chains of anti-γ-globulins showing cross-idiotypic specificities. *J. Exp. Med.* 139:128.
24. Brodeur, P. H., and R. Riblet. 1984. The immunoglobulin heavy chain variable region (Igh-V) locus in the mouse. I. 100-Igh-V genes comprise 7 families of homologous genes. *Eur. J. Immunol.* 14:992.
25. Yancopoulos, G. D., S. V. Desiderio, M. Paskind, J. F. Kearney, D. Baltimore, and F. W. Alt. 1984. Preferential utilization of the most J_H-proximal V_H gene segments in pre-B cell lines. *Nature.* 311:727.
26. Nemazee, D., and V. Sato. 1982. Enhancing antibody: A novel component of the immune response. *Proc. Natl. Acad. Sci. USA.* 79:3828.

17

Aging and Autoimmunity

Edmond A. Goidl

School of Medicine
The University of Maryland at Baltimore
Baltimore, Maryland

I. INTRODUCTION

Numerous contributions in this volume have amply documented the progressive decrease in immune reactivity seen in the aging process of the immune responses. I shall concentrate on the changes in the regulatory immune network which occur in aging. As proposed by N. K. Jerne (1), the immune response may be represented as an interacting network of antibody molecules. This network comprises anti-antigen antibodies (idiotypic antibodies or Ab_1) and anti-anti-antibodies (anti-idiotypes or Ab_2). This network of interacting elements is disturbed from its steady state by the introduction of antigen, and an immune response is generated. Following the production of idiotypic and anti-idiotypic antibodies, all elements then achieve a new steady state.

This network has been looked at as "positive autoimmunity" by Wigzell (2). This is to be contrasted by "negative autoimmunity," best exemplified by autoimmune diseases in which a number of autoantibodies (Ab_1) are produced against autologous determinants. In this chapter, I shall try to show how this balance between positive and negative autoimmunity changes during the life of the animal. I shall also produce evidence that changes in positive autoimmunity may be required to control the alterations seen in negative autoimmunity with respect to increase of age.

We have documented extensively the changes in the production of auto-anti-idiotypic antibody (auto-anti-Id) with aging of the animal. Using a murine experimental system, we have provided evidence that there occurs a progressive relative increase of auto-anti-Id production during the normal immune response of aged mice.

I shall review the experiments that have led us to dissect the cellular control of the increased production of auto-anti-Id antibody seen in the normal immune responses of aging mice.

II. MAGNITUDE AND CHARACTERISTICS OF THE AGED IMMUNE RESPONSE

The decreased magnitude of the immune response of aged mice is accompanied by a preferential loss of high-affinity antibody and by a decrease in the heterogeneity of antibody affinity (3). When aged BALB/c and C57L/J mice of different ages are immunized with 500 μg of dinitrophenylated bovine gamma globulin (DNP-BGG), the magnitude of the immune response of aged mice is considerably lower than that of young mice (see Table 1). The immune response of young mice is characterized by a maturation process that leads to an increase in average affinity and an increase in heterogeneity of antibody affinity with respect to the time after antigen administration. In contrast, the immune response of aged mice is characterized by a decreased average affinity of the antibody produced and also by a dramatic decrease in the heterogeneity of antibody affinity produced. This decreased heterogeneity of antibody affinity is preferentially seen in the loss of high-affinity antibody production. The aged immune response by its decreased magnitude and by its relative loss of high-affinity antibody may contribute to the increased susceptibility to infectious agents seen in aging.

Table 1 Magnitude and Heterogeneity of Affinity of the Anti-TNP PFC Response in Young and Aged Mice[a]

Strain and age	Direct PFC	Indirect PFC	Heterogeneity index[b]
C57L/J			
2 months	2,500	8,000	2.8
12 months	3,200	6,400	2.3
25 months	900	1,200	1.6
BALB/c			
2 months	9,600	11,000	2.8
24 months	1,900	2,000	1.8

[a]Mice were immunized with DNP-BGG in complete Freund's adjuvant and sacrificed 2 weeks later.
[b]Shannon function of PFC heterogeneity with respect to avidity.
Source: Adapted from Ref. 3.

III. SUPPRESSOR ACTIVITIES IN THE AGED IMMUNE RESPONSE

The advent and interplay of specific and nonspecific suppressor activities have been elegantly discussed by Gottesman, Thorbecke, and Walford, and by Segre and Segre in Chapters 12 and 13 of this book. I will therefore not discuss suppression in the aged immune response. Only within the domain of the immune network shall I bring up, in later sections of this chapter, some interactions that may be viewed tentatively by their efferent function as leading to specific suppression.

IV. PRODUCTION OF AUTO-ANTI-IDIOTYPIC ANTIBODY IN THE IMMUNE RESPONSE OF AGED MICE

We have been able to document the production of auto-anti-Id during the course of the normal immune response by the use of two different methods.

1. We have shown that in the presence of low concentrations of hapten there frequently occurs an increase in the number of plaque-forming cells (PFC) enumerated in a Jerne localized-in-gel hemolytic PFC assay (4). These potential PFC, which are hapten augmentable, represent cells whose secretion of antibody has been blocked by the binding of auto-anti-Id to cell surface idiotypic determinants. In this system we believe that the hapten may compete with anti-Id for binding with cell surface antibody molecules. In a very narrow window of affinity distributions involving both the affinities of idiotypic antibody for the hapten and the respective affinities of idiotypic and anti-idiotypic antibodies, hapten is able to displace bound anti-Id antibody, after which inhibition of secretion is reversed. We have also shown that the presence of auto-anti-Id in the serum can be assayed by its capacity to inhibit PFC formation in a hapten-reversible fashion (5,6).

2. We have also developed an enzyme-linked immunoadsorbent assay (ELISA) for auto-anti-idiotype antibody (7). This assay utilizes an enzyme-labeled, affinity-purified IgM from immune animals as the idiotype probe for anti-Id. This assay can detect both heterologous and autologous anti-Id. Results obtained by this assay have confirmed those seen using hapten-augmentable PFC as a measure of the production of auto-anti-Id.

These methods were used to determine the extent of the contributions of the immune network to the regulation of the immune response of aged mice. Several inbred strains of mice [C57BL/6, BALB/c, CBF_7 (C57BL/6 × BALB/c)F_1 and AKR/J] of ages ranging from 6 to 100 weeks were immunized with 10 μg of trinitrophenylated-lysyl-Ficoll (TNP-F). The magnitude of the anti-TNP PFC response as well as the percentage of hapten-augmentable PFC were determined at

Table 2 Effect of Age on Production of Hapten-Augmentable PFC[a]

Strain and age	Overall average of hapten-augmentable PFC (%: $\bar{X}$ = SEM)
C57BL/6	
2 months	39 ±16
3 months	12 ±9
20 months	532 ±256
BALB/c	
2 months	15 ±6
7 months	37 ±20
25 months	49 ±25
AKR/J	
2 months	17 ±6
6–7 months	110 ±21
CBF_1	
2–3 months	20 ±6
20 months	190 ±94

[a]Mice were immunized with 10 μg of TNP-F intravenously and sacrificed 7 days later.
Source: Adapted from Ref. 8.

several times following antigen administration (18). These studies (Table 2) showed that there is a relative increase in the auto-anti-Id antibody response with age. This production contributes to a greater down-regulation of the immune response of the aged animals. The increase in the production of auto-anti-Id in the aging immune response could be due to the recognition of a larger proportion of anti-TNP idiotopes or, alternatively, a reduced heterogeneity of clonotypes responding to the antigenic determinant assay could contribute to this phenomenon. It is not possible at this time to determine which of these two mechanisms is responsible for the increased production of auto-anti-Id in aging. Szewczuk and Campbell (9) also reported the increase of auto-anti-Id production in the aged immune response to thymic-dependent antigens.

The effect of age on idiotype expression was also determined (8). We used hapten-reversible inhibition of PFC formation as an assay for anti-Id antibody and Id-antibody-secreting cells. Sera from aged C57BL/6 mice (21–22 months old) immunized with TNP-F significantly inhibited plaque formation in a hapten-reversible manner by spleen cells obtained from 81% of TNP-F-immunized age-matched mice (Table 3). When the same sera were tested on idiotype-bearing spleen cells obtained from TNP-immune mice 6–8 or 3–weeks old, a different pattern emerged. Sera from aged animals inhibited plaque forma-

Table 3 Effect of Age on Idiotype Expression

Age of source of anti-TNP PFC[a]	Incidence of suppression (%) — Age of source of anti-Id: 3–4 weeks	6–8 weeks	21–22 months
3–4 weeks	<u>58</u>	15	20
6–8 weeks	0	<u>67</u>	50
21–22 months	10	7	<u>81</u>

[a]C57BL/6 mice were immunized by the intravenous injection of 10 μg of TNP-F.
Source: Adapted from Ref. 8.

tion in only 50% of the mice aged 6 to 8 weeks and in 20% of immature mice (3–4 weeks). Remarkably, sera from TNP-F-immunized mice inhibited preferentially idiotypic-bearing lymphocytes of the same age as the mice from whom the sera were obtained. This effect was also reinforced by the fact that sera from a given age group rarely inhibited plaque formation by cells from mice of other age groups. These data strongly support the conclusion that with increasing of age there is a gradual change in the catalogue of idiotypes expressed after stimulation by antigen. In this case the TNP determinant was presented in a thymic-independent carrier. These data also seem to make it unlikely that idiotype expression is purely a random event. This is shown by the preferential auto-anti-Id and Id recognition within the same groups. Also noteworthy is the finding that sera from one age group do not recognize the totality of idiotypes produced by age-matched immune spleen cells, indicating that syngeneic mice of a given age differ to a certain extent in idiotype expression.

The shift in clonotypic antibody production may reflect changes in the distribution and/or expression of clonotypes as a consequence of repeated exposure to common antigens and infectious agents in the environment. This shift in idiotypic antibody repertoire with age was analyzed at the level of expression only; these results do not imply that such changes stem from differences in the catalogue of idiotypes present at the genomic level.

In conclusion, the relative increase of the production of auto-anti-Id with increase of age is a general phenomenon as shown by elevated responses in aged mice of different inbred strains. Also, with respect to age, there occurs a gradual shift in the expression of the repertoire of idiotypic antibody. The precise nature of this shift has not been determined.

V. CELLULAR REGULATION OF AUTO-ANTI-IDIOTYPIC ANTIBODY PRODUCTION IN THE IMMUNE RESPONSE OF AGED MICE

To determine the cellular regulation of the production of auto-anti-Id in the aged immune response, we first established whether this increase was a trait that was stable upon cell transfer (10). Spleen cells were obtained from young or aged C57BL/6 mice. Cells were transferred along with 10 μg of TNP-F into lethally irradiated syngeneic recipients. Results (Table 4) showed that mice reconstituted with spleen cells from aged donors produced high levels of hapten-augmentable PFC, in contrast to mice that had received cells from young donors, which had low levels of hapten-augmentable PFC. Thus the high percentage of hapten-augmentable PFC that had previously been reported to be a characteristic of the immune response of aged mice (8) is also seen in animals that had been reconstituted with spleen cells from aged donors. The relative increase of auto-anti-Id production seen in the immune response of aged mice is therefore a trait that is stable upon cell transfer to syngeneic lethally irradiated recipients and is not a phenomenon dependent on the internal physiological milieu of the aged mouse.

The increased production of auto-anti-Id in the aged immune response (8, 9) had so far been a characteristic of the peripheral lymphoid system (i.e., spleen). We next decided to determine whether this characteristic extended to the lymphoid cells obtained from the central lymphoid organs (i.e., bone marrow) of young and aged mice. In a series of experiments (Table 5) 5×10^7 bone marrow cells obtained from young or aged mice were transferred into syngeneic lethally irradiated recipients. All recipients were immunized with 10 μg of TNP-F, and 7 days later their responses were analyzed for the presence of anti-hapten PFC and for the production of hapten-augmentable PFC. Bone marrow cells are able to reconstitute recipients, and these mount a modest anti-TNP

Table 4 Increased Auto-Anti-Id Antibody Response Is a Trait Stable Upon Spleen Cell Transfer[a]

Age of donors (months)	Direct anti-TNP PFC (PFC/spleen ±SE)	Percent hapten-augmentable PFC ($\bar{X}$ ±SE)
4	17,000 ±3,000	6 ±5
18	10,000 ±1,200	109 ±25

[a]Lethally irradiated mice were reconstituted with spleen cells from syngeneic donors of the indicated age. Recipients were immunized with 10 μg of TNP-F administered intravenously and their response assayed 7 days later.
Source: Adapted from Ref. 10.

Table 5 Transfer of Bone Marrow Cells from Aged and Young Mice Leads to Low Levels of Auto-Anti-Id Production

Age of bone marrow[a] donors (months)	Direct anti-TNP PFC/spleen ($\bar{X}$ ±SE)	Percent hapten-augmentable PFC ($\bar{X}$ ±SE)
2–3	4000 ±600	13 ±3
18	1400 ±200	7 ±5

[a]The 5 × 10^7 bone marrow cells from donors of indicated ages were transferred into lethally irradiated syngeneic mice, 2–3 months old, along with 10 μg of TNP-F. Assays were performed 7 days later.
Source: Adapted from Ref. 10.

PFC response. In no case did we find the recipients producing any significant numbers of hapten-augmentable PFC. Lymphoid cells obtained from the bone marrow of either young or aged mice are therefore indistinguishable from each other, leading to the production of low to undetectable levles of auto-anti-Id antibody.

We had shown previously that T-cell-deficient animals when immunized with TNP-F fail to produce auto-anti-Id (11). In these cases data obtained from young adult mice showed that the production of auto-anti-Id is a thymic-dependent phenomenon. We next examined the thymic dependence of the production of auto-anti-Id in the aged immune response. Thymectomized, lethally irradiated syngeneic recipients were reconstituted with spleen cells from aged or young donor mice. Pools of cells from aged or young donors were heated with complement alone or with complement and monoclonal anti-Thy-1.2 antibody to eliminate T cells. Resultant cell populations were injected into recipients along with 10 μg of TNP-F. The immune responses of the recipients were analyzed for the presence of anti-TNP PFC and for hapten-augmentable PFC

Table 6 Effect of Removal of T Cells on the Production of Auto-Anti-Id Antibody by Splenic Lymphocytes of Old Mice[a]

Treatment of cells	Direct anti-TNP PFC/spleen ($\bar{X}$ ±SE)	Percent hapten-augmentable PFC ($\bar{X}$ ±SE)
Complement	1500 ±250	42 ±13
Anti-Thy-1.2 + complement	2000 ±250	43 ±13

[a]Lethally irradiated thymectomized C57BL/6 mice were reconstituted with spleen cells from 18-month-old mice. As indicated, spleen cells were treated with anti-Thy-1.2 and complement to remove T cells, or with complement alone. Immunization has been described; see Table 5.
Source: Adapted from Ref. 10.

(Table 6). The results obtained showed that in contrast to the immune response of young mice, whose production of auto-anti-Id is a thymic-dependent event, with splenic non-T cells obtained from aged mice the production of auto-anti-Id is a relatively thymic-independent phenomenon.

The experiments described so far in this section point to the similarity of low levels of auto-anti-Id production between cells from bone marrow of young and aged mice. We also have documented a relatively low thymic dependency of auto-anti-Id production in the spleen of aged mice, while these cells give rise to high levels of auto-anti-Id antibody. Since lymphoid precursor cells arise in the bone marrow of adult animals and migrate to populate peripheral lymphoid organs, we next determined the identity of the cells responsible for the dramatic change in auto-anti-Id production seen between cells of the central and peripheral lymphoid organs of aged mice. Groups of lethally irradiated syngeneic young adult mice were reconstituted with cells from bone marrow of young or aged donors. It is important to note that so far all recipients are identical with respect to their capacity to produce auto-anti-Id. We have shown (Table 5) that bone marrow cells from aged or young donors are indistinguishable in this context. Next some recipients received B-cell-depleted spleen cells from either young or aged donors. The different mixtures of cells were allowed to reside for 5 days. At this time all recipients were immunized with 10 μg of TNP-F, and 7 days later their immune response was analyzed for anti-TNP PFC and for the presence of hapten-augmentable PFC.

Recipients of T cells from young donors had a low percentage of hapten-augmentable PFC, such as is typical of young mice, regardless of the source of the bone marrow cells (Table 7). In contrast, recipients of T cells from aged

Table 7 Influence of Splenic T Cells on the Production of Auto-Anti-Id Antibody[a]

Age of cell donors (months)		Direct anti-TNP PFC/spleen)	Percent hapten-augmentable PFC
Bone marrow cell donor	T-cell donor	($\bar{X}$ ±SE)	($\bar{X}$ ±SE)
2–3	2–3	2300 ±500	12 ±4
2–3	18	1200 ±200	55 ±12
18	2–3	2300 ±500	16 ±5
18	18	1500 ±600	38 ±12

[a]Male C57BL/6 mice were lethally irradiated and reconstituted by the intravenous injection of 2.5–3.5 × 10^7 bone marrow cells obtained from donors of indicated age, and 2–4 × 10^7 B-cell-depleted spleen cells from donors of the indicated age. Recipients were immunized 5 days following cell transfer by the intravenous administration of 10 μg of TNP-F. All assays performed 7 days following immunization.

Source: Adapted from Ref. 10.

donors had a high incidence of hapten-augmentable PFC, as is typical of old mice, and again regardless of whether the recipients had received bone marrow cells from young or old donors. In both cases the groups that received T cells from old donors had significantly higher percentages of hapten-augmentable PFC than did the groups that had received T cells from the spleens of young donors. In conclusion, the magnitude of the production of auto-anti-Id antibody is regulated by the non-B splenic cell population. Since this population was shown to be greater than 95% Thy-1.2$^+$, it seems likely that the increased production of auto-anti-Id in the aged immune response is regulated by peripheral splenic T cells.

The data presented in this section attest so far to the complexity of events leading to the increased production of auto-anti-Id in the aged immune response. First we have shown that lymphocytes arising from central lymphoid organs of both young and aged mice are indistinguishable in their capacity to form auto-anti-Id. That these two populations lead to the same low auto-anti-Id productions is consistent with the findings of Ogden and Micklem (12) and Harrison et al. (13) that bone marrow cells from young and old donors were similar with respect to stem cell activity. We have also shown that the increased production of auto-anti-Id in aging is a characteristic of the peripheral lymphoid populations and that the expression of this trait, which is transferable, is under splenic T cell control. Transferability, of course, implies that this trait is not dependent on the internal milieu of the aged animal. Once this characteristic has been acquired in the peripheral lymphoid system of the aged, it is, in contrast to young mice, relatively thymic independent. The dichotomy between the "young-like" bone marrow cells from old mice and the control exercised by the long-lived peripheral T cells allowed us to predict that if the peripheral lymphoid system of an old animal were acutely depleted of cells while the bone marrow were left intact (e.g., by means of irradiation with bone marrow shielding) and the animal allowed to reconstitute its peripheral lymphoid system from its own marrow, it should behave like a young mouse with respect to the production of auto-anti-Id antibody. Furthermore, this type of manipulation should be alterable by the transfer into such irradiated animals of peripheral T cells from donors of different ages.

The experimental results obtained confirm these predictions. Mice that were exposed to a normally lethal dose of irradiation while their bone marrow was partially shielded survived and within 6 weeks regained normal immune function. At this time, animals were immunized with 10 μg of TNP-F, and their anti-TNP PFC and hapten-augmentable PFC and ELISA titers for auto-anti-Id were determined 7 days following antigen administration. After recovery from irradiation, old mice produce low auto-anti-Id antibody (Table 8) comparable to the levels produced by young mice. This is true whether the production of auto-anti-Id is measured by the magnitude of hapten-augmentable PFC or by ELISA

Table 8 Concentration of Auto-Anti-Id in the Serum of Mice[a] After Recovery from Irradiation and Following Immunization with TNP-F

Age of mice	Treatment	Binding of anti-TNP antibody (A 405 nm)
18–24 months	None	0.400 ±0.07
18–24 months	Irradiation	0.290 ±0.04
8–10 weeks	None	0.270 ±0.04
8–10 weeks	Irradiation	0.280 ±0.04

[a]C57BL/6 mice of the age indicated were untreated or were exposed to 800 rads of gamma irradiation with their bone marrow shielded. Six weeks later the mice were immunized with 10 μg of TNP-F intravenously. Six days later the mice were bled and their serum assayed for auto-anti-Id by ELISA assay (7).
Source: Adapted from Ref. 15.

assay for serum auto-anti-Id from these animals. The magnitude of auto-anti-Id production is under the control of peripheral splenic T cells, as demonstrated by T cell transfer into such animals. When mice were irradiated with their bone marrow shielded and then received splenic T cells from aged donors, they produced high levels of auto-anti-Id antibody, while mice similarly irradiated that received splenic T cells from young donors produced low levels of auto-anti-Id antibody (Table 9).

These results are consistent with the hypothesis that the idiotypic catalogue is similar in the bone marrow B cells of young and aged mice. These

Table 9 Influence of Splenic T Cells from Donors of Different Ages on Auto-Anti-Id Antibody Responses

Age of irradiated mice	Age of T-cell donor	Average % (±SE) hapten-augmentable PFC
8 weeks	(None)	17.0 ±4
8 weeks	8 weeks	16.0 ±3
8 weeks	24 months	31.0 ±4
18 months	(None)	15.0 ±3
18 months	8 weeks	10.0 ±4
18 months	18 months	36.0 ±6

[a]C57BL/6 mice of the age indicated were untreated or were exposed to 800 rads of gamma irradiation with their bone marrow shielded. Seven days later they were injected intravenously with 2 × 10^7 splenic T cells from donors of the indicated age. Seven weeks after irradiation, mice were immunized with 10 μg of TNP-F intravenously; their responses were analyzed 6 days later.
Source: Adapted from Ref. 15.

two populations are thought to be similar in their stem cell activity potential (12,13); furthermore Zharhary and Klinman (14) demonstrated that the level of diversity of antibody repertoire for PR8 influenza virus is similar in young and old mice. The differences observed in the immune responses of young and old mice may be due to Id-anti-Id interactions that occur between cells arising from the bone marrow and the long-lived peripheral T cells.

VI. AUTO-ANTI-IDIOTYPIC ANTIBODY AND ANTI-SELF REACTIVITY IN THE AGED IMMUNE RESPONSE

Within the premise that shifts in clonal distribution of long-lived peripheral T cells are the consequence of lifelong interactions with internal and environmental antigens, it is appropriate to ask whether there is a beneficial component to the increased production of auto-anti-Id in the aged immune response. I shall discuss in this section some of the preliminary data obtained recently in my laboratory. The extent of by-standing or cross-reactivities toward self antigens that are generated during the normal immune response of aged mice has been determined. Aged mice have been immunized with 10 μg of TNP-F and their immune responses measured at different times following antigen administration. Their anti-TNP PFC responses were measured, as well as their capacity for plaque formation against self antigens. Three such self antigens were chosen: bromalin-treated mouse erythrocytes (Br-MRBC), mouse transferrin, and mouse albumin. A considerable degree of anti-self reactivity was generated in the immune response of both young and old mice (Table 10). These anti-self reactivities increased dramatically with age: at 24 months, 75% of the magnitude of the anti-TNP PFC response was found to cross-react with Br-MRBC; similarly 58% was cross-reactive to mouse transferrin. In these series of experiments, the level of cross-reactivity to mouse albumin was always very low (< 10%). One should

Table 10 Immune Reactivity Arising in the Response to TNP-F in Young and Aged Mice[a]

Age of mice	Anti-TNP PFC/spleen ($\bar{X}$ ±SE)	Percent anti-TNP response reactive with: Br-MRBC	Percent anti-TNP response reactive with: Mouse transferrin
6–8 weeks	9500 ±600	46	31
24 months	4000 ±300	75	58

[a]C57BL/6 mice of the indicated age were immunized with 10 μg of TNP-F administered intravenously. Seven days later single-cell suspensions obtained from their spleen were tested for plaque formation against TNP-SRBC, Br-MRBC, and mouse transferrin–SRBC.
Source: From Goidl et al. (manuscript in preparation).

Table 11 Effect of Removal of Auto-Anti-Id Antibody from Immune Cell Populations from Young and Aged Mice on Anti-Self Reactivity

Age (months)	Increase in anti-self reactivity after anti-Id removal (% for each of 12 individual mice)
2–3	0, 6, 10, 8, 10, 14
18–20	28, 33, 39, 34, 42, 31

[a]C57BL/6 mice of the age indicated were immunized with 10 μg of TNP-F administered intravenously. Seven days later single-cell suspensions obtained by teasing their spleen were plaqued against TNP-SRBC and an aliquot was incubated in vitro with 10^{-9} M TNP-ε-amino caproic to remove auto-anti-Id, and washed before plaquing versus TNP and versus self antigen targets.
Source: From Goidl et al. (manuscript in preparation).

emphasize that at this time it is not possible to distinguish actual cross-reactivity of the anti-TNP PFC response from the activation during immunization of by-standing lymphocyte populations with anti-self reactivity. Such differentiation will be determined at the level of monoclonal antibodies obtained from such immune cell populations.

One finding that supports the proposition that at least a proportion of the anti-TNP response is cross-reactive toward self antigens was obtained following the removal of auto-anti-Id from immune spleen cells obtained from old mice (Table 11).

After removal of auto-anti-Id, anti-self reactivity in the immune cell population obtained from young mice was found to increase modestly (< 15%). In contrast, removal of auto-anti-Id from aged immune spleen cells led to an increase in anti-self reactivity ranging from 28 to 42%. Still these results are as yet inconclusive in determining the exact origin of the anti-self reactivities.

VII. CONCLUSION

One of the dramatic changes occurring in the aging immune response is the increase in auto-anti-idiotypic production. This increased production is under the control of the peripheral splenic T cell—presumably a long-lived cell that has been influenced by lifelong interactions with internal and external environmental antigens. The capacity to produce high auto-anti-Id once acquired in the peripheral lymphoid system then becomes relatively thymic independent. The role of the increased auto-anti-Id response in aging may be to down-regulate anti-self responses that arise during the immune response.

ACKNOWLEDGMENT

This chapter was supported in part by USPHS grant AG 04042.

REFERENCES

1. Jerne, N. K. 1974. Towards a network theory of the immune system. *Ann. Immunol.* (Paris). 125C:373.
2. Wigzell, H. 1977. Positive autoimmunity. *In* Autoimmunity. Genetic, Immunologic, Virologic and Clinical Aspects. N. Talal, editor. Academic Press, New York. 693–707.
3. Goidl, E. A., J. B. Innes, and M. E. Weksler. 1976. Immunological studies on aging. II. Loss of IgG and high-avidity plaque-forming cells and increased suppressor cell activity in aging mice. *J. Exp. Med.* 144:1037.
4. Jerne, N. K., and A. A. Nordin. 1963. Plaque formation in agar by single antibody-producing cells. *Science.* 140:405.
5. Schrater, A. F., E. A. Goidl, G. J. Thorbecke, and G. W. Siskind. 1979. Production of auto-anti-idiotypic antibody during the normal immune response to TNP-Ficoll. I. Occurrence in AKR/J and BALB/c mice of hapten-augmentable anti-TNP plaque-forming cells and their accelerated appearance in recipients of immune spleen cells. *J. Exp. Med.* 150:138.
6. Goidl, E. A., A. F. Schrater, G. W. Siskind, and G. J. Thorbecke. 1979. Production of auto-anti-idiotypic antibody during the normal immune response to TNP-Ficoll. II. Hapten-reversible inhibition of anti-TNP plaque-forming cells by immune serum as an assay for auto-anti-idiotypic antibody. *J. Exp. Med.* 150:154.
7. Gibbons, J. J., E. A. Goidl, G. M. Shepherd, G. J. Thorbecke, and G. W. Siskind. 1985. Production of auto-anti-idiotypic antibody during the normal immune response. XII. An enzyme-linked immunosorbent assay for auto-anti-idiotypic antibody. *J. Immunol. Methods.* 79:231.
8. Goidl, E. A., G. J. Thorbecke, M. E. Weksler, and G. W. Siskind. 1980. Production of auto-anti-idiotypic antibody during the normal immune response: Changes in the auto-anti-idiotypic antibody response and the idiotype repertoire associated with aging. *Proc. Natl. Acad. Sci. USA.* 77:6788.
9. Szewczuk, M. R., and R. J. Campbell. 1980. Loss of immune competence with age may be due to auto-anti-idiotypic antibody. *Nature.* 286:164.
10. Goidl, E. A., J. W. Choy, J. J. Gibbons, M. E. Weksler, G. J. Thorbecke, and G. W. Siskind. 1983. Production of auto-anti-idiotypic antibody during the normal immune response. VII. Analysis of the cellular basis for the increased auto-anti-idiotype antibody production by aged mice. *J. Exp. Med.* 157:1635.
11. Schrater, A. F., E. A. Goidl, G. J. Thorbecke, and G. W. Siskind. 1979. Production of auto-anti-idiotypic antibody during the normal immune response to TNP-Ficoll. III. Absence in nu/nu mice: Evidence for T cell dependence of the anti-idiotypic antibody response. *J. Exp. Med.* 150:808.

12. Ogden, D. A., and H. S. Micklem. 1976. The fate of serially transplanted bone marrow cell populations from young and old donors. *Transplantation.* 22:287.
13. Harrison, D. E., C. M. Castle, and J. W. Doubleday. 1977. Stem cell lines from old immunodeficient donors give normal responses in young recipients. *J. Immunol.* 118:1223.
14. Zharhary, D., and N. R. Klinman. 1984. B cell repertoire diversity to PR-8 influenza virus does not decrease with age. *J. Immunol.* 133:2285.
15. Kim, Y. T., E. A. Goidl, C. Samarut, M. E. Weksler, G. J. Thorbecke, and G. W. Siskind. 1985. Bone marrow function. I. Peripheral T cells are responsible for the increased auto-anti-idiotypic response of older mice. *J. Exp. Med.* 161:1237.

Index